D0577933

The Great American Sex Diet

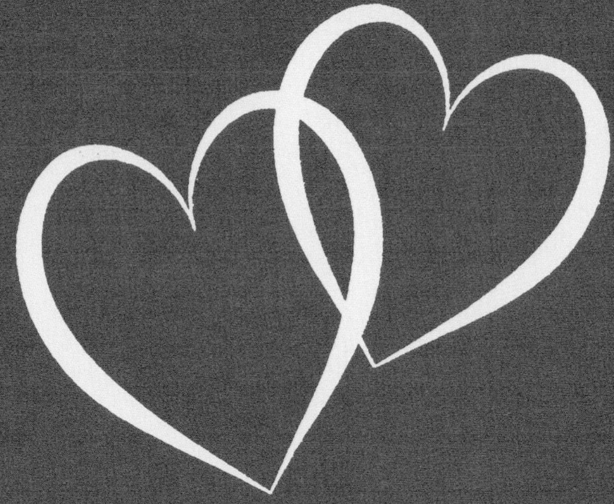

Also by Laura Corn

101 Nights of Grrreat Sex

101 Nights of Grrreat Romance

101 Grrreat Quickies

52 Invitations to Grrreat Sex

237 Intimate Questions Every Woman Should Ask a Man

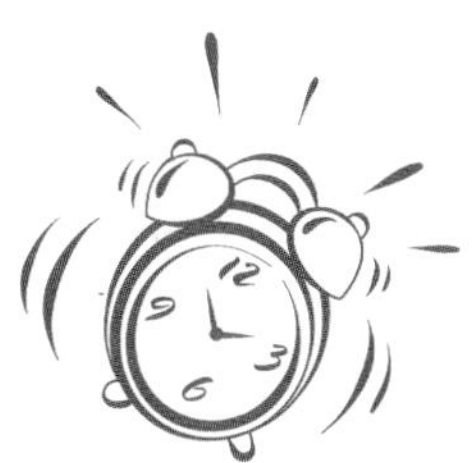

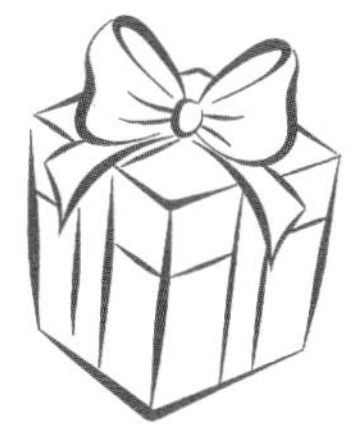

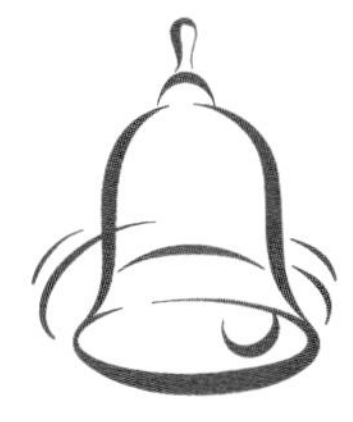

The Great American Sex Diet

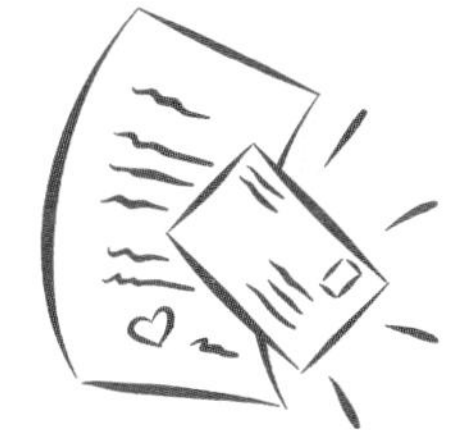

Where the Only Thing
You Nibble On . . .
Is Your Partner!

—

Laura Corn

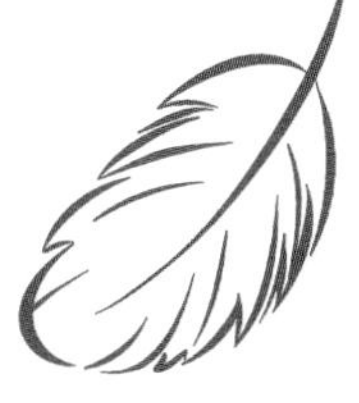
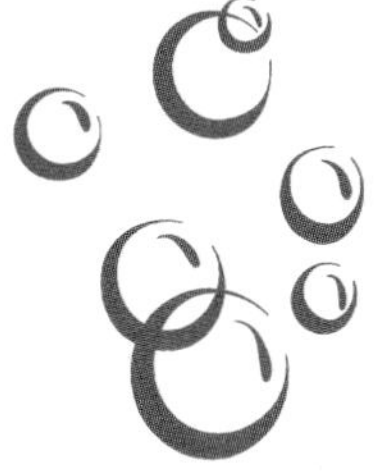

wm
WILLIAM MORROW
75 YEARS OF PUBLISHING
An Imprint of HarperCollins*Publishers*

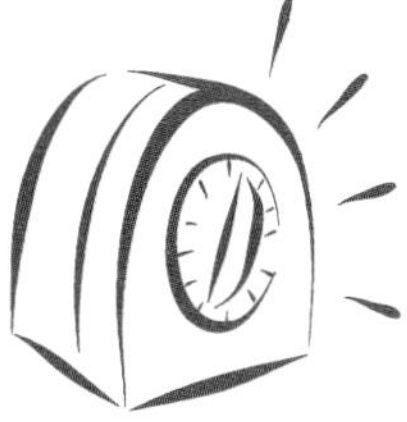

HarperCollins books may be purchased for educational, business, or sales promotional use. For information please write: Special Markets Department, HarperCollins Publishers Inc., 10 East 53rd Street, New York, NY 10022.

FIRST EDITION

Designed by 27.12 Design Ltd. NYC
All illustrations by Mona Daly

Printed on acid-free paper

Library of Congress Cataloging-in-Publication Data
Corn, Laura.
The great American sex diet: where the only thing you nibble on . . . is your partner! / by Laura Corn.
p. cm.
ISBN 0-06-621278-2
1. Sex instruction. 2. Intimacy (Psychology). 3. Sex—Health aspects. 4. Sex (Psychology). I. Title
HQ31.C824 2001
613.9'6—dc21 20010300438

01 02 03 04 05 ❖/RRD 10 9 8 7 6 5 4 3 2 1

Contents

Part III
Corn's Secrets of Sex-cess

Part IV
The Great American Sex Diet: The Secret Ingredients

Part V
The Magical Journey of Surprise

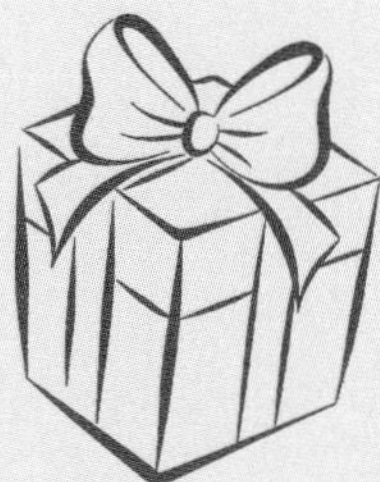

Heartfelt thanks to the wonderful couples who made up the research team, whose friendships I have come to treasure. I am in awe of your remarkable bravery. It took a lot of courage to open up your relationships and let the world see your hopes and fears, your secrets and fantasies. You have put a face to intimacy—and every couple who follows your example and tries the diet owes you a debt of gratitude. I do, too, for your stories and your trust . . . and for helping my own relationship flourish like yours.

My sincere thanks to Rick Dahms, the photographer whose brilliant portraits in this book reflect the true essence of the couples on the research team. Rick, your mastery of the photographic arts is unsurpassed—but even more impressive is your amazing ability to communicate so deeply with the people in your pictures. You made thirty-eight couples comfortable enough to open up their lives and secrets and innermost thoughts to you, and then, remarkably, you managed to capture those moments of emotional intimacy on film for the rest of us to share.

Rick Dahms is a freelance photographer. He's won numerous awards both as a portraitist and as a photojournalist, and was recently nominated for a Pulitzer for his work at the WTO police riots in Seattle. He lives near Seattle, Washington, with his wife, designer Kristine Anderson-Dahms, and their dog and cat.

Acknowledgments

My deepest thanks to:

Jeff Petersen—my love, and my strength. I could never thank you enough—for helping me find my way through a rough time, and for letting me share that story in these pages. There wouldn't be a sex diet at all if not for you.

Julie Taylor—whose words and style helped give life to this book. Julie, you're the sister I never had—smart, talented, funny. The best part of this project was throwing ideas at you, and finding them bouncing back fresher and brighter. Please thank your husband for letting me have so much of your time this past year. Julie is the author of *The Girls' Guide to Guys* and has been published in *Cosmopolitan* and several other national magazines.

Marty Bishop—my friend and partner through several books, and the Master Chef who helped me create the wonderful Spice Menus that are the heart of this project. My gratitude also goes to **Marcy,** for inspiring him and for sharing him with me. Let's do it again!

Bill Wright—my biggest supporter, who believed in me and my work from the very beginning.

Lorraine Day—my Girl Friday (and former assistant to the legendary Herb Ritz)! Lorraine, I don't think there's a single part of this book that didn't benefit from your insights and hard work. You really helped bring this vision to life.

Penny Maples—who helped put the research team together. Wow, and I thought I was organized! Penny, you're a marvel.

Frank Weimann—literary agent. People in this business are always amazed when I tell them how you spent all those years calling me, encouraging me, admiring my work . . . *before I was even your client!* There aren't enough gentlemen like you. Here's to the next level. . . .

Mona Daly—the illustrator who did all the lovely drawings scattered through this book. I love your work . . . and your spirit. Mona Daly has been a professional illustrator for ten years and resides in Reno, Nevada, with her husband and two-year-old daughter.

Amy, Jen, and Merideth Harte at 27.12 Design—who are responsible for the really striking layout of this book. I don't know how you three manage to create such beauty under such crushing deadline pressure!

Acknowledgments

Tim Hall—the very talented photographer who shot the portraits of David and Lucia.

Everyone at William Morrow. I'm so happy to be joining this powerhouse team! Special thanks to executive editor **Mauro DiPreta**: Your advice and suggestions made this project so much easier for me . . . and the astonishing number of hours you put into it made it clear how much you love your work, and this book. It's no exaggeration to say that it wouldn't have happened without you. **Joelle Yudin**: Your wonderful spirit and unflagging effort made the long hours easier to bear. My deepest appreciation also goes to design director **Lucy Albanese,** who worked hand-in-hand with the 27.12 Design crew, and whose creative talents are matched only by her dedication to perfection; executive managing editor **Kim Lewis,** who kept the whole team focused and moving forward (even in the face of staggering deadlines!); production editor **Christine Tanigawa,** who swears she will never let anyone know how many mistakes I made; art director **Richard Aquan,** who made the outside of this book far more beautiful than I had imagined it could be; director of marketing **Lisa Gallagher,** who ultimately was responsible for placing this book in your hands (Good work, Lisa!); **Kristen Green,** for making the book tour a simple pleasure; **Michael Siebert**: Wow, do you know a lot about printing! Thanks for making this all so flawless; and, of course, **Michael Morrison,** publisher of William Morrow, who saw what *The Great American Sex Diet* could be, and then gave me the resources to make it real. And, finally, to **Susan Weinberg**: Of all the things you did for me, the emotional support is what I value most. You made me feel like this will be the Book of the Year.

And to the rest of the publishing team: So, do any of you ever take a break??! You're the hardest-working crew I've ever been involved with, and your dedication is one of the reasons I know I picked the right publisher in William Morrow.

Ann Johnson—for helping me design this book. It's so nice to work with nice people!

David Wilk and Susan Shaw—my distributors for many years. You guys nurtured my tiny company and helped it take flight.

Sharon House and Laurel W. House—L.A.'s top publicists. I'm your number one fan!

Kristine Anderson-Dahms—a brilliant graphic design artist, who helped create the book cover... and who also serves as inspiration for her husband (and my favorite photographer!), Rick Dahms.

Michelle Faulkner—friend, supporter, and one of the reasons I've found as much success as I have.

And, finally, to the authors I admire—Paul Joanides, Lou Paget, Phil McGraw, John Gray, Greg Godek. You inspire me, and you enlighten me.

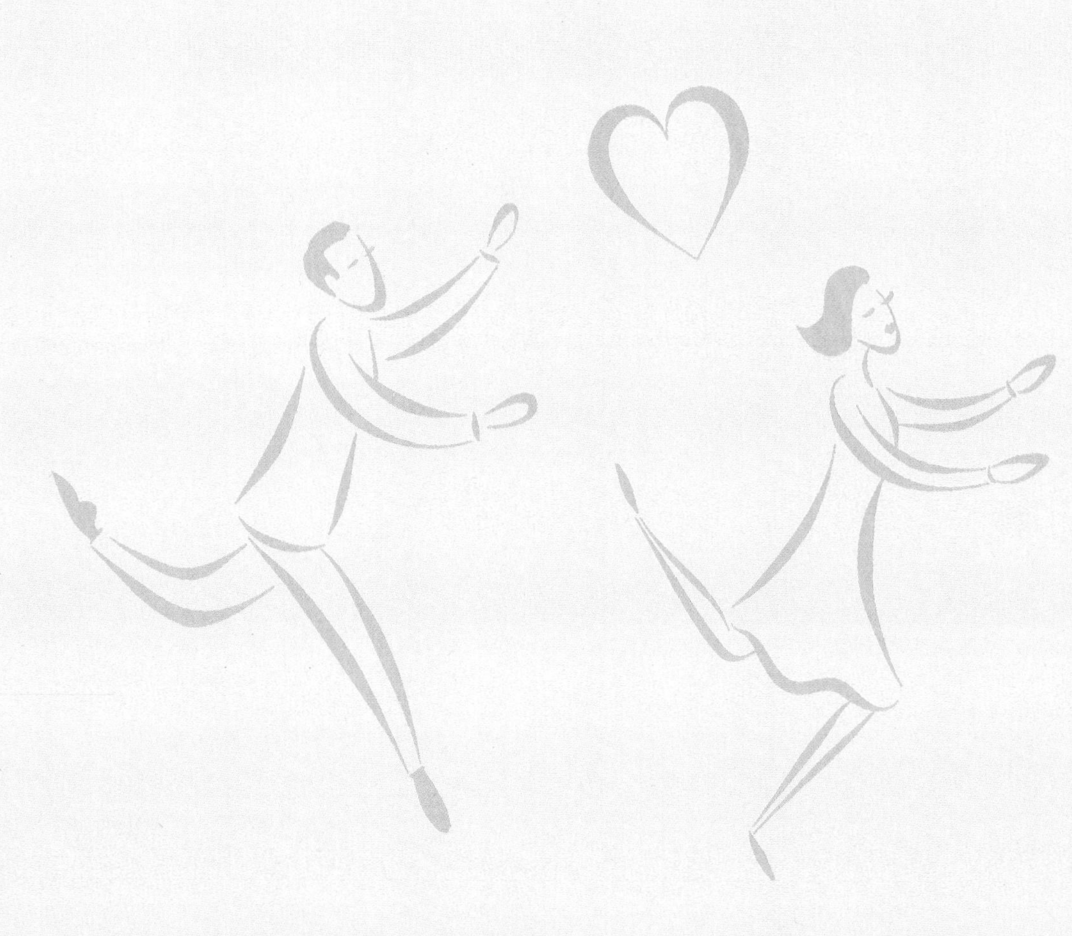

PART
I

In the Beginning

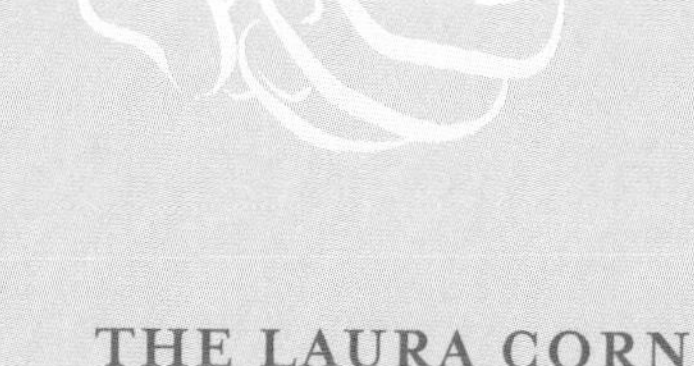

THE LAURA CORN CHALLENGE

—

A couple of years ago, I'd been going through a very rough period in my life and I was feeling extremely stressed. I was under a tight deadline for a TV project and used this preoccupation to let my relationship slide.

The more my boyfriend Jeff tried to comfort and support me, the more I pushed him away. The more I focused on work, the more depressed and listless I felt. I knew I was busy and stressed, but why was I turning away from my best friend and partner?

As always, Jeff was understanding and comforting. But I knew he was frustrated. One of his big frustrations was that we weren't having sex. I was aware of this, too, but there was nothing I could do to motivate myself to want to have sex. Jeff wasn't the problem. He was still the wonderful, sexy guy he'd always been. No, the problem was with me.

It had been two months since Jeff and I had had sex, and I was caught up in a vicious cycle: The more I didn't have sex, the more I didn't want to have sex. Here I was, an author of four bestselling books on sex, and I had become turned off by sex. I had always had low desire, but this was a record—even for me! What was wrong with me?

If I were to be truly, fully honest with myself, I would have to admit that like many women and men, I just stopped having sex. I know I'm not alone in this experience. In more than ten years of talking to thousands of men and women about their sex lives, one of the most astounding lessons I've learned is that, no matter how much in love they are or how healthy their relationship, they often stop having sex with any frequency. Sound familiar? Anyone you might know?

Why do we stop wanting sex? How does that thrilling fire of passion turn into weak embers? And in my case, what was I going to do about it?

One morning during this dry (pun intended) period of my life, I decided to have sex with Jeff. To be honest, I was feeling sorry for him. It wasn't his fault that I didn't want to have sex. He was still interested in love, romance, and passion. I was the one with the problem. Of course I still loved him deeply, but somehow these feelings weren't translating into me wanting sex. So, finally, I asked myself the question: How bad could it be to lie there and open my legs? Please excuse my crudeness, but I mean, really, wasn't that the least I could do for the man I love?

Although it began with me "going through the motions," I have to admit, once we got started, my body took over and, before I could say "abracadabra," I was into it. What a relief! What a feeling! It was as if floodlights of energy began to awaken my tired, stressed-out body, and my every cell surged with pleasure, reminding me of how great it feels to make love.

Later that day, instead of returning to my former morose, deflated state of mind, I realized I felt better than I had in months. This sudden and immediate change inspired me to make a promise, to Jeff and to myself: For the next week I would have sex with Jeff every day. And that's exactly what I did.

Needless to say, Jeff was thrilled and felt like he was walking on the moon. And me? Well, I just felt better and better with every passing day, energized in my body, relaxed in my mind, and completely in touch with myself at the core of my spirit. What was happening? Was this the power of sex?

On the seventh day, I was standing in line at Gelson's grocery store in Marina Del Rey, California, when a man behind me said, "You are so happy! What are you on?" I guess I must have been smiling. When I turned to look at the man, I didn't hesitate before I said, "I'm on the Great American Sex Diet!" And the whole line broke out in spontaneous applause.

Thus the idea for this book was born. Clearly, its inspiration was very personal. Does sex really make us feel better—in our bodies, our heads, in our relationships? This was the question that I sought to answer. I had remarkable evidence: I knew for certain that *I* felt better. One week had made me start to think of sex differently.

What I did next was to expand that one week into six months, during which I began to observe myself, Jeff, and our relationship. I was determined to see if the link between having sex regularly and feeling better—both physically and emotionally—was real. In that first week, I had sex every day. For me, knowing the number of times (seven) motivated and inspired me. Instead of feeling buried in *why* I should or shouldn't have sex, I kept thinking only of having sex seven times. There was something very powerful about the number. Then, over the course of the next six months, I decided to have sex with Jeff more often, as many as three or four times a week.

Immediately I saw results: When Jeff and I were having frequent sex, he became more attentive and passionate. He flirted more, made dinner, created romantic moments that just blew me away by their thoughtfulness. He was simply more affectionate and loving—all without me having to ask. And not only was I happily reciprocating, but I was also on a high. My body trembled with energy and desire. This was not just sexual desire; it was more than that. The sexual energy between Jeff and me spread like wildfire throughout my body. I was zinging with life whereas before I was empty and hollow.

Still, every once in a while, I would revert to my old ways. I would use one of my standard excuses of feeling too tired, not having enough energy for sex, having too much work to do. When I became aware of my relapse, I'd get back on the proverbial horse and start riding again!

Then I happened upon an amazing piece of evidence: the pictures taken during this six-month period. Jeff and I have always been big on taking photos of each other, but these photos were a revelation. I loved the way I looked; my vitality and health were obvious. Then there were the pictures of me when I'd fallen off the wagon, so to speak, and there I was, lethargic and listless, and anything but energetic. I was amazed at the difference, but there it was in Technicolor! I had stumbled upon further proof that sex not only makes you feel better, but you look better, too. I knew I was on to something.

The more I thought about the positive effects of having sex regularly, the more I believed that I should share what I'd discovered. I had this gut feeling that there were many—hundreds or thousands—of couples out there who had stopped having sex. Now, obviously, couples stop having sex for many reasons, sometimes completely out of their control. But I was interested in couples who are otherwise totally committed, in love, and wanting to have sex, but who have inexplicably lost their motivation. I started to think about how most of us think we have to *feel close* to have sex, without realizing that sex makes you feel close.

I began to see sex as a kind of nourishment that, when absent, left people feeling listless in body, mind, and spirit. It was my theory that, more than likely, this listlessness has a negative effect on a relationship: One or both people might withdraw, intimacy becomes stagnant, and the fun and energy that people feel early in the relationship (during the honeymoon phase) is gone. Who wants to live the rest of his life with someone he feels disconnected from and dispassionate about?

Sex, I began to understand, should be a staple of everyone's diet. Now, this diet has nothing to do with food or weight loss. Rather, it's about looking at sex differently: Instead of thinking of it as an extra in your life, an extra that often becomes an afterthought, sex should be an integral part of a healthy, well-rounded diet, not only for you as a person, but also for your relationship. Just as you need to include a good balance of water, protein, and carbohydrates to maintain a healthy body and mind, you need to include sex as a source of energy to make your life full, healthy, and vital.

Just as your body needs nutrients to stay healthy, your relationship needs sex to stay strong. Look at it this way: When couples are not having sex, the consequences are obvious. As I mentioned, when Jeff and I weren't having sex, there was more tension and stress between us. We just weren't getting along as well and we became more disconnected. These are real, concrete consequences.

Just as less sex has a negative impact on a relationship, more sex has a positive effect. Again, I would just compare the pictures Jeff and I took, and the difference between how we both looked was amazing. We were happier, healthier, and clearly more in love and at peace with each other when we were more intimate. Using the self-timer on our camera, I took a photo of Jeff and me in our clothes right after we had made love. Just take a look at the picture on this page. I call it the Afterglow because it captures the essence of what sex is: all those feelings that make people alive and connected to each other at a deep level. So now, when I reverted to my old ways and avoided sex, I recognized the slip and, within my innermost self, began to make a change. I started to want sex for me, even

more so than for him. This is what motivated me to get back to having frequent sex.

It's easy to see how sex is the deepest form of connection between two people. For me, to feel the man I love inside of me touches my soul. The combination of the electricity, vulnerability, tenderness, and closeness goes to the heart of what makes us all human, and its power is almost indescribable. When this spirit is awakened between two lovers, the world stops and you become the center of the universe.

Although it was clear that the diet worked to spice up our sex life, it also became clear that the diet greatly impacted another, altogether deeper level of our relationship, and Jeff and I both felt it. There was a passion between us, and we felt closer than we had in years. I also felt a renewed sense of confidence in myself. My work flowed better, I got more done, and I felt more generous in spirit.

My experience so overwhelmed me that I wanted to share it. I wanted to shout from the rooftop so that everyone out there could feel the same sense of miracle. But first I had to prove my theory. So when I came down to earth, I began a research project. I decided to see what other people would discover if they, too, committed to having sex a certain number of times each week. I contacted and queried over a hundred couples across America and signed on thirty-eight couples who would test out my theory. After speaking with them at length, I then had them commit to the Great American Sex Diet: twenty-eight days of sex four times a week. Through my own experience over that six-month period, I determined that four times would be enough to create the frequency effect I was looking for. I then gave each couple a seduction packet that contained the keys to their sexual kingdom: a calendar, two menus of spices (secret seduction techniques and suggestions—one for *his* eyes only, and one for *her* eyes only), and instructions on how to implement the "diet."

I explained to the couples that the Great American Sex Diet is about a healthy approach to sex. It gives you a tried-and-true formula for how to reinvigorate your sex life. It makes sex fun, adventurous, and filled with endless variety. It restores lost passion, gives you new tips on how to surprise your partner, and teaches you the tools to turn "no" into "yes."

All Jeff and I did was change *one* ingredient of our relationship and the entire dynamic transformed. And, I'm happy to report, Jeff and I weren't the only ones who experienced this kind of shift. Interviewing all the couples after the diet, I discovered *all* who had successfully completed the diet also felt their relationship had been transformed. If they were already having frequent though predictable sex, their sex life got hotter and more experi-

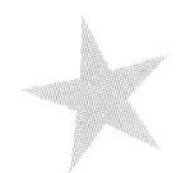

mental. If they'd been alienated and irritable with each other before the diet, they became closer and more connected. Many couples said that they had lost years, but now their relationship felt as it did in their early days together. To my great surprise, of the thirty-eight couples I interviewed, only two couples were unable to complete the diet successfully. One was for health reasons and the other due to one partner's lack of commitment.

The overwhelming results from the Great American Sex Diet were irrefutable! As one man said, "When we're having frequent sex, there's a difference in the way she looks at me. I can swim in her eyes at any given moment." A woman described the experience in this way: "Now we're closer than ever and we've never had so much fun!"

Physicians, psychologists, and sexologists have been saying for years that those couples that schedule sex have better sex. The Great American Sex Diet is the first program that actually gives you the tools to see the amazing truth for yourselves.

By now I was convinced that I needed to share these special couples' experiences with all of you. I had discovered a truth and it had been staring me in the face the whole time: The key to staying connected at a deep, heart level in a relationship is through physical intimacy. I may not be the first person to make this observation, but when it sank in, its sheer power swept me away. Your relationship with your lover is special. It is separate and different from all the other relationships you may have in your life. Why? Because you have sex with only one person, your lover. Sex is the only thing you do with your partner that you don't do with anyone else. How fantastic is that?

As I listened to my research team of couples over the course of their twenty-eight-day diet, I heard again and again about walls coming down and breakthroughs being made. Listening to their stories has made an enormous impact on me: Being on the Great American Sex Diet was not only their journey, it was mine as well, a Magical Journey of Surprise that will inspire me—not to mention people from all walks of life—forever!

THE FABULOUS CORN RECIPE

If you come to this book already familiar with me and my philosophy about sex, then you might remember my recipe for great sex. If you are new to me and my ways and are finding this book for the first time, then let me introduce myself. I believe that all couples can have great sex if they keep in mind a few simple ingredients:

Anticipation + Variety = Great Sex!

Each of my books, *101 Nights of Grrreat Sex*, *101 Nights of Grrreat Romance*, *101 Grrreat Quickies*, and *52 Invitations to Grrreat Sex*, is based on this formula. Why? Because it works. Thousands and thousands of men and women across this great country of ours have told me how this simple recipe led them to have amazing sex.

The heart of the recipe can be explained by a quick examination of its two vital ingredients: anticipation and variety.

Anticipation

When you create a sense of anticipation surrounding sex, you give your partner a route to recharge the lust factor. Remember when you first got together? You could barely wait to rip each other's clothes off. You pawed at each other, teased each other, and reveled in the waiting period as much as in the consummation itself because you never knew what was going to happen next. Your physical and sexual attraction was so palpable sex felt ignited and out of control.

Without anticipation, sex often feels predictable and we end up taking it for granted. *"Oh, it's you again."* The face and body that used to drive you wild with desire seems like the same old, same old. So how do we create this magical sense of anticipation? I knew that if my diet was to be successful, it *had* to include anticipation. But what was the best way to create it? It's actually quite simple, but you'll have to read on a bit for all the juicy details.

Variety

I'm sure you're familiar with the phrase "Variety is the spice of life." Well, this couldn't be truer in the realm of sex. Part of that same old, same old feeling is the belief that the partner we love and adore will not, cannot surprise us anymore. Haven't we done it every way possible? Why doesn't my partner surprise me and do something different? I knew this was an important factor. When I asked all the couples on the research team before the diet if they could predict what would take place if they made love that night, almost every person said yes. Their responses made me more determined than ever to shake up this rut of predictability.

Believe me, there are many tools and techniques of seduction on this diet that you'll be presented with that will rock your world! When you introduce a new position, technique, or toy, it not only adds to your sexual

Anticipation + Variety = Great SEX!

treasure chest, but also expands your sexual horizons and recharges the batteries of your sex life. It's obvious that if your sex life revolves solely around doing it missionary style, one or both of you will feel bored. So I challenge you: Open your door to variety and, I promise, you will infuse your sex life with energy!

So what is great sex? Well, for me, great sex changes all the time. Sometimes it's about having a wild, fun time. Sometimes it's more slow and romantic. And sometimes it's being able to connect with Jeff at the level of the soul. Great sex is what you believe it to be, whatever makes you feel good inside and out. But the common denominator for all great sex is that the two people sharing the experience are into it together.

BEYOND THE CORN RECIPE

Tighten Your Seat Belts, This Is Going to Be a Wild Ride!

—

Together, anticipation and variety create great sex. But what I discovered on the diet was another important factor in fabulous sex: frequency. Essentially, when couples commit to having regular sex, they will not only feel better, they will feel more alive. They will see this difference when they look in the mirror. (Remember those photos I took?) They will feel stronger physically and emotionally and they will also feel more connected. As I say above, *connection* is the key not only to great sex, but to great sex *whenever you want it*. This means that when you and your partner fall into a slump, you will have the tools to get back on track. You'll know how to reignite the spark. You'll know how easy and fun it is to stick to the diet and reap its many rewards.

For me and for many of the couples on the research team, the specific number of times that we scheduled sex worked wonders. I prescribed having sex on the diet four times a week for twenty-eight days because that was the number that in my experience worked best to create the benefits from frequency and was the most realistic and feasible. In almost every case, men and women responded to the idea of a number as a motivator for wanting sex. It gave them a goal to achieve, something special to strive for.

THIS IS FOR YOU!

—

The timing for this book seems serendipitous. In the past few years it seems we have been inundated with media reports about the sad, lackluster state of the American sex life. *U.S. News & World Report* stated that more than 40 percent of women were dissatisfied with their sex life, according to a survey of nearly 2,000 representative women. A study in the *Journal of the American Medical Association (JAMA)* estimated

24 million American women "aren't interested in sex," which means they are suffering from low desire.

As a result, both women and men are turning to their pharmacies for help. Some are trying dietary supplements such as ArginMa; others are testing Viagra, the little blue pill that has helped many men overcome impotence; and still others are using hormone creams or patches in hopes of feeling more sexually lively.

I have known all my life that I suffer from what experts call low desire. That is, I have a less-than-average physical desire for sex. This is why I got into this business—to help me come out of my shell. This condition is more common among women than men, and some women experience no desire at all. Low desire is real, but its exact cause is unclear. Scientists and sexologists studying this condition and its prevalence believe low desire is related to hormone imbalance (especially in women over forty), outside stresses, and perhaps unresolved emotional or psychological issues.

If you are someone who suffers from low desire, then the Great American Sex Diet will give you the tools to access your lust. If you and your partner already have great sex, the diet will give you an opportunity to make your sex life even better. Maybe you and your partner have great sex, feel close and incredibly

LOOK WHAT HAPPENED FOR THE VERY FIRST TIME ON THE DIET!

1. Over half of the men and women discovered new ways to bring their lovers to orgasm.
2. Seven women found their G-spot and several had their first G-spot orgasm.
3. Over half of the women tried sex toys for the first time.
4. One woman had a thirty-minute orgasm.
5. One woman became pregnant on the diet.
6. Several women had their first water orgasm.
7. One woman experienced her very first orgasm.
8. Several men had the best oral sex of their lives.
9. One woman watched (and enjoyed!) erotic videos for the first time ever.
10. One woman discovered the intimate pleasures of masturbation.
11. One woman experienced her first orgasm through oral sex.
12. Several men learned how to last longer.
13. One couple had sex nine times in two days.
14. One man had multiple orgasms.
15. One couple was able to climax together.

loving, but you want to explore your sexual options and add some spice to your sex life. Perhaps you and your partner love each other, but something has happened to that spark. Or maybe you haven't had sex in six months and are on the brink of a divorce or a breakup. No matter where you are on the sexual continuum, you will benefit from the Great American Sex Diet. The premise of the diet may seem simple at first, but its power is nothing short of amazing, as the accounts from my research team will attest. I believe it has the power to change your life. It has certainly transformed mine.

THE MIRACULOUS, MARVELOUS BENEFITS OF THE GREAT AMERICAN SEX DIET

Never in my wildest imagination could I have dreamed of all the truly remarkable and at times even overwhelming benefits that couples experienced on this diet. Listening to the stories of my research team made my heart swell with pleasure and pride, for this indeed was just more of my magical journey of surprise. At the outset of this project, I was already very familiar with the many concrete medical benefits of sex. I was also becoming more and more familiar with the other benefits to women's and men's self-esteem and confidence and to a couple's relationship. Jeff and I experienced many of these benefits, and as you will see as you read on and get to know the research couples who "tested" the diet, these results have been substantiated.

The Deep Rewards and Emotional Benefits

The emotional benefits of the Great American Sex Diet are many and varied. Across the spectrum of the research couples, I discovered that the diet has the power to:

- Rejuvenate your relationship, giving you and your partner a new lease on life.
- Jump-start your sex life and reignite the spark of lust.
- Recharge your desire for each other and make your lust tangible and throbbing.
- Strengthen your heartfelt commitment to each other.
- Increase the romance so you and your mate will be ringing bells and popping corks.
- Draw you closer to each other and improve your ability to communicate openly, honestly, and frankly.
- Intensify your emotional and spiritual connection so that your love feels deeper and wider than an ocean.

What was truly astounding is that couples walked away with their own unique breakthrough. Spicing up their sex life was definitely an all-around hit. These men and women experienced a ton of fun! They learned new tools and techniques and expanded their sexual treasure chests.

But it was at the deeper emotional level that couples seemed to experience the most positive change and growth. I was simply amazed at how much being on the twenty-eight-day diet helped all the couples to reconnect at the level of the heart and soul. When you read their individual stories at the back of the book, I'm sure you'll be blown away, too.

For me, one of the most powerful emotional benefits of the Great American Sex Diet is how it boosts self-esteem. I *know* the diet boosts self-esteem because it happened to me! Before I created the diet, before I had even considered the impact of having frequent sex, I was aware of the connection between having sex and feeling better about myself. When I was closer and more connected to Jeff, I would simply feel more relaxed, more confident, and more at peace with myself. When I added the element of frequency, my self-esteem was transformed. I was like a new person—energetic, in charge, and excited!

And I looked different: My eyes sparkled, my skin glowed, and I had a softness that simply made me look and feel more attractive. I've noticed these changes not only in myself, but in other women and men, too. A certain hardness disappears when someone is sensual and sexual. It's as if the tenderness and vulnerability that come to the surface when we make love take away the rigidity that is so often the result of carrying stress, harboring anger, or simply having bad feelings. Unleash these trapped feelings through sex and you will see the transformation. It comes shining through.

> *"I haven't seen my wife this happy in six years. This is the most confident, the most self-aware that I've seen her. To see her the way she is now, it's an awakening. It's rejuvenating. It's remarkable. I can't say enough about it."* —Conrad

This same connection between frequent sex and high self-esteem proved to be true among all the men and women on the research team. Like me, the women tended to experience this self-esteem at a deep emotional level and connected the feeling to the idea of confidence. They felt sexier, more desirable, more proactive. They let go of inhibitions and discovered their power as women and as sexual beings. Several women who before the diet had issues with their weight discovered a new way of looking at themselves. The diet let them embrace who they are, regardless of their weight or body shape. Many of the women who are now mothers voiced continual frustration with the fact that their bodies were no longer, as Julia said, "tight and hard." But during and after the diet, they felt better about their bodies. In some cases they lost weight; in other cases they changed their perspective. When I asked Sherry what her number one reason for not wanting to make love was, she admitted, "It's my attitude. When I had children, I would say, 'I'm tired.' But now it's my age or my hormones or something. I'm always in bitch mode about myself, about my husband, about so many things. It's all rolled up into one bad attitude." And with the diet that was something that went out with the trash!

Doreen sums up the change in her relationship by saying, "When we have frequent sex, I flirt and tease more, and I'm more playful. I feel better about myself as a person. I'm just so much more confident."

The men tended to experience this boost in self-esteem in terms of feeling empowered. Both Kirk and Brian felt this empowerment physically, accessing that very virile, male sense of physical strength and masculinity. Dwayne, who had been reluctant to put any pressure on Melanie, let go of his passivity and enjoyed fully embracing his lust and desire for her. He was even able to last longer—talk about empowerment.

Raul and Eric also felt a surge of male power and pride. "I could take on the world!" claimed Eric. Needless to say, the women on the receiving end of these boosts of power relished—in every sense of the word—their men.

Some men were more thoughtful and experienced the increase in self-esteem at a more emotional level. As Don said, "[The diet] is about rediscovering yourself." Isn't that the truth! After all, the best way to be in a relationship is by first loving and accepting oneself. The rest is a cakewalk.

The Power of the Physical

According to Michael F. Rozen, M.D., in his book *Real Age*, the average sexually active American has sex about once a week (fifty-eight times a year to be precise). Married people tend to have more sex than singles. Frequency also varies with age and economic, social, and ethnic backgrounds.

Since 1950, studies have proven a correlation between regular (frequent) sex and longevity. Other studies show that sexual satisfaction can be a predictor of cardiovascular disease: Both men and women who were less satisfied with their sex lives were more likely to have premature aging of the arteries.

A recent study in Great Britain suggests that men who have sex considerably more than once a week have lower rates of mortality. What does this mean? The more sex a person has, the longer he or she will live. "This study is the strongest proof we have that sex can actually help us get younger and stay younger," confirms Dr. Rozen.

Dr. Rozen further estimates that "if the numbers from this study prove true, we can say that having sex twice a week (twice the national average) can make a person 1.6 years younger. And if we extrapolate linearly, something the early evidence suggests that we can do, the person who has sex almost every day (350 times a year) and is happy with his or her sex life could have a Real Age as much as eight years younger." I don't know about you, but I'm all for this particular benefit!

Graham Masterton, a well-known sex educator, captures the essence and power of having frequent sex when he says in his book *How to Make Love Six Nights a Week*:

Having frequent sex does very much more than release tensions. It raises your self-esteem; it re-establishes your closeness with your partner; it defines your status as a woman; it demonstrates that somebody needs you and desires you . . . not just every now and then . . . but all the time. Frequent sex is good for your self-confidence. Frequent sex is good for your physical fitness and general well-being. Frequent sex gives you a more positive and creative attitude toward life and will have a direct beneficial effect on anything that you're trying to achieve, either at home or at work. Frequent sex makes you more calm and less irritable. . . . Frequent sex improves your self-image. Frequent sex helps you to explore the full potential of your emotions, your body, and your imagination. Without any exaggeration, frequent sex can change your life from top to bottom.

As if that doesn't say it all, here are some other benefits of frequent sex:

- Regular sex has a therapeutic effect on the body's immune system, keeping it strong and healthy.

- Regular sex can help you sleep better, relieve menstrual cramps, and even improve digestion, according to Dr. Ava Cadell, a Los Angeles–based sexologist.

- Women who remain sexually active through menopause typically avoid some of the physical problems associated with menopause that can make sex painful, explains Mary Jane Minkin, M.D., clinical professor of obstetrics and gynecology at Yale School of Medicine.

- Sex helps you to learn better and remember more. Studies show that intense stimulation, like the kind sex provides, can produce chemicals in the brain that help brain cells grow new dendrites—the filaments attached to nerve cells that allow neurons to communicate with one another. The more dendrites you have, explains Lawrence Katz, Ph.D., professor of neurobiology at Duke University Medical Center, the more capacity you have to learn new things.

- Regular sex makes it easier to have more and possibly better sex. A recent study out of the University of California at Berkeley found that sex may cause certain brain cells governing sex to fire longer and become stronger.

- Lots of lovemaking may cut stress-triggered bingeing. Sex can dramatically lower the levels of cortisol, a hormone that increases during stress, which can trigger fatigue and cravings.

If all of these very real benefits haven't yet convinced you of the remarkable merits of frequent sex, then consider some of these highlights from the research couples after they completed the twenty-eight-day diet.

- A man and woman on the verge of breakup not only reconnected on a totally new level but also had the best sex of their sixteen-year marriage!

- One woman who had suffered severe depression before the diet experienced a radical shift in mood, and most of her depression symptoms disappeared.

- A woman went from having absolutely no sexual desire to craving sex!

- One woman experienced her first orgasm on the diet and was amazed by her body's ability to experience pleasure.

- One man went from feeling too inhibited to ever initiate sex to becoming a Don Juan of seduction!

- Both men and women experienced a huge increase in sex drive. Most said their sex drive actually doubled!

- The diet's secret menus inspired couples to be creative and break sexual boundaries. Some couples found themselves in marathon sex sessions; others found themselves on wild, sexual adventures!

- Couples became more romantic, flirtatious, and playful. They did things for and to each other they hadn't done since they were dating!

- Several women experienced radical shifts in self-esteem. Before the diet, they were plagued by poor body images; during and after the diet, they were buying lingerie and doing stripteases for their lovers!

The Romance Factor

We tend to associate romance with the early years of our relationship, yet the diet is further proof that while romance may fade a little, it never completely disappears.

Inspired by the diet's creative zeal, Christie and Glenn (as you can see from their after photo on page 147) resumed a wonderful tradition they hadn't experienced since before their kids were born: a night out on the town.

As Christie remarked, "It reminded me of being back in the beginning of the relationship. Now we get dressed up and have nice dinners together and have little dinner parties." The thrill and excitement that comes from romantic gestures cannot be underestimated.

Romance has the power to make both of you—the giver and the receiver—feel special.

Other couples exchanged love notes, arranged picnics, wrote poems—Jordan even wrote Reneé a song! The connection the couples felt made them more flirtatious and willing to express the tender feelings of romance.

When you read the Magical Journey of Surprise, which contains all the stories of the research team, you will be able to see and hear how moved these men and women were by their experience. It's my hope that these stories not only entertain you (some will make you laugh out loud with hearty recognition, I'm sure), but also provide insights into your own relationship. You may be totally different from these people, but by reading their comments and experiences, you may gain a better sense of how to look at and evaluate your own relationship. I know I have. Every couple on my research team taught me an invaluable lesson. I want to share with you these lessons, along with other wisdom I have gained throughout this entire project. Remember, this book is for you!

My Spectacular Research Team

The thirty-eight couples on my Great American Sex Diet research team vary in age; length of time together; and general social, economic, and ethnic background. Some couples are married, some are living together, some have kids, and some are well into their retirement. They are teachers, nurses, bus drivers, store owners, software developers, writers, interior decorators, construction workers, CEOs, housewives, and business owners. They also range in age from early twenties to late sixties and represent a wide range of interests and personalities, and I must say I came to love them all.

I interviewed both members of each couple before they started the diet and after they finished. I asked them such questions as how is the current state of their relationship; how frequently (or infrequently) they were having sex; and how they would describe their level of love, commitment, and connection to each other.

I used these questions to open the dialogue with them about the diet and also to prompt them to start observing and evaluating their own relationships. As I say above, any real change begins simply with becoming more aware of your interaction with your partner—sexually, emotionally, and spiritually.

I also sent Pulitzer Prize–nominated photographer Rick Dahms to photograph the couples before and after the diet. Rick is an extraordinary talent and I immediately knew he had a real feel for the project. These photos are included in the stories that appear in the Magical Journey of Surprise, where you'll find the couples' profiles. This section is my special gift to you. It's a scrapbook and includes their stories, mementos the couples sent to me from their diet experience, and the photos.

For me, the photos are one of the most dramatic aspects of the diet. I asked each couple the following question: If you were to take a photograph of your relationship right now, what would it look like? I wanted them to think about this and make their own decision. The couples then chose their own pose or scenario that best captured the main feeling of their relationship before they went on the diet and then after they completed the diet. These photos swept me away with their honesty. They showed couples vulnerable and open. They showed couples loving but disconnected sexually. They showed couples clobbered by their responsibilities, kids, and work.

Immediately following the before interview and photos, the couples then began their Great American Sex Diet adventure. After twenty-eight days, I reinterviewed the couples and listened to their very changed voices, and Rick returned to capture these remarkable transformations in the after photos. Again, they were asked what their relationship looked like and they then chose their pose or scene.

The after photos are incredibly telling, and contrasting them with the before photos said everything about the value of the diet. Look at Andrew and Stephanie on pages 140 and 141. In their before photo, their distance and alienation from each other is absolutely blatant. In the after photo, they are not only smiling broadly, they are attached at the hip in the hot tub together.

On pages 166 and 167, the before and after photos of Kirk and Sherry show a more subtle kind of transformation. Their before photo shows that they are close and very much in love, but their after photo shows the spark of wild sensuality that has been ignited. Kirk is empowered to be Sherry's jungle man, ravishing her with his desire.

These photos and their accompanying stories are a testament not only to the very vivid rewards the couples reaped from being on the diet, but also to their tremendous satisfaction as they changed their relationship. Sex is a vital, powerful force that has the capability of saving a relationship or sending it to the moon. I challenge you to harness this power and make it work for you!

PART
II

The Diet in Action

THE DIET THAT WILL BLOW YOUR MIND

The Great American Sex Diet will enlighten you, enrich you, and empower you. You will learn to use the tools for having (and keeping on having) great sex now and throughout your relationship. The diet is a tried-and-proven recipe that shows couples how to achieve fabulous sex throughout their relationship—not simply at its passionate beginning.

"This diet is wonderful because it puts you in a happy, fun frame of mind all the time. You're 'in the mood' continuously for twenty-eight days!"
—Donna

As the research has proven, when couples commit to having frequent sex, they will not only feel better physically and stronger emotionally, but they will feel more intimate, trusting, and connected to each other. You will be able to break the patterns of not having sex. Just like an exercise program, you can fall off the diet and get right back on—that's reality. We live in a complicated world and most of us have very complicated, busy lives. But sticking to the twenty-eight-day diet will not add more complication to your already taxed lives; it will add more fun!

If you and your partner commit to the goal of the diet and keep your eyes on the prize, then I promise you will be successful. Trust me.

I've found that one of the keys to this success is giving yourself permission. As you will see later, many couples made very intense and exciting breakthroughs on the diet. Some of these breakthroughs were emotional. Melanie and Mo were able to voice pent-up feelings that had been getting between them for years and found themselves discussing topics they had never been able to talk about before. Another couple broke down the thick walls of taboo: Both partners not only got wild with the spices, the woman actually masturbated for the very first time!

Again, since sex is so powerful, it seems only natural that it can bring to the surface powerful emotions and feelings. When you commit to the diet, you naturally create an intimate space with your partner. You will be amazed by how close you will feel to your lover. Your trust and comfort with each other will know no bounds.

Let's Get Started

Remember the Corn recipe?

Anticipation + Variety = Great Sex!

The diet is based on this recipe, plus the added factors of commitment and frequency. Before you begin the diet, I think it's important for you and your partner to take stock of where you are in terms of these four components. As you read through the sections below, think about your own relationship and what you'd like to improve upon.

Step One: Commitment

If great sex throughout your relationship is something you want to achieve, then you simply have to agree and commit to wanting better sex. This first step is more mental and emotional than physical. You and your partner have to agree to go on the diet for twenty-eight days. Sound easy? It is. Many of the couples on the research team were amazed at how just making the commitment to be on the diet together gave them the incentive to complete it. That initial decision created a palpable momentum that made the couple's experience on the diet successful! Believe me, the twenty-eight days will fly by because you will be having so much fun.

"We made the commitment to each other that we were going to stay on the diet. When I made the commitment, I said, 'Okay, I'm going to do this. No matter how I feel, I'm going to follow through.' And then right away I saw the rewards coming back to me."—Christine

Step Two: Frequency

An essential key to having great sex is in the frequency. The research supports my conclusion that the more often couples have sex, the better their sex will be and the better they will feel as a couple. But you have to have frequent, regular sex, and a great way to accomplish this is by scheduling sex. I understand that some couples may shy away from this approach. Isn't scheduling the opposite of spontaneous, fabulous sex? Absolutely not. Scheduling sex means two things: (1) it's a priority in your life; and (2) it's going to happen (i.e., you're going to get some!). Remember to use the number. I chose four times a week as the target for the diet. Keep this in mind as motivation and as inspiration—accomplishing a goal has never been this exciting before!

"When we're having frequent sex, I feel security from him and I feel love. I feel that everything is going to be taken care of. Any insecurities you have just vanish."—Robin

Step Three: Anticipation

Without spice, without the power of suggestion, surprise, and seduction, sex can and will get predictable, even boring. You know by now that anticipation is critical to a relationship's success, and creating anticipation involves piquing your lover's curiosity, keeping him guessing, and giving him something to look forward to.

Think about how excited you are the days before a big event like Christmas or Hanukkah, a big birthday or Valentine's Day. As you're counting down the days, your anticipation mounts. You fantasize and imagine what kind of surprises you'll get and how special you will feel—thinking about the day is almost as fun as the occasion itself!

This is how your partner should feel about your relationship. When the anticipation is there, the passion grows, and when the passion grows, the sex—and the relationship—gets hotter and hotter.

Scheduling sex is a great way to build anticipation and that's what the Spice Calendars are for (more on them later). Use this diet tool to drop hints about what you've got planned—believe me, her curiosity will skyrocket! With anticipation you've got the power to create drama, excitement, and intrigue. All it takes is a few minutes and, presto, you're having the time of your life!

"One of the most exciting things about the diet is the anticipation. You know something is going to happen when you get home, but you don't know what it is. It's like you're a kid in a candy store—'I can't wait, can't wait!' I was close to getting speeding tickets on the way home!"—Burnie

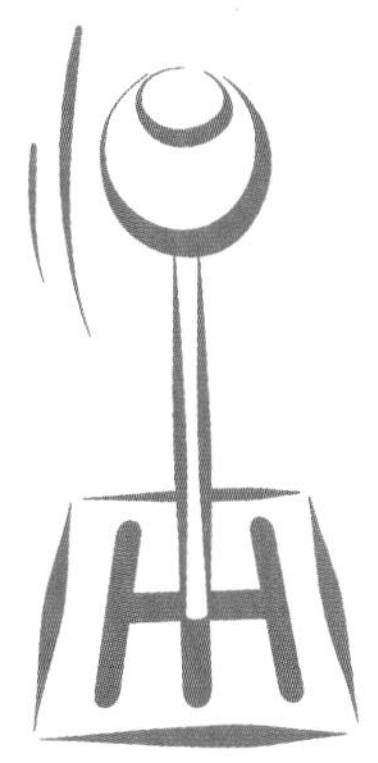

STEP FOUR: VARIETY

Without surprise and diversity, sex can become boring and predictable. The key to turning the predictable into the passionate and seductive is in the secret His and Hers Spice Menus, which provide specific spices so there's no chance of a dull moment. These spices are Corn showstoppers! The research team actually tested all of them. Those that didn't work or didn't appeal, I threw out. So what you have here are the crème de la crème of techniques and suggestions that will arouse men and women and quickly send them over the edge. In general, the spices include techniques for foreplay, oral sex, intercourse, fantasy, and ways to arouse more than one erogenous zone at a time. Bon appétit!

"The menu gives you options, gives you ideas, and gives you choices. For couples that aren't very adventurous, this gives you easy things to do. It offers great ideas for the beginner and great ideas for the more experienced!"—Casey

Once you've made a commitment to go on the diet, you are ready to begin! You have received the same materials that the research couples received in their original packet of information and instructions. Those sealed envelopes are just waiting to be torn open and enjoyed. But no peeking just yet!

The Essential Ingredients:

- His and Her Secret Spice Menus
- The Spice Calendar

And some extra treats—the envelopes:

- His and Her Diet Secrets
- His and Her Extra Spice Menus
- His and Her Anticipation Teasers

USING THE SECRET SPICE MENUS

Your Ticket to Surprise and Adventure

—

Spices are my specialty and the Secret Spice Menus are the keys to opening the door to explosive, wild, and adventurous sex. Each spice offers you a seduction suggestion, position, or technique to surprise your lover and wow them in bed or out of bed, as the case may be. The menus are what will bring you and your partner endless sexual and sensual variety and allow you to create mind-blowing anticipation. As Christie and Glenn point out, the menus made them "look at the [diet] as a great adventure." Let the adventure begin!

The Spice Menu was designed to give BIG variety in a SMALL space. I've taken a few of the most popular spices from my other books and introduced them in a new, quick way, plus I've come up with lots and lots of new ones. When you start mixing and matching the spices, there are virtually endless combinations.

My accountant even did the numbers: If you combine spices from just one menu, you can actually create almost half a million spice combinations. Combine four spices from two menus and you'll have almost 8 million spice combinations. And if you mix in all the extra spices, you'll get a mind-bending number of possibilities. Think of how many sleepless nights that will give you!

The two secret His and Hers menus are divided into types of spices: Foreplay, Oral, Intercourse, and Toy Spices, as well as a few extra categories you won't discover until you open your sealed envelopes. The men's menu ("For His Eyes Only") offers hundreds of ways you can seduce the love of your life. Does she like long, sweet foreplay that makes her body tremble? You'll find the foreplay spice that

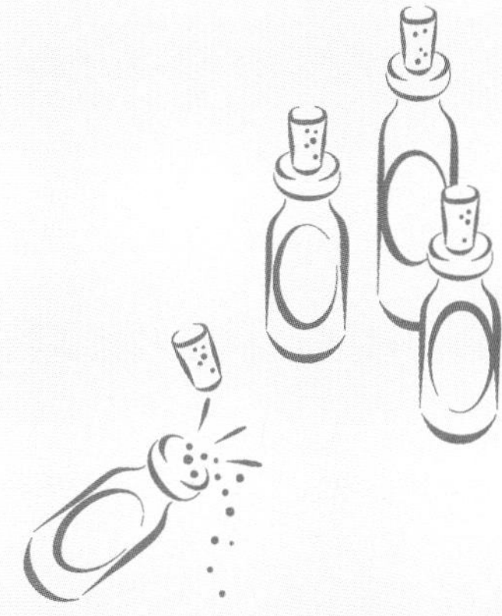

gives you the tools. Does she like to be pleasured by your roving tongue? You will be able to choose from a variety of oral spices that will make her beg you for more, more!

The women's menu ("For Her Eyes Only") is running over with techniques to bring your man to his knees. Want to know a creative way to use your lingerie? Check out the intercourse spices! Want to treat him to a sexual experience he'll never, ever forget? Wait until you read the Heat Is On! in the oral spices. Or, add a foreplay spice with a fantasy spice for an unforgettable combo!

"When you're reading through the menu, you can visually fantasize about doing each one of these things to her. I mean, talk about getting all hot and bothered just reading through these spices! I liked that there were so many choices on the menu. It gave me the opportunity to do two or three spices at a time, which was a lot of fun!"—Doug

Since I've made the seductions "short and sweet," you can read them in thirty seconds and gain some great ideas. All of them are on one page that you can take with you to work or hide in a secret place. Easy and convenient, the Spice Menu is something you can always pull out at a moment's notice. You can have sex 365 days a year (!) and still surprise each other with the menu's limitless variety. And, I promise, even after you finish your twenty-eight-day diet, you will continue to use the menus for years to come.

All of the thirty-eight research team couples said the Secret Spices made them feel more experimental and provided totally new spices that worked like a "sex refresher course!"

She's going to be curious and wonder, "Did he pull out his menu today?" He'll wonder, "What spice is she going to try tonight?" It's a fun, fabulous way to flirt with each other. When he asks, "Honey, what's for dinner?" she can say, "I don't know, let me pull out my menu!" I truly believe that this one page will add years and years of excitement to your love life.

If you're going to be successful on this diet—if you really want frequent sex and its benefits—then you need to inject variety and build anticipation. And the Spice Menu will help you do that. The fact that your partner knows something a little different is going to happen in each encounter will create more desire, anticipation, and mystery.

You can use the menus in whatever way you choose. The research team used the menus in all sorts of ways. Some couples tried a different spice each night, and others looked at the menu for inspiration and then went on their merry way, creating their own spices and sexual fantasies together.

For instance, one night Heather surprised her husband, Lars, with a six-spice combo. Talk about becoming a chef in the bedroom! They both said that their secret menus really inspired them, and the variety and anticipation really turned them on. You may want to find out which spices Heather used in her famous combo!

Other couples did four or five spices the way

they are described in the menus and then improvised. This was the case with JoAnn and Jerry, who went to town with one spice. She wrote "don't forget your Vitamin C" on the calendar and then did a spice called Passion Fruit. Talk about getting the juices flowing!

A few couples referenced the menus for ideas, but didn't follow the exact directions of the spices. Frank explained it this way: "I used the Total Control spice and came up with my own version." Wouldn't you like to know how he used the chocolate to bring Julia to her knees?

Some couples, like Sara and Scott, got into changing the time and location of when and where they had sex. These slight shifts in their routine were enough to make them tremble with sexual energy.

Angela and Jeremy went into the diet wanting to be more experimental and watch less TV. The Spice Menus really worked for them. As Jeremy said, "We got off on being creative . . . it was like a new workout program." And although Angela had already done a few spices on the menu, she was still excited to try all the other different options.

Before the diet, Kara had never experimented with toys. Bob had always wanted to introduce them, but Kara had resisted. Once they were on the diet, the sheer momentum and excitement of having sex felt like a game and together they made headlines!

Use the menu in whatever way works for you. As you read through the spices, think about what you know about your partner. Does she like to be romanced? Does he like hard and fast sex? By focusing on what you already know about your partner, you can predict what he or she might like. Then again, if you try something new and unexpected, you'll be in for some big surprises!

Though most of the spices on the menu will be completely new and tantalizing, there's no doubt you will encounter a few spices that you may have done before. Just combine them with another spice, and they take on a whole new meaning. Prepare for the wild world of combos!

And although I think it's important to introduce a new technique, position, or toy with care and respect, I also think it's worth the risk. Sure, trying something new can make you both feel a bit vulnerable. But what about the payoff? The spices give you permission to introduce something new and become creative and imaginative. I was amazed at how many women and men on the research team responded to this permission. They were no longer afraid or hesitant to be adventurous. Because both of you have your own menus, the whole process becomes interactive, opening the doors to possibility in a whole new way. The endless variety provided by the menus gives you the power to surprise your partner.

Isn't surprise the antidote to boring, predictable sex? Of course! The Secret Spice Menus are your keys to surprise, seduction, and sensational sex.

"Ohmigod, I read the menu a hundred times! I'd just keep going over it and over it. On my breaks at work, I'd take the Spice Menu out and decide which spices I wanted to surprise Scott with. Then I'd kind of pick and choose and say, 'Okay, tonight I'm going to do this one!'"

—Annette

Extra Spices

I always like to give my readers something extra, and since I couldn't fit everything I wanted on one menu, I've added a bonus. These sealed envelopes—one for her eyes only, one for his eyes only—of Extra Spices will not only add to the sense of anticipation and mystery, but will also give you more spices with which to surprise each other. Who knows, you may even create your own additions to the Spice Menu by the time you're done!

Spice Bonus

Wondering what the three most popular spices from each menu are? See your Diet Secrets envelope!

USING THE SPICE CALENDARS

The Route to Great Sex Four Nights a Week

I can't emphasize enough how miraculous the calendars are for most couples, including Jeff and me. I'm a typical type A personality and pretty much a workaholic. I'm driven. I like to organize my day, my week, and my month. I like to stick to schedules. At the same time, like many people, when it came to the idea of scheduling sex, I was suspicious that planning sex would take away the element of spontaneity. But what I found was that nothing could have been further from the truth. When Jeff and I would sit on the couch on a Sunday night, glass of wine in hand, to fill in our calendar for the upcoming week of sex, we'd start

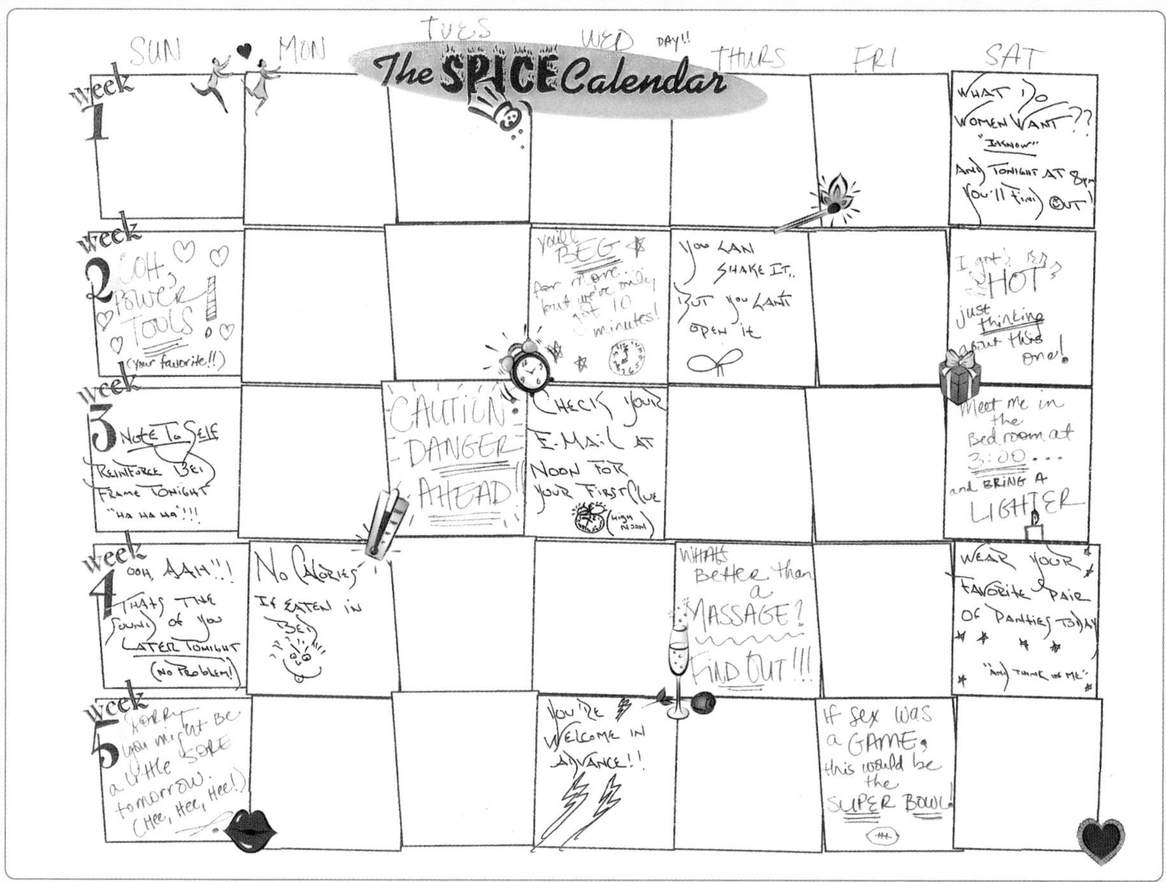

to get excited right then and there. We were giggling, flirting, and the double entendres were flying. The thrill of the chase was on!

You can fill in the calendar in any way that seems to elicit excitement or curiosity from your partner. And let me tell you from experience, filling out the calendars is fun! Sunday night is a great time to sit down with your sweetie and plan your lovemaking for the week. You might want to use a pencil because there's bound to be some changes along the way, but that only adds to the excitement. In honor of the "ladies first" tradition, let's say the woman goes first. She looks at her Spice Menu and then fills in her two days for the upcoming week. When she's done, he fills in his two dates. Be prepared for some bartering: "You've got a spice scheduled for Monday, and that's when I watch *Monday Night Football!*" You'll banter and barter for prime times and that's half the fun.

Take a look at the calendar above, which we sent to the research team as a sample. Are you curious about what danger may lie ahead? Or what kind of Power Tools you might be using on the diet? And what's better than a massage? These are just a few examples of how you can tease your partner with the calendar by using the Anticipation Teasers provided. You'll find a list of these tantalizing and playful turn-ons in your sealed envelopes that will help you tempt and torment your lover. Or you can make up your own prompts to create anticipation. Some of the couples simply wrote in the name of the spice; others used their own special code. It's all up to you.

I've offered you the Anticipation Teasers as suggestions, but feel free to go to town. Do you and your partner have your own special language for sex? If so, then use it to whet each other's appetite, and remember, making your lover wait adds to the excitement. Think about how the billion-dollar entertainment industry thrives because it creates anticipation: It teases us with advertisements, trailers for movies, or an "upcoming special." By the time the movie or TV show arrives, we are dying to see it. That's the power of anticipation. The same theory applies to lovemaking: You've got to keep things interesting and keep your partner on his or her toes, and the easiest, hottest way to do this is to build anticipation.

And how do you do that? It's as simple as writing down one or two sentences on your Spice Calendar. Imagine how excited your partner will be if he or she reads what you've written: "You'll ache with pleasure," or "Meet me in the bedroom at nine, but not a second sooner!" These simple sentences have the power to create all sorts of fired-up feelings—curiosity, excitement, fascination, and arousal! You'll find these and more Anticipation Teasers in your sealed envelopes.

The calendar works because it helps you schedule sex and makes sure it happens. That said, couples used the calendars in a variety of ways. Describing his and Elizabeth's experience with the calendar, Jeff said, "Scheduling sex was so much more fun and spontaneous than we thought it'd be. We liked using the calendar. We both had our menus and we'd get ideas and then just write them down. We kept the calendar right on her mirror in the bedroom so if one of us wrote something down as a surprise, the other person would walk by and be inspired to write down two more notes!"

The calendar helps to make sure that you plan sex. As Cameran said, "I really like to schedule sex because if it's not on my to-do list, it might not get done. It was easier to make it a priority because it was a commitment and it was something to look forward to. I knew it was going to happen, so I could plan accordingly."

Like Jeff and me, Heather and Lars also had a "workaholic mentality," and as a result, scheduling sex and planning on it made total sense to them. If you look at their photos on pages 154 and 155, the after photo includes the clock: It's 7:30 P.M. and it's time for their preplanned sex break! Before, they would have both worked through the evening. Now they know they've made time for sex. If they want to return to the computer after sex, so be it. But work won't get in the way of their intimacy any longer.

Many research couples got a kick out of filling in the calendar. Donna said that she and Casey taped the calendar to the inside of their bedroom closet. "Every time Casey or I went in the closet it was kind of funny. He'd go in to write something on the calendar and he'd have to shut himself in. So every time we saw each other in the closet, we'd run in there afterward and read the calendar!"

At the beginning of the diet, Reneé and Jordan thought the idea of scheduling sex was "kind of dumb." They thought it would feel "way too formal . . . but it's actually fun. It's exciting, like a game." I like to think that by using the menu and calendar together, couples will feel more creative. As Reneé points out, "Even if you are a creative person, sometimes you get stuck in the rut of life and you just need that extra little push to get you to go a little bit further. . . . It opens the door to creativity."

The calendar ensures that you will set aside the time at least four times a week for intimacy with your partner. Penni and Burnie used the calendar religiously. As Penni said, "This caused us to plan for ourselves. Everything else was secondary—with certain exceptions. We finally had time together that we enjoyed." As Burnie explained, "The more we planned it, the more excitement we generated, and the more inhibitions melted away."

Casey got turned on just by the thought of it. "The calendar makes you know that something is waiting for you. It's always a turn-on for a man to be wanted. Just the thought that your partner is taking the time to plan something for you is a major turn-on."

Christie and Glenn made filling out the calendar a romantic, intimate moment. "We'd actually both have our menus and sit on opposite sides of the bed, so we couldn't see the other one. We took turns filling in the calendar—it was fun!"

Couples like Angela and Jeremy didn't really need the calendar to guide them on the diet. Though they began the diet with the intention of having sex four times a week, they couldn't stop. Angela and Jeremy ended up having sex almost seven days a week—clearly the record! And I say, why stop when you're having fun!

As you can see, the calendar can be used in many different ways; it's all up to you. But what's important is that it clearly shows your

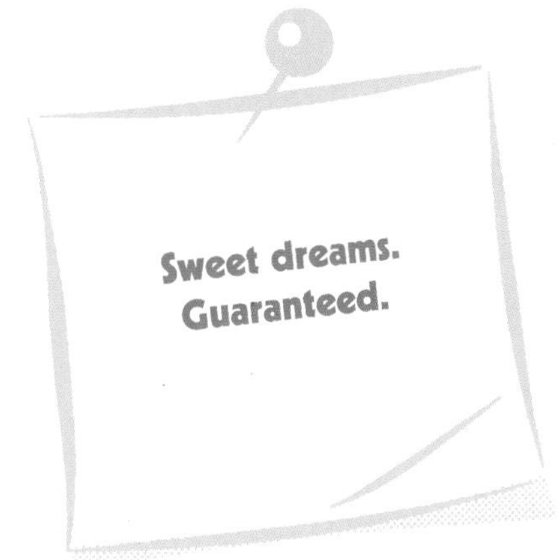

commitment to the twenty-eight-day diet. Whether you see this commitment as a challenge or as a goal to achieve, once you are on the diet and believe in its results, you will automatically make the time for intimacy and sex with each other. You can use the calendar as a way to schedule sex four times a week, carving out those special times in advance, or you can simply use it as a fun way to interact with your lover and get each other revved up. There's nothing complicated about using the calendar or being on the diet—it's all fun!

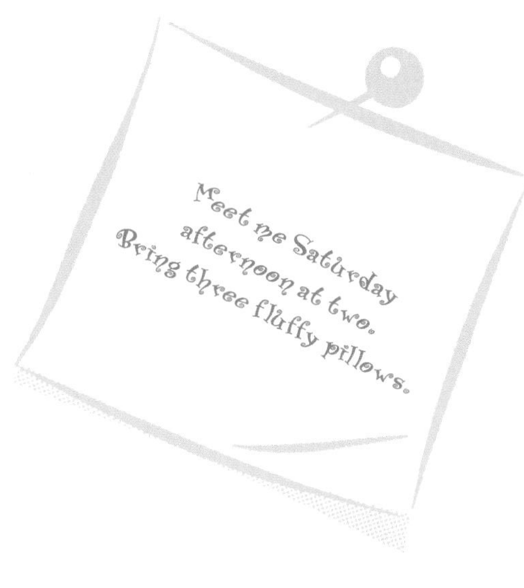

It is my opinion that if you don't schedule sex, chances are you won't have sex. Don't you want a little more excitement in your life? Stop and think about where making love is on your to-do list right now. I bet it's not even there. But if you plan on it, you'll make it happen. Scheduling sex is a great way to tell yourself—and your partner—that sex is just as important (or even more so) as everything else on your to-do list. If you make it a priority, it will become one. Write it down and make it happen!

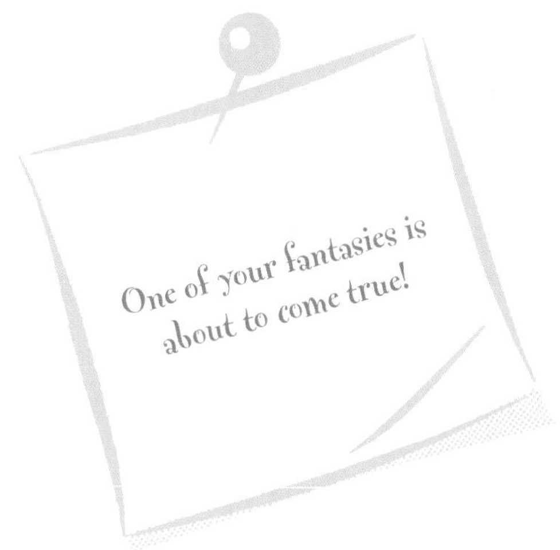

PART
III

Corn's Secrets of Sex-cess

IN THE MOOD FOR *YOU*!

We are busy! If it's not kids, it's work. If it's not work, it's something else. In this day and age, everything we do seems to happen at warp speed. The constant rush makes you want to return to horse and buggies and the Pony Express. I think most of us would agree that this focus on doing everything quickly develops into a form of pressure, and with this kind of pressure to keep speeding ahead, I ask you, how can we slow down enough to get sensually aroused? How do we find the time to wrap our arms around our honey and give him or her a squeeze? How can we fit in a long, slow kiss on the couch or in front of a blazing fire or in the front seat of the car? Getting in the mood for love is the first major secret to sex-cess on the Great American Sex Diet. At this point, you may have already imagined the wonderful suspense and mystery that the calendar and the Secret Spice Menus can bring. You and your lover will not only be ready for romance, but out of your minds with anticipation for sex. However, if these tools of seduction haven't yet pushed all of your buttons, all you have to do is consider these four essential tips that will put you and your lover in the mood for the rest of your life. With these, you'll be able to create your own rhapsody of desire in no time flat:

1. Turn "no" into "yes" and never turn down sex again.

2. Put aside distractions such as work and make time for you and your sweetie to get physical!

3. Kiss your bad habits good-bye and get into a rhythm that includes sex as a priority in your life.

4. Learn how to navigate differences in desire and alternate initiating, so each of you has the pleasure of playing seducer.

When you follow all these tips, not only will you be one step closer to diet success, you will ensure that you will both be in the mood for lovin'. And that's lovin' that includes fabulous, mind-blowing sex!

Turning "No" into "Yes": Let Me Count the Ways

One of the biggest challenges to succeeding on the diet and achieving a lifetime of great sex is learning how to say "yes" instead of "no" to sex. Consider these top ten excuses and their snappy comebacks!

"I'm too tired."
"How much energy does it take to open my legs?"

"I don't have the time."
"I know I'll have the time of my life!"

"I have too much work to do."
"Sex will make me more productive."

"I don't have enough energy."
"I'm going to feel like the Energizer Bunny after this!"

"I have too many responsibilities."
"Sex is my responsibility . . . or it may become someone else's."

"I can't . . . the kids."
"The more the kids are surrounded by happy, connected parents, the better off they'll be."

"What's the point? It's always the same thing."
"If I throw in a few spices, it's never the same thing!"

"After a long day, all I want to do is watch TV."
"If I turn off the tube, I can turn on my partner!"

"I never seem to turn you on."
"Now I have endless ways to surprise you!"

"I'm tired of always being the one to initiate. It's your turn."
"Whose turn is it? Just take a look at the calendar!"

These are not earth-shattering proclamations, but they are very real truths once you experience their power. Try them and you'll see for yourself. Also, keep your magic number in mind and use it as a motivation and an inspiration for sex. It worked for Jeff and me and for the other couples, so I bet it will work for you, too. After you get into the habit of turning no into yes, the next step to staying in the mood is overcoming work issues. So let's go work it out.

Work It Out!

Our lives are complicated and any responsibility, task, or commitment outside of the relationship can keep the flame of romance from burning bright. How do we manage it all? Work is a necessity for all of us. Like most Americans today, many of the men and women who make up the research team work not only full-time jobs but also additional jobs, after hours or on weekends. We are busy, busy, busy!

Tired of your job?

You may not like your job, but you can still leave work with a smile on your face. As Christopher said, "I still don't like my job, but I enjoy knowing that I can leave there and come home and all that affection will be waiting for me!"

Work at home?

Your coffee breaks are about to get real hot! Christie learned how to shift around her priorities to make room for the diet. "I didn't get as much work done as I normally do, but it was okay. It took a good month for that to happen. But I figured that if I wanted to [make sex a priority], I would have to look at work in a different way. Now after sex Glenn goes to bed at 10 P.M. and I stay up and get my work done."

Leave work at the office.

Shelli and Dan not only live together but work together. "One of my major complaints when I started the diet was that because we have a business together, we didn't really have any connection time," Shelli says. "But now we make the effort and spend thirty minutes together a night focusing on us. I really looked forward to that half an hour a day. It made all the difference." When you work together and live together, there is an immediate and undeniable challenge to keep the boundaries clear: Where does work end and the fun of the relationship begin? You've got to do what it takes to leave work at the office.

Keep your work in perspective.

Scott, who had gotten into the habit of putting work before Sara, made a huge shift in attitude. Being on the diet was "a real culture shock. Now in the evening, I don't continue working on my computer. Now we eat dinner together, and I spend time with Sara. I can always work later, after she's gone to bed. Everything seemed to come together on the diet."

Work is real, and there's always more to do.

But the precious, passionate, playful time you spend with your lover will make all the difference in the world! Work will always be there, ready to distract and preoccupy you. If you learn to leave it alone while you tend to your relationship, I guarantee you'll not only feel better, you'll probably be more productive the next day.

It comes down to changing your attitude toward work and making sure that your intimate time with your partner is just as important a priority as your job. We must find the time to relax, for the sake of our mental, emotional, and physical health. Reneé explains the consequences of work in this way: "I think work has a lot to do with my low desire because when I get home from my job, I'm mentally exhausted and it's hard for me to get myself into a sexual mood toward him." And what better way to relax than in the arms of your lover? What better way to get recharged—in body, mind, and spirit—than through sex?

Navigating Differences of Sexual Desire

In most relationships, mine included, there is usually one person who wants sex more than the other. That is, there is one person with the higher sex drive and one person who usually takes responsibility for initiating sex and making the first move. You know who you are! In Jeff's and my case, I suffer from low desire, and Jeff doesn't. In 70 percent of the couples who made up the research team, the men had a higher sex drive. Thirty percent of the women told me they had the higher sex drive, and these numbers reflect the national average. The third tip for getting yourself and your partner in the mood is learning how to navigate these differences and make sex fun and exciting, instead of a battle to overcome. The more you understand about yourselves as a couple and the more in tune you are to your own sexual desire, the easier, faster, and better you will be at getting in the mood. And if you learn that by alternating which one of you initiates, you create an equal playing field that inspires trust and creativity.

Many women on the research team can relate to the battle to overcome low sexual desire. For Rana, it came down to scheduling sex. In order to get in the mood, she says, "I have to simmer, and just knowing that we were going to do it later that night helped me do that."

I heard again and again how the key to getting over low desire and getting in the mood for love was in the scheduling. And I know this for myself, too! I still have to battle with this, constantly reminding myself to check in and think about how often I've had sex in any particular week. As Christine said, "Sexual desire is tied to your emotions; it's a cycle. And if you don't break the cycle, if you don't pull yourself out of it and say to yourself, 'Okay, this is going to be fun and I'm going to play this game,' then you won't find the rewards—not only the pleasure but the emotional rewards in your family, your relationship, your bond with your partner—everything."

The anticipation and the scheduling helped many women to conquer their low desire. Melanie got "psyched for sex." On the diet, "the spices and the little Anticipation Teasers that you write down on the calendar got me excited because I would have time to think about it and plan on it and that adds to the fun." And, of course, when she got excited, Mo, her partner, did, too. Melanie continued, "It helps in two ways: helps me get excited and helps him to just relax and know it's coming. I thought that was awesome!"

Low desire and hesitation to initiate sex are clearly linked. Because of Shelli's low desire, she always resisted sex and resisted initiating. She and Dan were stuck. Dan could have sex every day, and before the diet, all they were managing was sex once or twice a month! Once they became more regular, Shelli was able to get into sex more and feel more sexual herself. "I think it was a big thing for [Dan] as I was actually the one who wanted to have sex. He didn't have to beg. He didn't even have to mention it. I was just the one who did it." In the end, she changed her whole attitude toward sex: "Now sex is something I need to do because it's right for *us*."

A number of men expressed grateful relief when their wives began to initiate sex. As Jeff said about him and Elizabeth, "For the past few years, it seems like I was the one doing all the foreplay and all the seducing. And if it's not me who gets it started, then it won't happen at all. Instead of her just grabbing me and saying 'Come on, honey' or giving me the look in the eye, she waits for me to make the move. I get tired of it. I think a lot of men fantasize about a woman who just takes control of the situation and does it." So how did they do on the diet? Jeff said, "It was nice that she initiated twice a week and I initiated twice a week. It really leveled things out, and took the responsibility off me."

Men who in general experienced a lower sex drive than their wife or partner were also motivated by the idea of scheduling sex. But more than that, they seemed to tap into the options provided by the menu. For instance, at the outset of the diet, Doug felt too inhibited to initiate sex with Sally for fear of rejection; on the diet, he used the permission granted by the hundreds of scintillating seductions on the menu to let loose. He felt inspired, emboldened, and surging with confidence. As Sally said, "Some nights were his nights, some nights were my nights. I think that puts all the romance back into the relationship." Many men were able to overcome their hesitation to initiate by fixing on a goal: to wow their lover and rock her world!

The fear of failure, so often an inhibiting force behind men's difficulty initiating, all but disappeared for the men on the diet. Now that they didn't have to worry about not pleasing the women or doing something wrong, they were able to go for it. Brian used the variety of the menu to jump-start him. "Now it's like I have no problem approaching her to do something . . . I look at my list and she looks over hers, and I'd say, 'Any problems with these?' No. Okay. Then it was fair game."

It goes without saying that initiating and navigating low desire are huge issues between the sexes and often mirror the roles that men and women play in their relationship. Usually one person feels that he or she is getting the short end of the stick because he or she is the one who is always doing the seducing. The seducers (initiators) often end up feeling cheated, resentful, even taken for granted.

All of us want to be seduced and surprised and it's not fair to rely on one person in a relationship to carry this responsibility. How do you put things on a more equal footing? Well, the diet does that naturally by stipulating that each person selects two times a week to do a spice or seduction. This way, the initiating is evenly split. As you can see from the testimonials above, couples raved about this!

When it comes to overcoming low desire, most couples found that the frequency and the scheduling helped them over the hump. And once they were into sex, they never looked back. Low desire became more desire! As Julie said so succinctly, "The more I have sex, the more I want to have sex." It can be that simple for you, too.

Getting Out of a Rut and into a Rhythm

We all need and want affection and relaxation time. But what if the typical way we relax has nothing at all to do with our partner? Getting in the mood also means becoming aware of habits that may be getting in the way of romance. It's time to change a bad habit and surprise yourself and your partner. Seducing your lover may never be this easy again!

Do you clean at night?

Many women on the research team say they get easily distracted by doing chores around the house, including caring for the kids, cleaning the house, or making sure that all the day's phone calls are returned. As Penni said, "I clean the toilets, I mop the floors, I dust, I vacuum, I fold the laundry, I change the sheets, I pay the bills, I take care of social obligations, I water the plants, I pick off the dead flowers. There are always a million things I could do!" Like Penni, before the diet Melanie (of Melanie and Dwayne) and Jayme also had a penchant for cleaning at the end of the day. As Melanie recalled, "Before the diet, it seemed much more important to do the laundry and make sure the dishes were done. But now I've learned that having sex is a lot more fun. After all, what do I have to show for those years of cleaning besides a sparkling kitchen and dishwater hands?" But the diet enabled these women to focus on their relationships, and all three of them forgot about cleaning and started using their downtime to romance and seduce their partners instead. As Penni said, "Sex is more fun. We're not in a rut anymore!"

Turn off the box.

Several of the men and women on the research team used to be reliant on the television as a way to relax before bed. KaeCee figured out that she needed to steal Paul away from the TV. "He comes home, takes a nap, and then watches the news and his little shows for the evening while I do all the kids' stuff. So I began to steal him away from the TV and the diet allowed me to do that because he had an obligation." Angela agreed, "When Jeremy and I get home now, we end up spending two hours together in the bedroom instead of watching TV. Our relationship is closer and a lot more fun." So why waste all your time in front of the TV? Take a little time to get in between the sheets instead!

Look your best.

Nothing turns on your partner more than letting them know you did something special for them. This is especially true about taking the time to care about your appearance. A number of women found that if they took the time to look their best, their men responded in kind. As Julie said, "In the last month Jay really noticed that I paid a little more attention to my appearance. He noticed that I wore more perfume. I put on makeup and fixed my hair. I really dolled myself up more." And it certainly hit the mark with Jay. Julia also took the time to make Frank feel special. "I would call Frank at the office and ask him when he thought he'd be coming home. Then I made sure I went and took a shower and did my hair. It definitely reconnects you; we feel like we're dating again."

Navigate that special "time of the month."

As Julia said, "We just got creative during that lovely time of the month because we didn't want that to stop us. Before, we would avoid sex." But not anymore. Most of the women on the diet felt the same way, and if they didn't feel comfortable having sex, couples like Melanie and Dwayne "planned cuddle time."

Get sexy.

Many women fall into the rut of wearing sweats at home, especially at the end of a long day. But with the diet, they started wearing lingerie! A number of women said that wearing lingerie not only turned on their men, it also made them feel more attractive. JoAnn agreed, "When I wear lingerie, it just makes me feel sexy, which I think is really important for a woman. You've got to feel good about yourself." Heather said, "Wearing teddies makes me feel more confident."

Surprise your lover.

In any long-term relationship, it's easy to fall into a sexual routine in which sex becomes bland and boring—same old, same old. As Roxanne says, "Before we started the diet, our sex life was the exact same thing over and over again. And it was like, '*This is really boring! No wonder I have no sex drive!*'" On the diet, it's just as easy to introduce surprise and seduction as it is to settle for the tried-and-true. How? By using the endless variety of the Secret Spice Menu. You will see how to surprise and delight each other in ways that will banish the boring forevermore!

Getting out of a rut and into a new rhythm is simple. It's about acknowledging old habits and taking the time to change your routine. It doesn't have to take a lot of effort, but it does have the power to get you both in the mood for a fabulous evening.

"That's the first thing that popped into my head: The sex is more fun. We're not in a rut anymore!"

—Penni

Quick Checklist to Get in the Mood

I can't tell you how many couples—especially women—need to feel relaxed in order to get turned on. Burnie knows this about Penni and put it to the test one night on the diet. "When she came in the door, I undressed her and took her to the bathroom. I had already lit candles and put the wine in there. It was on Wednesday, hump day, so, joking around, I said, 'Okay, now hump this!' I started with a little rubdown here and there and then she was ready to go!"

Women need to relax. So, guys, this requires taking note of how your wife or girlfriend likes to relax. In addition to those tips that come in your Secret Spice Menus, here are some scintillating suggestions culled from the research team favorites:

- Draw her a warm bath by candlelight.
- Give her a massage and be sure to use plenty of oil.
- Clean the house before she arrives home.
- Hand her a glass of wine in the evening.
- Plan to make dinner (or make a dinner reservation at her favorite restaurant) and e-mail her the invitation at work.

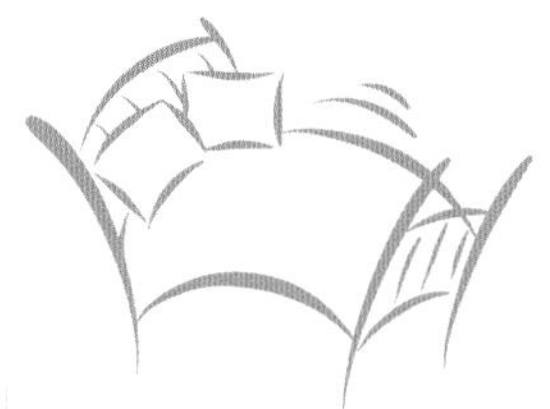

Remember, you know her best, and if you're not sure, ask her. And keep in mind that you'll benefit from how deeply she relaxes.

And what do the men need to get in the mood, girls? Well, you getting naked, of course. But here are some other ideas:

- Be affectionate.
- Take time to pamper yourself, which will pamper him.
- Buy some new sexy lingerie that's a little daring.
- Surprise him with a romantic weekend getaway.
- Treat him with a massage when he falls into bed at night.

Getting in the mood is absolutely paramount to having great sex! In addition to these tips for getting in the mood, you will find other wonderful ways to romance your lover inside your sealed envelopes and on your menu. They will definitely add fuel to your fire.

The reality is that our responsibilities are not going to disappear or dwindle in number. Rather, they are going to keep on increasing and life is going to continue to become more and more complicated. So the challenge is to prioritize intimacy and clear the path to a romantic, special evening when all you have to do is enjoy each other.

FUNNY DIET MOMENTS

As you can imagine, the couples on the research team encountered some hilarious moments on the Great American Sex Diet.

Sally remembers, "There was a time early on in the diet when we were walking past Victoria's Secret and I saw a sexy black nightie in the window and said, 'Ooh, I think I need that.' And he said, 'Yes, I think you do.' So he went in, bought it, and walked out. Then I said, 'That is going to be so perfect for this spice I have for you.' And he said, 'Oh, you bought it for one of yours? 'Cause I bought it for one of mine!' There was just this sexual playfulness between us."

Stephanie and Andrew had such intense sex for so many days (at one point they reached seven days in a row!), she could barely walk, her legs were so sore. But that didn't stop her from grinning from ear to ear!

When Kirk and Sherry invited Don and Donna, friends who were also on the diet, to join them for a weeklong sailboat cruise during the diet, they never knew how rocky things might get. They not only watched each other get excited, running for private time belowdecks, but they also felt the waves. As Sherry recalls, "Don would make this announcement each night, 'Well, I've got to go tuck in Donna,' and pretty soon the whole boat would be rocking!" Kirk has his own details to add: "We were sleeping in the back underneath the cockpit and Don was sleeping right above us. We could hear him snoring, so we thought, well, it must be cool, you know. So I did a combination of spices on Sherry—what I called the aft cabin quickie. She was singing by the time we were through. The boat was definitely rocking."

—

One night Eric was in the midst of doing a secret spice on Robin when the seduction went a little haywire. "He had tied me to the hook on the back of the bedroom door," she says. "He was in the middle of getting me all excited when the hook snapped off and I fell to the floor! We both cracked up laughing and couldn't help but wonder if someone in the house had heard us."

THE POWER OF COMMUNICATION TO CROSS BOUNDARIES AND FORGE INTIMACY

—

Sex gets tongues wagging in more ways than one. And on the Great American Sex Diet, you're going to be talking about stuff you have never talked about before. One of the most important secrets to sex-cess is open communication. Although this holds true for relationships in general, it's especially true in the area of sex. Some of us (like myself) are used to and comfortable talking about sex. I ask for what I need, tell Jeff my fantasies, and show him how I like to be touched and stimulated. He also shares his needs and desires with me, and as a result, we get along great in bed.

However, in my years of talking to hundreds of women and men, I know that some of you are not comfortable talking about sex. The diet will make that easier. First, by using the calendar, you will automatically be bringing sex out into the open and talking about it. One of the many lessons I've learned over the years is that a key to having great sex is to share what you need and want with your partner. If you're honest and share how you like to be aroused and turned on, then not only will this kind of communication bring you closer, it will also bring you more pleasure.

So much of what I discovered as I observed the couples on the diet had to do with communication. As clichéd as it may sound, communication is key to keeping a relationship growing, fun, and passionate. Many of the research couples made communication breakthroughs on the diet. This made the partners feel closer to each other than ever before. They also became more playful with each other, teasing each other by sharing their sexual fantasies. All in all, they learned how the power of words can create more intimacy, which in turn creates more sexual desire. When you're really talking to each other, instead of trading information, you know the other person cares about you. And what's more of a turn-on than knowing you're loved?

On the diet, Eric and Robin found themselves more open and communicative overall. Robin describes the change this way: "Now we are real in tune with what is going on with the kids and with work—everything that's going on in our lives right now. We spend fifteen to twenty minutes a night just talking and holding each other. Whereas before, a lot of times we didn't know what was going on. And we'd have to say, 'What are you talking about?'" As any couple knows, staying in touch and in tune is a huge component to intimacy. If making love helps these communication channels stay open, then why not just get in between the sheets!

Valerie said her conversations with Cesar didn't even have to be that special to make the moment special. "They could be just ordinary, how-was-your-day conversations. But I was more open as far as talking about things that I ordinarily wouldn't share with him. I just have more of a desire to talk and share my feelings. You just feel the other person cares about you more." Sex has the power to make even the most mundane conversation magnificent!

Partners also began to flirt more with each other, building the anticipation and suspense. Julia said that she and Frank "started doing little things like e-mailing each other. One day I e-mailed a little note from a secret admirer and another time he called me and asked, 'So are you going to wear that red thing tonight?'" This kind of verbal intimacy has now become part of their routine.

On the diet, Sally found the gumption to share her sexual fantasies with Doug. "In years past, I used to cringe when my lover would ask me what my fantasies were. I wasn't even sure if I wanted to know his. I got really good at avoiding those kinds of questions. But on the diet I found myself asking Douglas what his were and I wouldn't let him stop at his Top Three! He had me going, too! I feel like this is territory that we should all explore and how wonderful it is to feel this comfortable doing so." I say explore the territory and stake your claim!

Couples also learned how to let go of more serious baggage. One night, while Melanie and Mo were having wild, passionate sex on the bathroom floor, Melanie did something that brought things to a boiling point. Mo couldn't take it any longer and he finally vented his anger. Because of their closeness, they both accepted his anger and were then able to talk about all the issues. Their fight had become a catalyst for healing. As Mo said, "I learned more about our relationship in the last twenty-eight days than I've learned in ten years."

Kevin said that he and Christine totally changed their relationship on the diet because of more communication. "Our life is very different because of this diet. What I think was so important was that in the midst of doing this, we were talking and we were communicating. And we were listening to each other and being sensitive. And I was changing inside—realizing things and valuing her again."

Couples learned how communication about sex connects partners at a deeper, more satisfying level. I can't urge you enough to explore and expand your communication skills in your own relationship. Don't be afraid to share—after all, this is the person you are closest to in the world. Women and men love to talk and to be heard—it's a total turn-on. If sex is the element of your relationship with your lover that separates it from all the other relationships in your life, then you owe it to yourself and each other to blast the doors wide open. And just imagine how exciting it will be to discover what *you* might be talking about—in and out of the bedroom.

TRAVERSING THE KID FACTOR

If you have kids and think their very existence makes it impossible for you to go on the diet, then think again! Thirty-two out of the thirty-eight couples on the research team are parents and thirty-one of them succeeded. That's why learning how to traverse the kid factor is a crucial secret to sex-cess. By fostering an open connection with your kids and learning how to distinguish between your role as good parent and great lover, nothing will get in between you and diet success.

> *"When you're having frequent sex that's like the ultimate way of showing your affection, and it seems to be able to bring down the walls afterward so you're able to talk. It's definitely a way of connecting, emotionally, physically, and spiritually. It just opens you up and takes away the inhibitions."*—Julia

When I first approached many of the couples who were parents and asked if they'd be interested in doing the diet and becoming part of my research team, their first response was, "Oh, I can't do it—I have kids." I just want to say at the outset, kids are wonderful but they do not have to prevent you from having wild, passionate sex! In fact, the research team proved that to be true time and time again.

As we all know, once you become parents, your entire life changes, not the least of which is your relationship. Sure, those bundles of joy can bring extraordinary happiness to your life, but there are some very real consequences that affect your primary relationship with your partner. Most parents I've spoken with over the years mourn the fast, inevitable disintegration of their love life. The challenge seems to be: How can you embrace these new (or growing) bundles of joy without wreaking havoc on your love relationship?

"Before, we were more like roommates and partners in raising kids, and our focus was all on them. But now the focus is more on us first. If we're happy and we're healthy, the kids pick up on that and they're happier and healthier."—Julia

Some of the parents on the research team are young couples who only recently became first-time parents, some have two or three or four young children—some still in diapers, others saddling on backpacks for elementary school—and others have teenagers, whose emotional demands can often feel perplexing. The research team also contains thirteen couples who have what they call "blended families," when couples have had previous relationships and enter the new one with children.

Yet despite the built-in stresses of caring for children, no matter what their ages, you can bring romance, intimacy, cuddling, kissing, and of course more sex into your relationship. If you are a parent, I am sure that like the research team couples, you, too, do not want to give up your love life just because you've become a parent. And you don't have to.

Look at how these research team parents coped with and overcame the challenge of kids.

- Marie and Michael, who have a six-month-old, said scheduling sex allowed them to make the time. "It helped us get that spark again. If you make the time, there is always time for it. Then you realize what you've been missing."

- Donna and Casey, who have two sons in elementary school, used to spend most of their "spare" time shuttling their kids to school and all their other activities. As Donna said, "It's horrible. You run your life by the clock. And it just seems during the school year with sports and school and homework from 6:30 in the morning until it's dark, all we do is run and run. By the time we get home and get the kids to bed, we're out of time for each other." So how did they turn it around? The calendar allowed them to schedule sex and make time for themselves. As Donna explained, "With the calendar we make the time to follow through with the plan, so now we get the kids into bed on time instead of half an hour later."

- Melanie and Dwayne also made a scheduling adjustment with her young daughter. When I asked her what kind of advice she'd give other parents, she said, "From my experience it would be having him make sure she is asleep so I have that time to unwind for a moment." Sound simple? It is and you should try it.

- Robin and Eric are another couple with obstacles galore. With four kids of their own (the baby still in diapers), they also care for Eric's teenage sister. And for the past year, they have been living in Robin's parents' house, sharing one bathroom with all their kids. Privacy? I don't think so. Alone time? Only if they make a very conscious effort! And that's what they did while they were on the diet.

- Christine and Kevin have six kids between them—all teenagers. Christine explained, "We had issues with the kids all the time. Some of the conflicts would make every day seem like World War III. As a result, Kevin and I weren't connecting and our bond was chipping away." Then they made a conscious choice for each other and things changed. Kevin said, "Some nights, we couldn't wait for the kids to go to bed so we could be together. It seemed like there was a lot more freedom and playfulness." In other words, the diet gave them permission!

I encouraged the parents on the research team to be openly affectionate with each other in front of the kids—and the results? In every case where the parents hugged or kissed, their kids responded positively. I believe strongly that the more parents kiss, hug, and show affection, the more kids will be comfortable with these feelings when they grow older. As Eric said of himself and Robin, "She'll be lying on the couch and I will come up and lie beside her or kneel down to kiss her. And we'll kind of look up and there are the kids watching. It's fun!" As you will read in the stories that come in the Magical Journey of Surprise, many couples discovered the joy and fun of sharing this part of their intimate relationship with their children. It's healthy. So please, don't hide your excitement from them. Let them see how thrilled you are to be spending some intimate time with your partner. Expose them to the flirting and laughing and hugging that goes along with a healthy marriage or relationship. Remember, you are their most important role models. They're going to model their future relationships on yours.

"Even our three-year-old son noticed the change. One day he said to Glenn: 'There you go, falling in love with Mommy again!'"
—Christie

Kids can bring tremendous joy and satisfaction to your life, and I know many a woman and man who say they wouldn't trade the experience of parenthood for the world. However, kids—without a doubt—can complicate your love life. Without making a conscious, concerted effort between the two of you to carve out the time for romance and intimacy, sex will just not happen. So make the time. Not only will your kids understand, they'll probably thank you for it.

ADVENTUROUS SEX-CAPADES

As you can imagine, many couples on the diet got carried away by their passion. For many, the spices alone took them to a place they had never before ventured. Whether these were new positions for intercourse, location, oral, foreplay, or toy spices, the newness and surprise of these seductions gave couples permission and license to cross over boundaries and explore new sexual territory. I like to think of these special adventures as the sex-capades because of how they show the wild, magical potential of the Great American Sex Diet!

Some women experienced a G-spot orgasm for the first time, another couple shared the intense pleasure of climaxing together—something they'd been trying to do for years. One woman discovered the erotic satisfaction of pleasuring herself for the first time. All of these accomplishments were experienced as mini-adventures.

Couples made love on kitchen counters, on the steps, in the backyard under a tent, and in a hot tub. No location was off-limits. These changes in location gave spark and freshness to an already heated moment, adding to the sense of adventure that the diet delivers.

Other couples became so inspired by the diet's variety, they created adventures that will just blow you away and, who knows, maybe inspire you!

- Annette and Scott, who claim to have reinvented their hot tub, spent an entire weekend in bed. Rather than go away for the weekend, they decided to stay at home, in the cozy comfort of their empty house—yes, all the kids were gone! In one day they had sex four different times!

- Sally and Doug had their own adventurous sex-capade—in a car! "We went to a Sea Hawks game, and beforehand we were running around doing a million things . . . do this, do that, get the kid to a baby-sitter, and we were all stressed out. So we were in traffic on the 520 Bridge and I said, 'You know, I'm not wearing any underwear.' Doug looked over and said, 'Well, that's a good thing to know.' Then I handed him the remote control to the dolphin vibrator I had on underneath my jeans. It was very fun!"

- Julie and Jay had their own wild time on the diet. As Julie describes it, "We were having this really intense lovemaking session, but we didn't even have intercourse. I think it lasted about an hour. We were in this beautiful hotel room, atop this huge four-poster bed. It started out by Jay telling me a naughty story in my ear. Something he said led me to do this thing where I was kind of pulling his hair. I became very dominant, and he was really into it. And then we'd kind of go back and forth between who was the dominant one and who was more submissive. It was one of the wildest nights we'd ever had!"

A few couples discovered the titillating pleasure of inhabiting alternate personas. As you will read in the individual stories of the Magical Journey of Surprise, one of these divas of the night was Amber Rose. Before the diet, Ralph had not seen his Amber Rose in quite some time, but when he went to meet his partner Doreen at a restaurant for a date, it was Amber Rose who showed up instead! Just wait and see how Amber Rose pricked Ralph's skin! Julia decided to surprise Frank by donning the fearless wig of Lola and transforming herself into the sexy woman of the night who had Frank begging for more. The real surprise came when Frank created a twist. But I don't want to give away their secret—read their story and find out!

My point here is to show you how the diet gave couples permission to let their hair down and run wild. They became creative, inspired, and adventurous. So I dare you: Create your own sex-capade and find your own impossible limit to pleasure!

SEX-CESS FOR A LIFETIME

Transformations

The Great American Sex Diet is something for you to enjoy and return to again and again. This is a gift; indeed, it's my gift to you. The diet has the power to transform your relationship. I do not exaggerate here. My relationship was transformed through the diet and so was every single couple's on the research team. Some relationships were on the brink of a divorce or a breakup. Others went from great to greater. Still other relationships went from mediocre to fabulous. Regardless of the degree or type of transformation, enormous breakthroughs were made on the diet, and you have this opportunity as well.

Christie, who rediscovered the wonderful romantic nights of her early relationship, said, "It was one of the best things we've ever done for ourselves in a long time. We got more connected, spent more time together, and flirted with each other more." In short, they both found the diet to be simply miraculous.

Stephanie and Andrew said, "It was the best sex in sixteen years!" Just look at the before and after photo of this particular couple: They went from being totally alienated from each other to embracing their love!

Ten months before the diet, Christine and Kevin were living in two separate houses. When they decided to give their marriage one more try, they moved into a new home for a fresh start. But it was the Great American Sex Diet that became their vehicle to nirvana, enabling them to overcome the complicated tensions of raising a blended family of six children.

Where there's a will, there's a way. The enormous changes this couple experienced on the diet nearly moved me to tears. I saw the same degree of transformation between Robin and Eric. They have five children to care for and live under the same roof as Robin's parents. They had always been a very close and committed couple, but they took their relationship to a whole other level on the diet.

You, too, have the power and the ability to take your relationship and yourselves on a journey—a Magical Journey of Surprise. A transformation awaits you as soon as you begin the diet!

After the Twenty-eight Days, Another Adventure Begins

The Great American Sex Diet is built to last, and after this incredible journey, you will never look at sex the same way again. But what do you do after the twenty-eight days is up? *What do you think? Keep on truckin'!* Again, I'm a realist and understand that four times a week may be hard to maintain, but most of the couples came up with their own magic number for how many times a week they can have sex and remain in that blissful fever the diet created. This number was something that the couples found themselves striving for. Before the diet, they'd never attached a number to sex, but it was so easy and doable, they said the magic number has changed their lives forever.

Remember how important the magic number was for me when I created and developed the concept of the diet? Well, that still proves to be true. I have to constantly pay attention to my sexual frequency. Sometimes Jeff and I will make love four times a week; sometimes we will make love only once a week. Sometimes an entire week goes by and we haven't been intimate a single time. The difference between now and then is that I am aware of the number. I am aware of how often I am practicing intimacy. And I am aware of the amazing benefits of having sex regularly and frequently.

Fifty percent of the thirty-eight couples told me that three times a week is what they'd like to strive for. That was the magic number for them, and this is now their goal. It's one I wholeheartedly recommend to you. Three times seems easy because it allows for catch up on the weekend (sex at least twice) and sex at least once during the week. But you and your partner may come up with something different. Essentially every couple has its own magic number. Deciding that number and keeping track of how often you make love will keep you having the strongest, greatest, healthiest relationship ever. I promise! On the diet, women and men found themselves motivated by their magic number, and this was only reinforced when they began to see the very tangible benefits of frequent sex. It's my belief that once you try the diet and reap the rewards of sex four times a week, most of you will not need further convincing. You will then find the number that best suits you, whether that number is seven, four, or three.

One of the miracles that the couples experienced being on the diet came from one simple fact: When they scheduled sex, it happened. Like anything else we want to do or commit to do, unless you make it a priority, it just won't happen. After a few months, if you find yourselves in a rut again, don't worry. The diet is full of fresh ideas to jump-start that fabulous seductive energy. As Andrew discovered while on the diet, "Now you can look back and say, 'Hey, let's do the sex diet again and see if we can beat our record from the last time! We had sex twenty times that month, now let's go for twenty-five!' You can do this diet for the rest of your life." And you can! Mo had another idea: "I am going to order a twelve-month calendar and make my own Spice Calendar. I'm serious. What's the difference in doing it for twenty-eight days or doing it your whole life? Let's put lovemaking on the calendar like every other event!"

And don't be afraid that the spontaneity of sex will disappear with a schedule. Remember all the benefits. The diet is meant to recapture closeness and get you to look at sex from a different point of view. Instead of thinking of it as an extra, think of sex as a necessary part of a healthy relationship. Every time you make love, you are practicing intimacy. And let's not forget about that wonderful afterglow: You can take 1.6 to 8 years off your Real Age!

So, without further ado, let's get started. You're ready to tear open the Great American Sex Diet in the next section. As you become familiar with these pages you'll also want to read the couples' profiles. These stories will surely enhance your experience as you embark on your very own Magical Journey of Surprise!

PART
IV

The Great American Sex Diet: The Secret Ingredients

Quick Tips

1. Find and remove two Secret Spice Menus . . . but do NOT read the one intended for your partner! Follow the perforation marks along the spine, bend, and detach. Keep your own copy safe and hidden from your partner. For the next twenty-eight days, the Spice Menu will be your road map to renewed passion.

2. Find and remove the secret sealed envelopes—there are three For His Eyes Only, and three For Her Eyes Only. (No peeking at your partner's pages! That would only spoil the surprises you have in store.) The envelopes contain special Diet Secrets, Extra Spice Menus, and Anticipation Teasers. With these hot tips and your Spice Menu, you are now ready to begin filling in your calendar.

3. Find and remove the blank Spice Calendars. One is for you to use during the first twenty-eight days of the diet. The other is for your future use—and I hope you'll end up making *lots* of copies over the years!

4. Once a week, sit down with your calendar and pick out your two special Spice Days—that is, two days during which you will take responsibility for seducing your partner with some of the items from the Spice Menu. Then hand the calender over so your sweetie can do the same. Use a pencil! There's almost always some bargaining and rescheduling involved (and that's half the fun!). Once you've decided what kind of erotic surprise you want to spring on your partner, write down a sexy little hint with one of the Anticipation Teasers. Post the calender in a place where you can both be inspired by it—but where it won't be too obvious to little eyes or visiting neighbors.

5. Remember this simple goal: *have sex four times a week for twenty-eight days*. It's my philosophy that the more times you make love in these twenty-eight days, the more you'll improve all aspects of your relationship. You'll have deeper intimacy, greater respect, increased desire, and more communication.

And, needless to say, *lots* more fun!

First tear page out of spine. Fold and remove perforated edge.

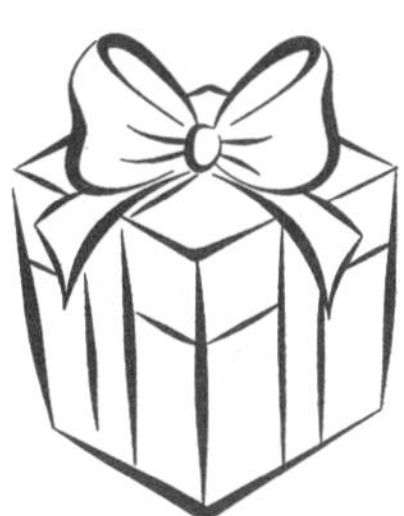

DIET SECRETS

For *Her* Eyes Only

Fold and remove perforated edge.

First tear page out of spine. Fold and remove perforated edge.

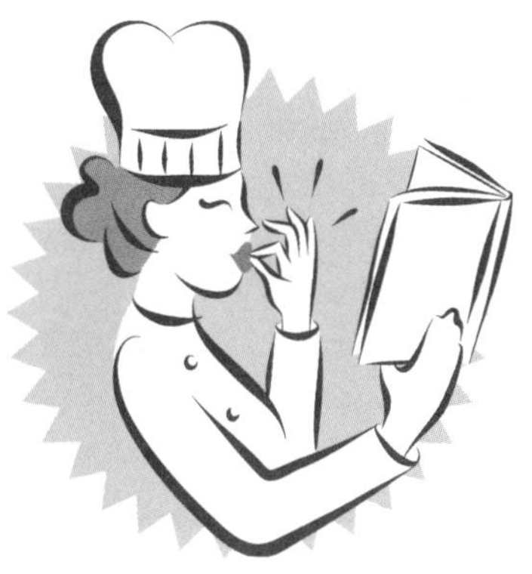

THE EXTRA SPICE MENU

For Her Eyes Only

Fold and remove perforated edge.

First tear page out of spine. Fold and remove perforated edge.

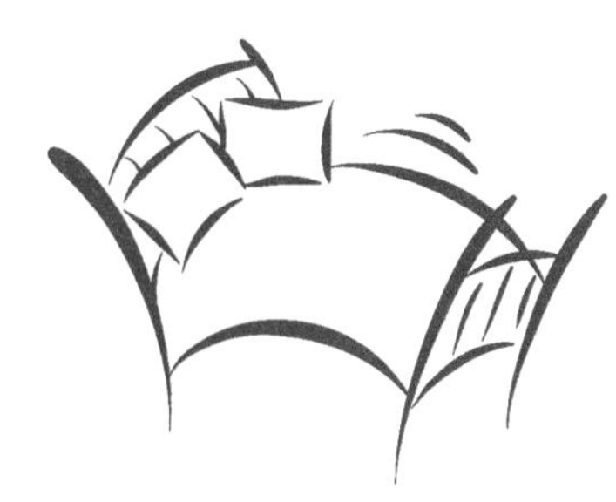

ANTICIPATION TEASERS

For Her Eyes Only

Fold and remove perforated edge.

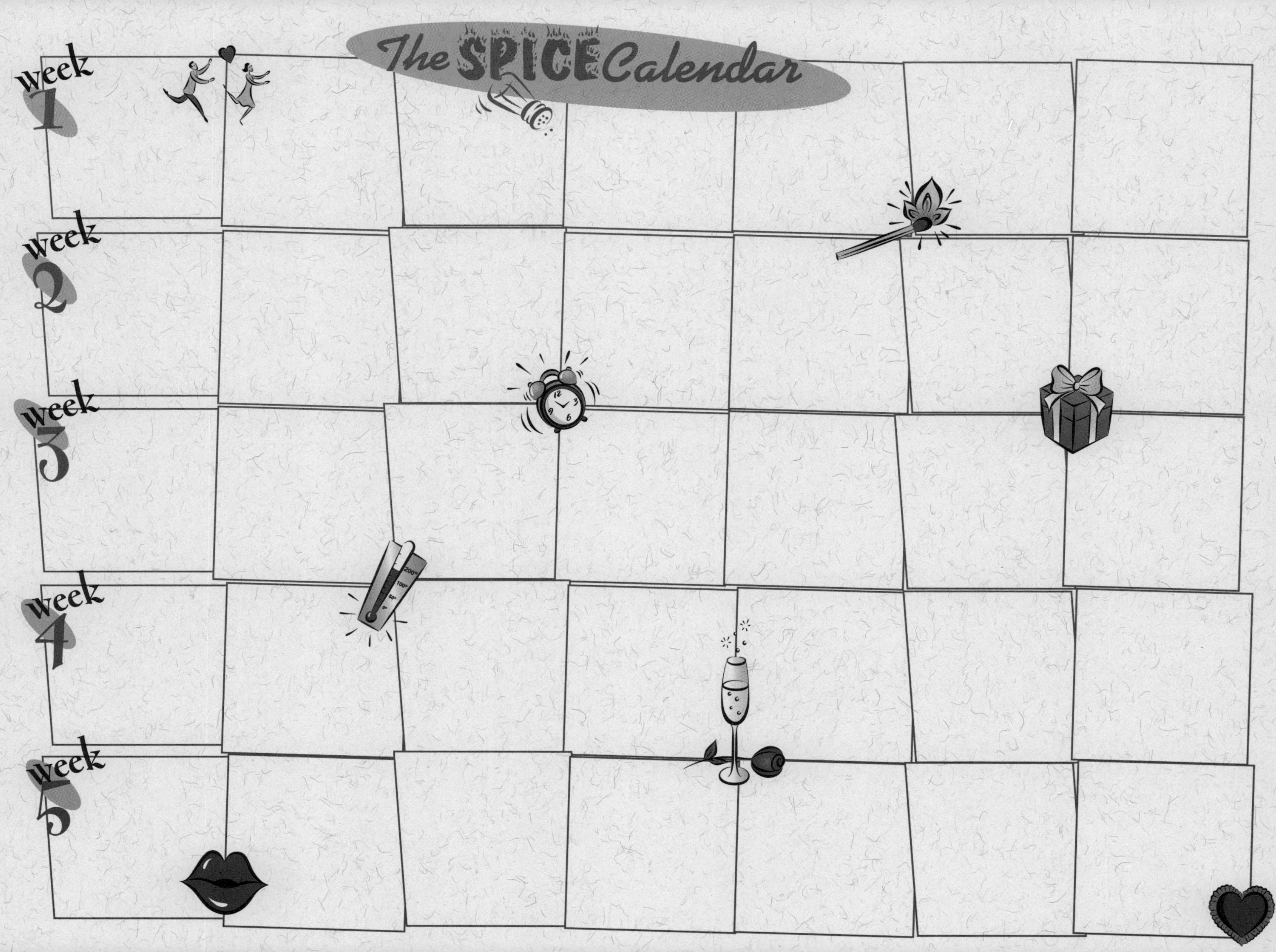
The SPICE Calendar
week 1
week 2
week 3
week 4
week 5
200°
100°
50°
0°

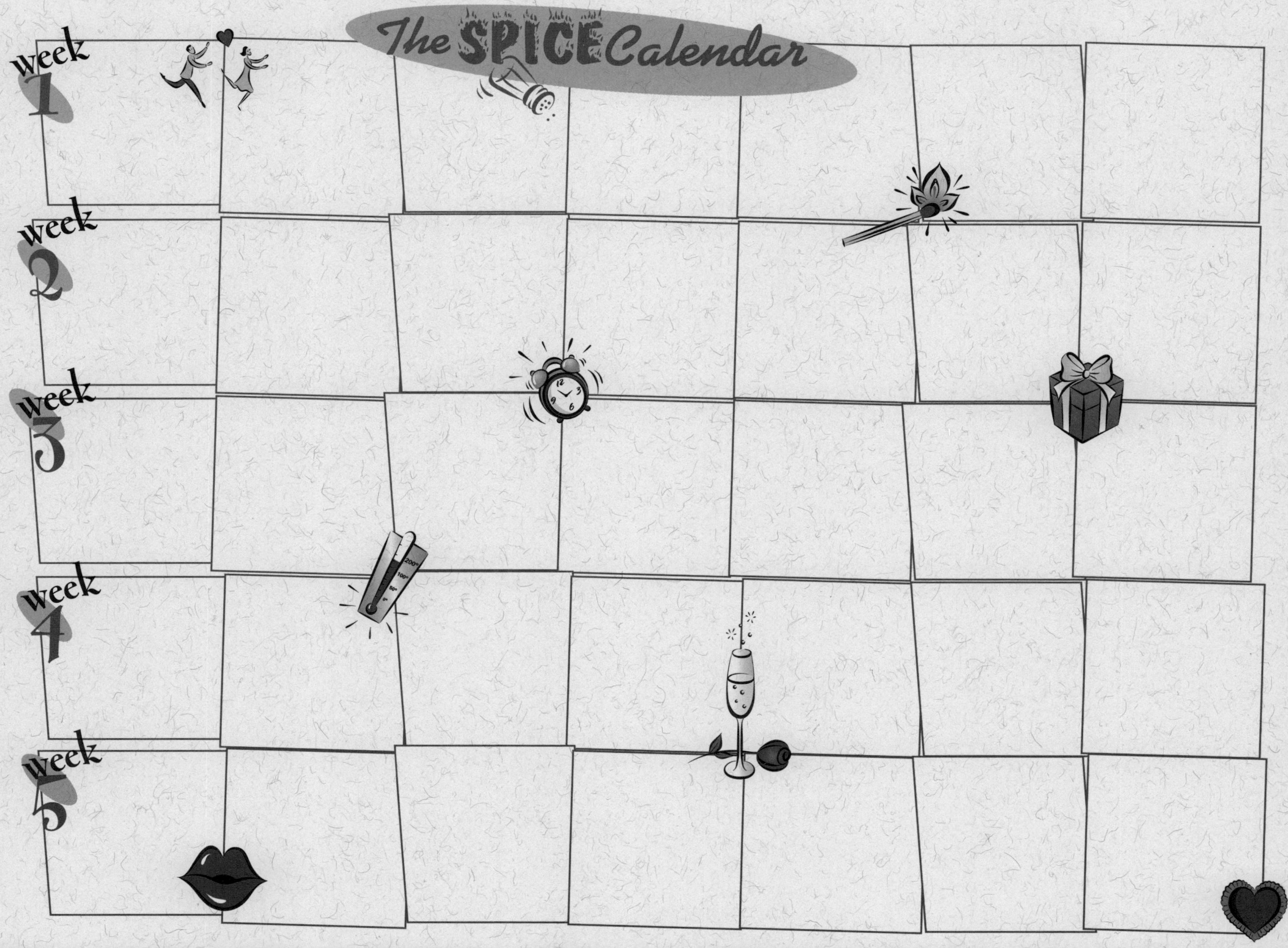
The SPICE Calendar
week 1
week 2
week 3
week 4
week 5
200°
100°
50°
0°

PART
V

The Magical Journey of Surprise

An Invitation to a Journey

♥

By now you probably know that the Great American Sex Diet is much more than a book for me. It changed my life in many ways—it transformed my vision of myself, inspired wonderful growth and closeness in my relationship with Jeff, and it introduced me to over seventy-five people who shared their experience of the diet with me. When these men and women opened their hearts and souls to me, describing how the diet impacted their lives, I was moved in profound ways. The experience of the couples on my research team not only shaped the contents and spirit of the book you're reading, but also inspired me to share their unique, fabulous, funny, multifaceted stories with you.

Listening to their stories has been my Magical Journey of Surprise. And it's my deep hope that when you read about these couples in all their idiosyncratic glory, you will enjoy their obstacles and their successes. And that as you shake your heads in wonder, surprise, and delight, you too will feel inspired as you embark on your own Magical Journey of Surprise.

Mel's Great American Sex Diet Journal

Before you get to the couples' profiles, I'd like to share with you an up-close-and-personal account of a couple's experience on the diet. I have included a special treat. The following is the transcript of the diary that Melanie (of Melanie and Mo) kept of her twenty-eight days.

Though the diary speaks for itself, I would just point out that it is a fascinating portrait of the emotional, sexual, and spiritual journey of a couple who dared to embrace their passion.

Thank you, Melanie!

Day 1, Wednesday, August 23

TRANSITION NOW!

Today Mo and I started the Great American Sex Diet. Mo has always been a die-hard romantic at heart: very free with his feelings of love for me. I've read many books on romance, and how to keep married sex hot. We have a respectable sex life, but it's definitely time to spend 28 days in the kitchen, tossing out the leftovers and seeing what new creations we can cook up. This afternoon Mo was holding tight to his Spice Menu, and I had mine. Although we both agreed to try the Great American Sex Diet for 28 days, I wondered if I would have to be the one to make sure we stick to this deal. After all, I am the planner and he is so spontaneous. I heard Mo tell his mom and dad (visiting) and [our children] Chris and Alex that he was going to take a nap for one hour . . . did not want to be disturbed. That was a first! He is usually so sensitive to being a good host. I was totally surprised he would bail on his host duties, but did I complain? He whispered in my ear, "Grab your 'spicy menu' and meet me upstairs." We lay on our bed and he started to read through the menu "For His Eyes Only," reminding me not to get too close; not to peek at his folder. He seemed to relish the idea of having his OWN set of instructions that were not available to me or to my comments. (Too many cooks, I guess!) I think just READING the menus serves as foreplay! I was excited to see many ideas that were new to me on the Spice Menu (after fifteen years I thought I had heard them all . . . I was WRONG!!!) Mo asked if I wanted to take the Spice Calendar and schedule the sessions for the week first, or if he should. Again, quite amazing, considering Mo does not even OWN a calendar. It made me excited that he was scheduling . . . filling me with hope that this would be a two-sided endeavor. I was also excited to see him acting counter to how he usually operates. It added a sense that after so much togetherness, I do not know the total of the person he is, or what he might do. We scheduled spicy encounters for the next two weeks, following the diet prescription of four times per week. Then (I guess after having enough) he threw the calendar and his menu on the nightstand and said, "Forget the schedule for now, I'm trying out one of these right now . . . just for pregame practice!" I realized how charming this man really is: all of a sudden we were in a sporting event. Very male, very cute! Truthfully, even though reading the menu made me kind of ready, I was distracted by this late-afternoon-kids-and-parents-downstairs kind of encounter. But I decided to junk all of those mental stoppers, just throw it all aside, and GO FOR IT. This was a really nice, albeit fast, encounter. Pretty much standard intercourse fare, but really close and nice. I don't think some of the more unusual spices had time to marinate into the experience yet. I remembered reading that each partner should be open to the other's advances/tries while on the diet. So I did it because I made a commitment to do it, whatever the time or place, scheduled or not! (A big advance for me, I must admit.) I'm thinking that this motivation to stick to my commitment will last during these next 28 days, and during that time I will realize so many benefits that THEY will become my NEW motivations. Right??????

Day 2, Thursday, August 24

FASTED

The "no action" status was mutual; neither one approached. Mo did not work yesterday, so he worked late tonight, catching up on things. I was busy entertaining our houseguests, supervising homework, etc. Busy as usual. I did, however, think about the diet throughout the day, planning in my head for the "meal" I had scheduled on the calendar for tomorrow! That was a novel thought. I mean, I do think about sex often, and what we might do, or how it might be, or which scented candle I'll light this time. However, I can't remember the last time I actually planned all of the details like I found myself doing now. It was like getting ready for a Halloween party, or Christmas. Something fun to anticipate!

Day 3, Friday, August 25

YEE-HAW!

I am sure Mo did not look at the "Yee-haw" I had on the calendar for tonight. He is just not used to looking at a calendar in anticipation of upcoming events. We store the Spice Calendar in the nightstand drawer in an attempt to keep it from the children's view (and the houseguests . . . you never know!). Chris and Alex know we are on the diet, and I do not hide the fact that their father and I are intimate. I want them to know, and I believe they DO know, in a very healthy way that sex, intimacy, and romance are all parts of a successful marriage. I just do not want to carelessly sexualize their lives by leaving a Spice Calendar in full view. The "Yee-haw" calendar entry might be a little TOO much information for them! Anyway, tonight I was going to be bold; try something new and a bit out of character for me. (I've always considered myself a sensual person. Never thought I needed props.) Anyway, I whipped up the Giddy Up spice. Actually, I decided to mix the Giddy Up spice with the How to Start a Fire Without Matches spice. We did not have a lot of alone time the couple of days preceding this encounter, so in the car together that morning I just replied a sexy "Yee-haw!" in answer to one of his questions. Mo looked at me kind of funny, but smiled. A few minutes later I answered another question with a more suggestive "Yee-haw!" He picked up on it this time! He said, "Yee-haw, bee-yah!" (Bee-yah is Mo's native language for "come here.") "Ooooohhhhh, I LOVE cowboy girls!" Mo rolled down his car window and shouted out, "Woo-hooooo!" He just loved this and kept on teasing me, knowing that something was up for tonight. That was a lot of fun! He broke into a playful mood so quickly it made me realize how much he really NEEDS to play, just like I do! When the kids were in bed later that evening, I called him up to the bedroom . . . everything was ready! I put on the Garth Brooks tape, donned a "cowboy girl" hat, a bandanna around my neck and a rope around my waist. It started off great, we were both really into it, then Mo said something that bugged me (so insignificant that I cannot even remember it now), and suddenly everything STOPPED. It was a really quick drain. We finally resumed, but with less fervor. The stop was definitely a symptom of a problem. Have to think about that one. Something needs to be worked out. The GOOD thing is that we eventually continued on instead of ending with a bad taste in our mouths.

Day 4, Saturday, August 26

FASTED

Errands, cleaning the house, sports practices. Another busy day. I looked on the calendar and saw that Mo has a "meal" planned for 7:45 tomorrow evening. It makes me chuckle anticipating what he means by "Cleaning the Fan." I am realizing what an important role humor and laughter play in our relationship. When we take ourselves less seriously and really enjoy being us; crazy ideas, imperfections and all, life is a real hoot!

Day 5, Sunday, August 27

CLEANING THE FAN

Totally funny and awesome. I had no idea where he was coming from or where he was going. (I am not convinced HE knew either, but that was okay, and made it even more hilarious!) Mo served me a portion of the Foreplay Gourmet (odd piece of furniture was a ladder, under the guise of needing to clean the ceiling fan) with a side dish of Heads or Tails. This was one dish I had never tried before! At one point during our time together he told me to stand up and hold my arms out to the side. He placed a coin on the back of each wrist, and told me that whatever happens, I cannot let the coins fall. Having a competitive spirit, I was determined. The coins fell a few times, due either to pleasure (I forgot to hold up my arms) or to pain (my arms became very tired). And guess what???? Our fan is STILL dirty!

Day 6, Monday, August 28

ICY-HOT FOOT FREAK MASSAGE PLUS! . . . TURNED BLAND: BLAH

I had dessert planned, but we were out of the house this evening and arrived home so late that we were too tired to do anything. Decided to move it to Tuesday (mutual). I've been thinking lately that this whole sex diet plan has been a lot about discovery. I am already humbled, hit with the question, "How can I think I already know all of who he is? What he wants? What he needs?" He changes. I change. Remain fluid. Keep discovering. The Joy of Cooking.

Day 7, Tuesday, August 29

WHO STOLE THE COOKIE FROM THE COOKIE JAR?

Yesterday I planned to introduce a spice combo I named the Icy-Hot Foot Freak Massage Plus! but Mo and I started looking through the tackle box of sex toys we have collected (the "Cookie Jar") and the evening took a different direction. I'm learning to throw PLANS out of the window and take advantage of the opportunities for romance and intimacy that are before us at any given time. This seems to feed Mo's appetite for spontaneity, and it is helping to get us out of our "sex-at-night-when-the-kids-are-asleep-and-we're-really-too-tired-but-let's-have-sex-anyway-for-the-release" rut. A good, stay-slippery lubricant, glow-in-the-dark condom (turn off the lights and he runs around the room), and a pair of foreplay dice are always good for some fun . . . and it was!

Day 8, Wednesday, August 30

CHANGE OF PLAN: NO TIME TO EAT

Mo had "The Gentleman at 9 P.M." written on the calendar. Although the meal was planned, we had an impromptu, large family gathering at our house which ended very late. We love our big family and we love to entertain. So this night we settled for secretly whispering about what we WOULD NOT be doing that night, and just enjoyed the delay and let the anticipation build. Decided to sample "The Gentleman" tomorrow.

Day 9, Thursday, August 31

DEAD STOP

Tonight was to be "The Gentleman" makeup session. Just as we were finishing up the dinner dishes, I received a call from my mother. My stepfather had just suffered what she thought (and was later confirmed correct) was a major heart attack. Tragic loss . . . he was gone. This was my poor mother's second husband (and my second father) to die this way. Vanished in a minute, and our lives changed forever. Needless to say, no makeup session this night. The family and I packed up and made that very sad ride to the hospital. What a love for life he had. *Really live, and really love, and really enjoy and make each moment count.* We never know how many more minutes we have left!

Day 10, Friday, September 1

LOST APPETITE

Mo had "Going Fishing" scheduled for 5:30 P.M. this day. Fate twisted our path and instead we were at Mom's taking care of her, accompanied by my sister and her family. No action. No desire for action . . . far from my mind. I still wonder, however, and am determined to find out, what the fishing trip was going to be about. I know that man loves to fish.

Day 11, Saturday, September 2

NOT EATING

Nothing on the calendar for this day. Just as well: We traveled back to our house today with Mom. Twenty-five other family members gathered in our home to lend their love and support. Taking care of Mom, guests, and details. No action. No desire for action on my part or on Mo's part. We were both sick, and sad, contemplating deeply what life is all about, and how we are living the days still before us. I am conscious of, and truly thankful for, Mo's deep love and support for me. True in general of human nature, it's easier to love me in "the good times" than in "the bad times." And he has loved me just as well during this bad time, which makes my love and appreciation for him even deeper.

Day 12, Sunday, September 3

NOT EATING AND KNOWING THIS IS NOT HEALTHY

Last week I planned a spicy encounter for this night. I chose the Shirt off His Back combined with the Attack! spice. On the calendar I had written "ATTACK! At 9 P.M. Wear an old T-shirt, old shorts, and no tighty whities [not a boxer man]." I was planning to get a little rough and aggressive, and rip his clothes off for a start. I know he wishes I would initiate sex more often, and I know he would love to be attacked! During the day Mo works in his business outside the home. In addition to taking care of the kids, the home, and running my own business, I was now so concerned about Mom and her grief. Not that I could DO much about it. In fact I felt very deeply sad and so helpless. I wondered if I would ever regain a drive for sex. I was always in a semi-tired, low-to-medium sex drive kind of funk anyway. Now the hunger was nonexistent. I had to start intellectualizing this. I knew if I left it up to my FEELINGS, I would not want sex for a REALLY long time, and that would build walls between Mo and me. Our marriage would crumble, no doubt about it. That's how important I know in my head that good sex is to our marriage. My body, my feelings, on the other hand, would just need to be hauled along with what my head knew was best. Mo and I discussed this. He was still in mourning, and was a bit appalled that I was even bouncing this around. But the more I talked, the more he started to track with me (or maybe I just pushed him into thinking it: typically me!). Regardless, we both acknowledged the need to start up again, and acknowledged that if we acted in the way we knew was good/right to act, then our feelings would follow. This night, we went to sleep holding hands. Feeling connected.

Day 13, Monday, September 4

KISS ME

On the calendar today was "Kissing 101 at 9 P.M." I planned to try the spice For Every Woman Who Loves to Kiss and to concentrate heavily on the mouth. Now, this was going to be a stretch for me. I remember when we first met, kisses were long and passionate. It seems, though, that I have evolved into something of a nonkisser. Wet kisses just exploded in my mind into slobbery, gooey exchanges of mess. In an effort to keep our kisses as dry as possible I think, no I KNOW, I squelched the most intimate act we could share together: mouth kissing. I read on the Spice Menu, "The power of a kiss should never be underestimated. If you and your lover aren't connected to one another's kisses, there will always be limits to your passion." Maybe I was subconsciously limiting our passion. Without Freud to help me figure it all out, I replayed my husband's simple pleas in my mind, "I wish you would REALLY kiss me!" Anyway, I was thinking about this and knowing that Mo and I needed to kiss. I know I'm a nerd, but I asked him to brush, floss, and gargle with mouthwash before we started. I did the same. Totally unromantic, but I was stretching here and I needed every opportunity for success! Mo did not seem to mind AT ALL! Then, starting at his feet, I worked my way up to his mouth. It was actually the mouth kissing that was the most exciting, and it was VERY exciting sex . . . because of the kissing! Sex without kissing is an emotional disconnect. I am most assuredly back in the kissing scene, although I will still probably have to psych myself up for a while just to conquer the spit phobia.

Day 14, Tuesday, September 5

PREPLANNED FASTING: NO ACTION

A lot more hugs and sexual touch without ending in intercourse is going on now. We have stopped thinking so much about THE BEGINNING and THE END of a sexual encounter. We are enjoying more the moment, with relaxed expectations. Savoring, together, the moments. Mo and I are also remembering, regaining touch with, the reality that everything we SAY and DO in our family affects the other members. Mo and I, by being our best for each other and for ourselves, are positively affecting our family. I believe our sons have a great chance to become wonderful loving husbands and fathers, and have hopes to marry a loving soul mate because of the examples Mo and I are setting for them. That is a huge honor for me as a mother. (Watch, they'll be in therapy along with everyone else.)

Day 15, Wednesday, September 6

STEW MEAT

To get to somewhere good from somewhere tough, slow down the process and let it cook. Slowly. Continuously. For a really long time. Stew meat. It starts out tough, but if you let it cook on low heat for a long time, it breaks down, becoming tender and delicious. It's not expensive. It just takes time. Try to stir-fry or microwave it and it stays tough and miserable. Good sex: it's like cooking stew meat. Where we were at the beginning of this diet was not our ideal happy place regarding sex. We were looking for improvements. Now, with the help of this diet, little by little, continuously cooking, we are stewing out the toughness, the imperfections in our sexual relationship, and are tenderly making progress toward a delicious end result.

Day 16, Thursday, September 7

IF YOU FALL OFF, GET BACK ON!

Tonight is a week since we received the bad news that spun us into a trip that led us away from intimacy with each other . . . away from the diet. We've had sex only once in the last week. After anticipating and planning four meal encounters each week, it seems like it has been AGES! Time to start something rolling again. In an effort to try to create a new mood in the bedroom, I bought a red lightbulb for the bedside lamp. Decided fairly quickly that we much preferred candlelight to red light . . . so switched to the standby candles. It was midnight when we sorted out the lighting. Mo and I reached out for each other from our exhaustion. I put my "Kissing 101" plan to work again, and it felt so good, SO healing. The kissing definitely connected us. I had to choke down a couple of freaks when I thought it was getting too liquid, but I just refused to let that get to me. It was unspoken that we still did not feel like having sex, but we cautiously anticipated the positive end results and pushed on. We ended up with a version of the Sweet Lazy Love spice. This is one spice that will be a staple for us, particularly when there is no time or will for extensive creativity. The result, the release was there. Worth the effort. Necessary. Wonderful.

Day 17, Friday, September 8

LIQUID ECSTASY

Time to reread the menu for some new ideas. I was tempted at first to agree with a random thought that told me I already knew what the menu said. Must be the same part of me that hates to see movies twice. I started thinking about Mo and what kind of sexual experience he might like tonight. I know there is one thing Mo loves, and that is a great massage, sometimes as much as good sex. I chose the spice Liquid Ecstasy, and wrote it on the calendar. Knowing again that my "visual" (noncalendar reading) partner would probably miss the whole "Liquid Ecstasy" note, I lined up three massage oils on the dresser in the bedroom: pineapple (my favorite), cinnamon and spice, and strawberry and champagne. Massage oils are not strangers to us. I like to use the edible/lickable oils for a sexual massage (as opposed to a "serious" my-muscles-are-aching massage). True, the edible oils still taste like oil, but somehow they are palatable in small doses, just in case you get the urge to kiss or lick a spot with oil on it. I really wanted to use the Now *This* Is a Massage! spice tonight. I just KNOW Mo would go crazy for it, but I need to build up some nerve for that one. I don't want to crack up right in the middle of it and spaz out that I'm doing something crazy. Then I might make him feel stupid, especially if he is really into it like I expect he will be. I absolutely have to be able to maintain composure through the entire ordeal! I can do this!

Day 18, Saturday, September 9

NOTHING SCHEDULED: FAST FOOD . . . AGAIN

Nothing is on the calendar today. I have noticed, however, that in little spaces of time, Mo and I are more physical than before. I guess these times would be considered "snacks" on this diet. Mo gets out of bed first in the morning. He used to jump out of bed when the alarm sounded and head directly for the shower. Today, and more often lately, he has been lingering in bed after the alarm goes off. He wants to body hug me, and squeeze me, and play with me. He rolls on top of me, or pulls me on top of him, and just fools around. Very lighthearted, very playful, with no end or finale expected or even wanted. I have a million things starting to roll through my mind the minute I wake up, and I usually get right up and start writing things down like a neurotic lunatic. But these brief "fast food" encounters have made me feel so desired, loved, appreciated, and happy that I have just chilled and basked in it all. These times are the best and I can't believe we have not done this every morning of our lives together. It feels THAT good!

Day 19, Sunday, September 10

SURPRISE! SURPRISE AGAIN!!

Mo surprised me tonight with a bubble bath. I learned later that this was the Our #1 Bestseller spice. My guy KNOWS what he's doing because he has done this for me many, many times over our years together. This time it was a little different, however. The bubble bath, candlelight, bit of incense, and champagne were the same. With prior baths he drew for me, he left me alone to read. I love to read and I love having time by myself. But this time he stayed. He did not intrude, or touch, or suggest. He just sat by the bathtub watching me. There was no way I would trade THAT for a book, so I did my thing and he did his thing and we ended up doing our thing together. Before tonight I had this bath thing all wrong.

Day 20, Monday, September 11

THE FOOD CHAIN

I'm watching Mo and admiring his wellspring of creativity. It's like my actions are fueling his actions, and when he acts then his actions fuel my actions. I'm starting to see a cycle of reciprocity. He becomes inspired and tries something, which in turn inspires me and I try something. I guess we have always been like that together, whether we are helping each other achieve career goals, raising our kids, dealing with our two families, or whatever. We never drew a line, figured out who had contributed which percent. We have always understood the value of each giving 100% plus to our situations together, always realizing great results. Somehow, though, it was taking on a new meaning with our sex life. We have always been about pleasing the other person. I think our problem, or more specifically MY problem, has been accepting all of the giving. Really letting go, relaxing, and accepting myself . . . allowing Mo to give to me. Also, focusing on each other's pleasure TOO much leads to an end result of focusing on the end result. We needed to relax. To enjoy our own ride and not focus on the starting or the stopping. Focusing more of our time and energy on intimacy this month is really paying off. It is going so much deeper than better sex. I am thankful for him every time I look at him. We laugh more together. We are judging each other less; understanding each other more. As long as we are two individuals living together, things will never be perfect. But life can be wonderful, and it is right now. There is no way I want to go backward, to lose ground after these 28 days are over. I guess after the 28 days we will be in "maintenance" mode . . . just like real Weight Watchers . . . monitoring our sex habits to make sure we don't fall into the bad-habit traps from which we have managed to pull away. This sex diet is a good thing, because for a period of time it bombards us with ideas . . . shakes us up. A maintenance mode will be the time we keep practicing the new habits until they become permanent fixtures in our lifestyle.

Day 21, Tuesday, September 12

HELIUM BALLOONS

Today is Mo's birthday. I arranged for lots of surprises for him at work today. (He puts up with me.) Later, after celebrating his birthday, Mo took me upstairs with six red helium balloons that previously decorated his birthday party. He tucked the string of each balloon between the mattress and the box spring, equally spaced apart, forming a circle of balloons around the bed. Okay, I was curious, to say the least. During our lovemaking he put a soft, fuzzy blindfold on me, and stopped every once in a while to pop a balloon with his lighter (made me scream and jump, not knowing at first that the "pop" was coming, then after the first, not knowing from which direction the "bang" would come). Mo said later that this was a twist on the original spice (How to Turn Burning Curiosity into Burning Love). Since these were already inflated when he received them, he modified the spice. I think he got a real kick out of making me jump . . . like he was ten years old again pulling a prank or something. I must admit, the balloon popping was weird but added a bit of strange excitement.

Day 22, Wednesday, September 13

DESSERT

A little Lingerie Parfait mixed with some Eye Candy and a dash of Body Heat . . . yummy! My big lap dancing debut! Sure, I've mini-stripped; a shirt, a bra, panties . . . just to tease . . . many times. I've stripped full-on, for the entire length of a song . . . a few times. But lap dancing??? Never . . . until now. I know this phenomenon is intriguing to men, and my man is no different, I'm sure. I would hate it if he ever had a lap dance in a strip joint. So I practiced and decided to perform a lap dance myself. I had it all: lots of bold stripper makeup, big stripper hair, stripper lingerie with holes in interesting spots, high heels, long pearls, gloves. Needless to say, I was kind of embarrassed at first, looking at myself in the mirror thinking, "Girl, what ARE you doing?" I think I would have DIED if he started laughing. Fortunately for both of us, he took it pretty seriously: his eyes opened wide and his jaw dropped. He was trying to act cool, but it was obvious that he was totally blown away and totally excited by the whole scene! I don't think I was that smooth, but he did not seem to notice. He was SO completely into it! I actually got into it, too. It was fun teasing him and only giving him what I wanted him to have. The control was kind of a high. I made up my own "House Rules," I think I could have told him any crazy thing and he would have done it just to keep that experience going. He was sweet and SO easy!

Day 23, Thursday, September 14

FLASH FRIDAY ON THURSDAY

Sometimes we flash each other. It ALWAYS makes us laugh, especially when the flasher makes a funny face or strikes a stupid pose. I often flash Mo (top half only) when he waves to me from his car as he drives off to work in the morning. I am discreet, making sure there are no neighbors, gardeners, or garbage men in sight. Sometimes, if there is a danger of being caught, I just PRETEND like I am going to flash. Now THAT makes him nervous. Today I was more creative, flashing different body parts at different times. Mo started flashing, too (always ready for a party!) in his usual funny style. He starting by making a thong out of his Fruit of the Looms and dancing around; too funny! I think it was Mo who first inspired me to flash him. I can't recall ever flashing anyone before him. Maybe because he is hands down a people person, an extrovert; gleaning his energy from interactions with the outside world. He does not spend a lot of time alone, reading, etc. (things I love to do, more on the introverted side, gleaning energy from introspection). He just loves to share himself with the world. I learn a lot from him, because my shoes-off self is the opposite. He knows, however, that flashing HIM is as far as it goes!

Day 24, Friday, September 15

WAITING . . . AND THAT IS OKAY NOW

Scheduling our intimate time together has taken the "when are we going to have sex again/when do I HAVE to have sex again" edge off of our days. B.D. (Before Diet) we could go one day without sex, getting edgy on the second day without sex, and trouble started on the third day without sex. With the schedule, we know that sex is going to happen, and plenty of it. This knowledge has taken the edge off even when we've gone a few days without sex. Interesting.

Day 25, Saturday, September 16

WRITING SOMETHING FOR ME

Scheduling sex has been an exercise in self-discipline. Just as exercising one's body, even after a long day of work, keeps the body fit. Just as putting wholesome foods in one's mouth, even when "fatter," sick-making food is more convenient, keeps a body functioning well. Just as thinking positive thoughts, even when the world bombards us with negative information, keeps our mind full of love, hope, peace, and goodwill. Scheduling sex has been a big deal. Listen to me, I'm solving the world's problems by scheduling sex. Wait . . . there is more to explore here. Scheduling sex is helping me develop the habit of controlling and replacing a natural, first-response or animalistic action (for example turning away from sex because I am too tired, or not aroused, or preoccupied) with what I know is good . . . better. This is refinement. This is the gift of reasoning given to a human being, and separating us from animals. Most simply it is doing the thing you don't want to do but you do because you know it is good for you, to obtain positive results. It's basically like Listerine: the taste you love to hate. After all of that . . . no sex today. Still mourning and still sad, but feeling really great at the same time. Working to restore our physical relationship through this hard time of a family crisis has helped to heal us and keep us strong. We, in turn, are our best selves and in the best position to help others who need us.

Day 26, Sunday, September 17

NO RULES. NO DENIALS. NO DOUBT.

Our breakthrough. This morning was some of the best sex I can remember having with Mo. Oddly enough the morning began without a hint of that great sex . . . quite the opposite actually. For some reason we have had terrible Sunday mornings lately. I think it has to do with Mo's new business, working six twelve-plus-hour days most weeks, and wanting just to do NOTHING or do whatever comes up or whatever HE wants to do on his one day off: no plans! If I have planned nothing else for a Sunday (a rarity, but I'm working on it), church is a priority with me. It always has been with him, too, except when there is not enough downtime in his life. Anyway, after lounging around in bed for a while, I initiated sex with him. He flatly refused with some kind of an attitude. I quickly became offended and emotional (not my normal self, of course) because I hardly EVER initiate sex, and he denied it when I did. Not a good plan. Amazingly, argument turned to discussion when I remembered to step outside my emotions and check out what issues were lying under the actions. Mo explained his own feelings of rejection many times when he tried to initiate sex with me, and I refused HIM. (I never thought much of it myself until now!) The situation began to gel. We pretty much decided then and there that we would both try our best not to reject initiations for sex from the other, and there would be no rules during sex (besides the obvious: don't hurt anyone and try to please), all inhibitions left at the door. I made the deal, knowing this would be easier for him than for me, but intellectually I know the benefits of the deal and I'll do my best. The sex Mo initiated after our talk was what he described later as the Panty Roulette spice. On the bathroom floor, passionate, long, and totally exhilarating. I let everything go and just absorbed myself in the moment. I guess the key to mind-blowing sex is the relaxation, the meditation ridding the mind of any thought. This seems simple as I write about it, but I know it takes concentrated effort (at least to learn on my part). That was a HUGE lesson for me, like I was the Road Runner, and Wile E. Coyote dropped an Acme anvil on my head. It was that heavy. SIMPLICITY RULES! Later, Mo packed the kids and the moms (his and mine were visiting) in the car to go to brunch, and he also threw in a large blanket and some cold drinks and fruit. Still, after all of the revelations with which Sunday morning gifted me, I still had to swallow the urge to know, to control. The words "Where are we going? What are we doing?" never made it out of my mouth alive. And the day was splendid. I actually felt like I was walking on air, meditative air . . . just going with the flow.

Day 27, Monday, September 18

CHANGE OF PACE

After all of this time scheduling our "meals," I noticed that most of them were scheduled for 8:30 P.M. or later. It struck me that we are together for sex at the end of the day, late. That has been the practical time for sex since we are apart during the day, and late afternoons/evenings are busy with kids, extended family, and other obligations. We know we need to lead ourselves to battle against predictability: the boring bed at night. We need more time together, alone and away from the house at various times during the day/night. We need to GET OUT! We need to schedule dates! Even if during the outings sex is not possible, at least it will build back more quality time with each other. Time when we are at our brightest and best, instead of at the end of the day when we are wound down and ready to sleep.

Day 28, Tuesday, September 19

THE ICEMAN COMETH

"Let's celebrate, it's been a month!" He was hiding something behind his back as he spoke with a sly look on his face. It was dripping down between his legs. It was ice . . . melting. It was the Ice, Ice Baby spice and it was nice, baby, nice. He's obviously been thinking about our intimate time together, trying new things, and having a blast. I really don't want this diet to end, so I bought a "write on/wipe off" calendar and hung it on the inside of the linen-closet door in our bathroom. (Our children have no reason to go there. And if they happen to, they will see only sweet, romantic reminders/anticipations from their parents to each other.) We have come to love the surprise of the other person's plans: The anticipation of the encounters are too much fun not to have a part in our lives. I think I'll thank Mo for all of his love and attention by taking him out to dinner. I'll wear this wicked pair of wireless, remote-control leather panties . . . and hand him the remote control right after the hors d'oeuvres. I'll let him figure out the rest. Should not take him long.

Yee-haw, bee-yah!

BEFORE THE DIET

"With Doug working two jobs and us living sixty-five miles apart, we're always running in two different directions."

—SALLY

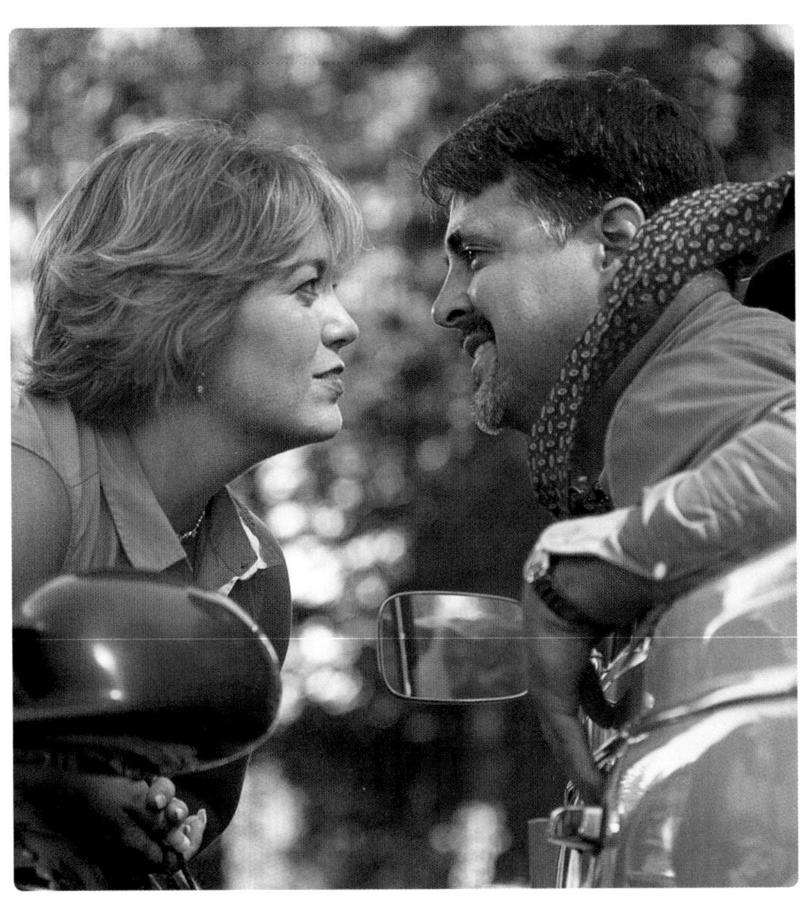

Fasten Your Seat Belts!

SALLY & DOUG

SHE: 30s, office manager

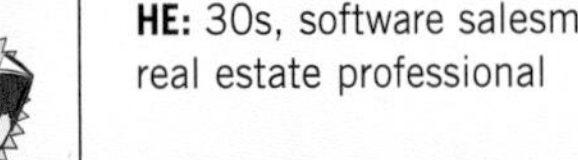

HE: 30s, software salesman and real estate professional

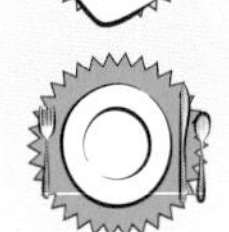

STATUS: together 2½ years, engaged; 1 daughter from her previous relationship

From the first minute I spoke with them, I could tell that Sally and Doug are a match made in heaven. A perfect stranger meeting these two people can feel their connection—it's in their eyes, their smiles, the energy coursing through their bodies. These two are live wires!

When they got involved more than two years ago, Sally had been out of a marriage for a

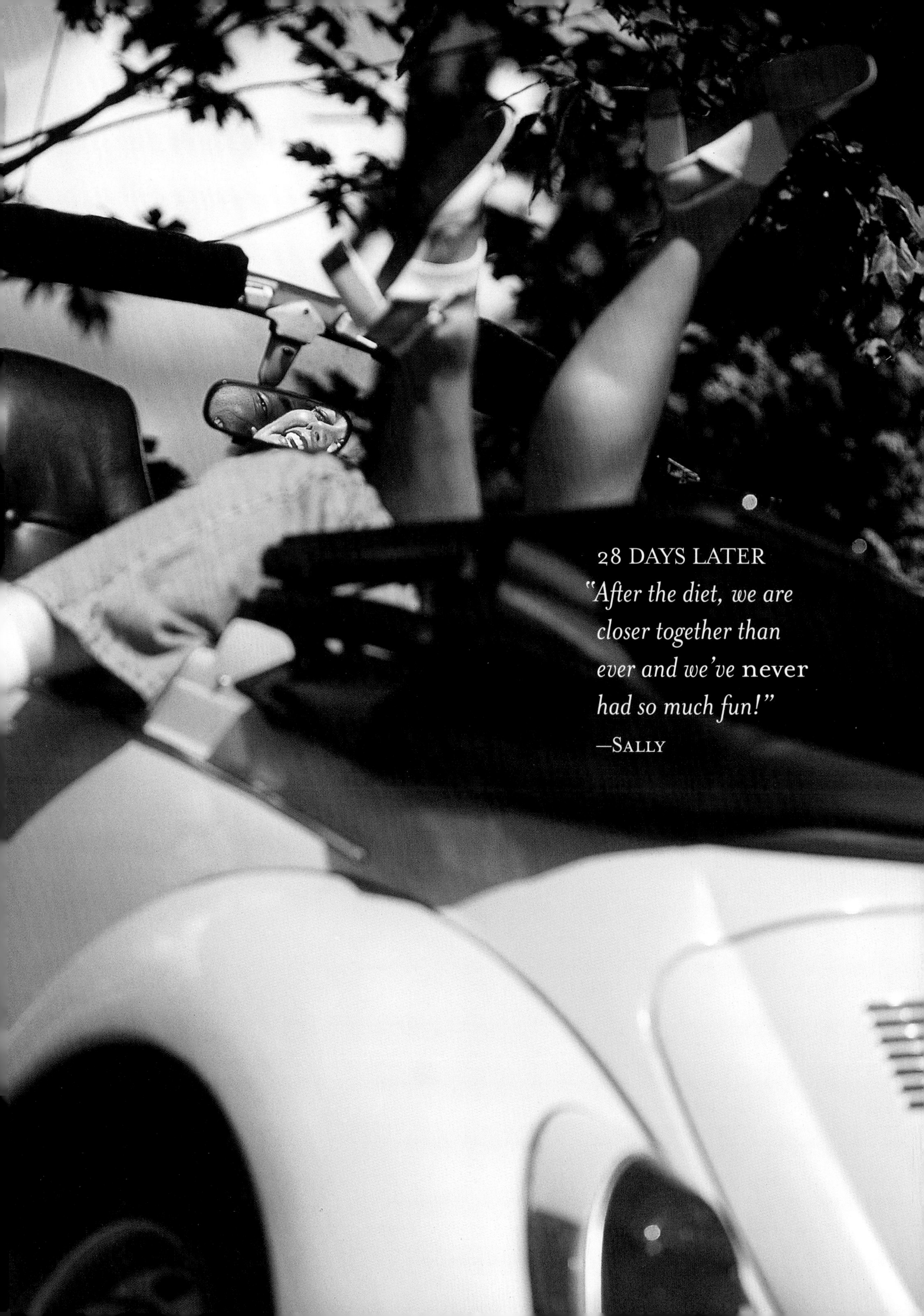

28 DAYS LATER

"After the diet, we are closer together than ever and we've never *had so much fun!"*

—Sally

number of years. Her daughter was then seven years old and Sally was reluctant and nervous about starting a relationship. Then she met Doug: "He's different from the rest," she says. "I love his energy and his positive outlook on life. I've never heard the guy say one negative thing."

At the time, Doug not only lived sixty-five miles away, but he also spent a great deal of time on the road for work, clocking as many as seventy-five hours a week. Clearly he was a very busy man! This inherent stress, however, did not stop them from wanting to go on the diet. In fact, they wanted to dig into their relationship and root out its problems. Though their sex life had always been pretty satisfying, their biggest issue was that Sally was tired of doing all the initiating. "As far as making the first move goes, I personally think I made all the effort," Sally explains. "I can't think of a time he seduced me other than the first time that we met. And that's the only thing I worry about in the relationship."

"When we have frequent sex, there's a difference in the way she looks at me. I can swim in her eyes at any given moment."
—Doug

At the same time, and possibly in an unconscious reaction to her growing disenchantment with Doug's trouble initiating, Sally stopped working out and put on weight. "Before we started the diet, I'd been feeling overweight and worrying that I was letting myself go," she says. "And I love this guy—I didn't want to let myself go. But he wasn't pursuing me. And when we're not having as much sex, I don't feel good about myself. It's a vicious cycle. Once we have sex again, then I feel beautiful, and I'll start working out."

The root of his not initiating had nothing to do with not being attracted to Sally. He says, "I'd like to lose my shyness about seducing Sally and just go for it." His trepidation was related to unresolved feelings of rejection from his previous relationship. His ex-wife consistently rejected his sexual advances, to such a degree that Doug internalized the rejection and stopped risking initiating.

But once Doug and Sally began the diet, all these problems disappeared and they rediscovered their original passion for each other! They were both ecstatic to split the responsibility of initiating, and Sally was blown away by Doug's total 180-degree turnaround. As

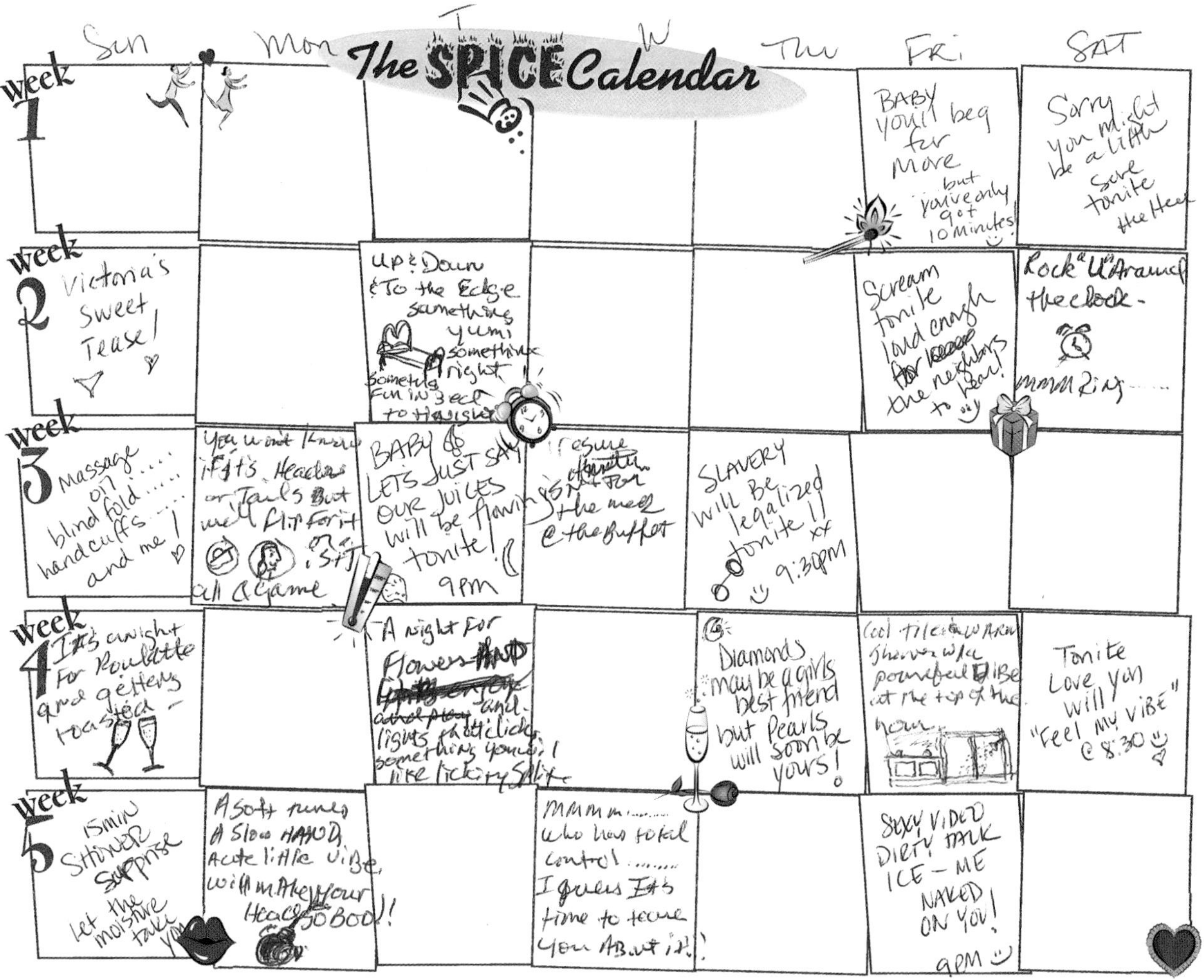

"Some nights were his nights, some nights were my nights. I think that puts all the romance right back into the relationship."—Sally

Sally points out, "Now I feel like Doug's sexual fantasy." And Doug says, "The diet really made me more excited to initiate, which I had always been kind of slow about. But this time I knew I had to have the floor, so I felt like it was completely and totally acceptable to experiment and have fun." He continues, "In my past relationship, I had the wind

"I combined these three spices: the Clock Technique, the Gee! Stroke, and Feel the Vibe. She didn't know what hit her! I liked that there were so many choices. It gave me the opportunity to do two or three spices at a time, which was a lot of fun."—Doug

blown out of my sails, but this has put the wind back."

Both Sally and Doug could feel the diet bring them closer. Doug explains, "Instead of walking hand in hand, we walk with our arms around each other. We walk closer together, step by step, in every way."

One of the aspects of Doug and Sally's story that really surprised me was how Doug went from zero to sixty in the initiating department. The diet gave him the permission and the freedom for total abandon! But that wasn't all that surprised me. Three weeks into the diet, I received the following e-mail:

Subject: And I used to think dieting was difficult!
Date:
From: Sally and Doug
To: Laura Corn
CC:

Wow!!!!!!!!!!!! Are we ever having FUN! "Thank you" is about the only response we can think to say to you each and every night. It's like, "Wow, I love you, babe." "I love you too." "Good night, Laura Corn, we love you too!"

Loved doing the Want to Hear Him Beg? spice the other night with the candles, and wowwiiee did I ever enjoy your helping hand in the Around the Clock spice. Douglas said he put a few of your other ideas together with that one and, yes, it did blow me away. The funny thing is we were having a midafternoon spice last week and with the warm weather these days, I had my bedroom window open and when we were in "complete bliss," I heard a neighbor from afar yell *"Right on!!!!"* And we had to laugh out loud! In the past . . . years back, I used to cringe when my lover would ask me what my fantasies were and not be sure if I even wanted to truly know his. I got really good at avoiding those kinds of questions.

I found myself asking Douglas the other day what his were and wouldn't let him stop at his top three. He had me going, too, and well . . . thank you, because I feel like this is territory that we should all explore, and how wonderful it is to feel this comfortable doing so.

Your biggest fans,

Sally and Doug

After reading Sally's e-mail, I couldn't stop smiling for days! And I got an even bigger smile on my face a week later when I received another e-mail, this time from Doug:

Subject:
Date:
From: Doug
To: Laura Corn
CC:

Dear Laura,

Just wanted to say thank you for this wonderful diet!! Sally and I really enjoyed each other on this diet and look forward to taking the after photo this weekend. You have afforded us so many choices, when typically on a diet you are very limited. Thank you so much, Laura, for letting us participate—giggles and all.

Your faithful 28-day diet junkie,

Douglas

Needless to say, both e-mails touched my heart. The fact that the diet has the power to give so much to people, make them happy, and even transform their lives is more than I could ever ask for.

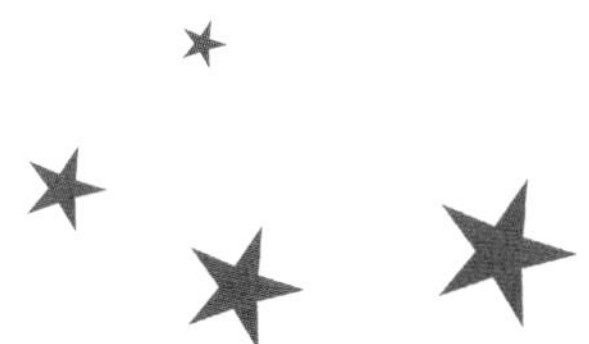

"In past relationships, I've always felt like the guy was looking at every girl and he was liking the girl in the sexy video more than me. I felt so insecure, because I knew I had all that potential inside me, but I just didn't know how to release it and feel like his fantasy. And now I feel like I can do that with Douglas."—SALLY

BEFORE THE DIET

"We have a great sex life, but we also have a lot of down time—reading and watching TV. We need a little more variety."

—ANGELA

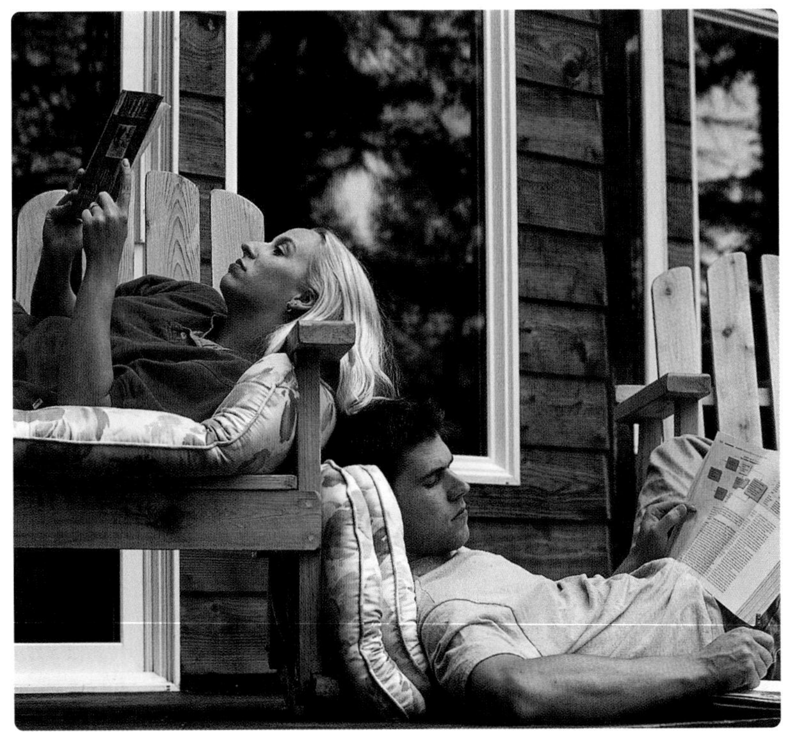

From Down Time to Boogie Time!

ANGELA & JEREMY

SHE: 20s, works at a credit union

HE: 20s, cabinetmaker and full-time student

STATUS: married 6 years

Angela and Jeremy were no strangers to turning their bedroom into a fun zone! When I spoke with Angela, it was clear that she'd done wild stuff with Jeremy before, but nothing compared to what the diet inspired.

Married six years, Angela and Jeremy had started dating in high school, and though they immediately felt attracted to each other, they

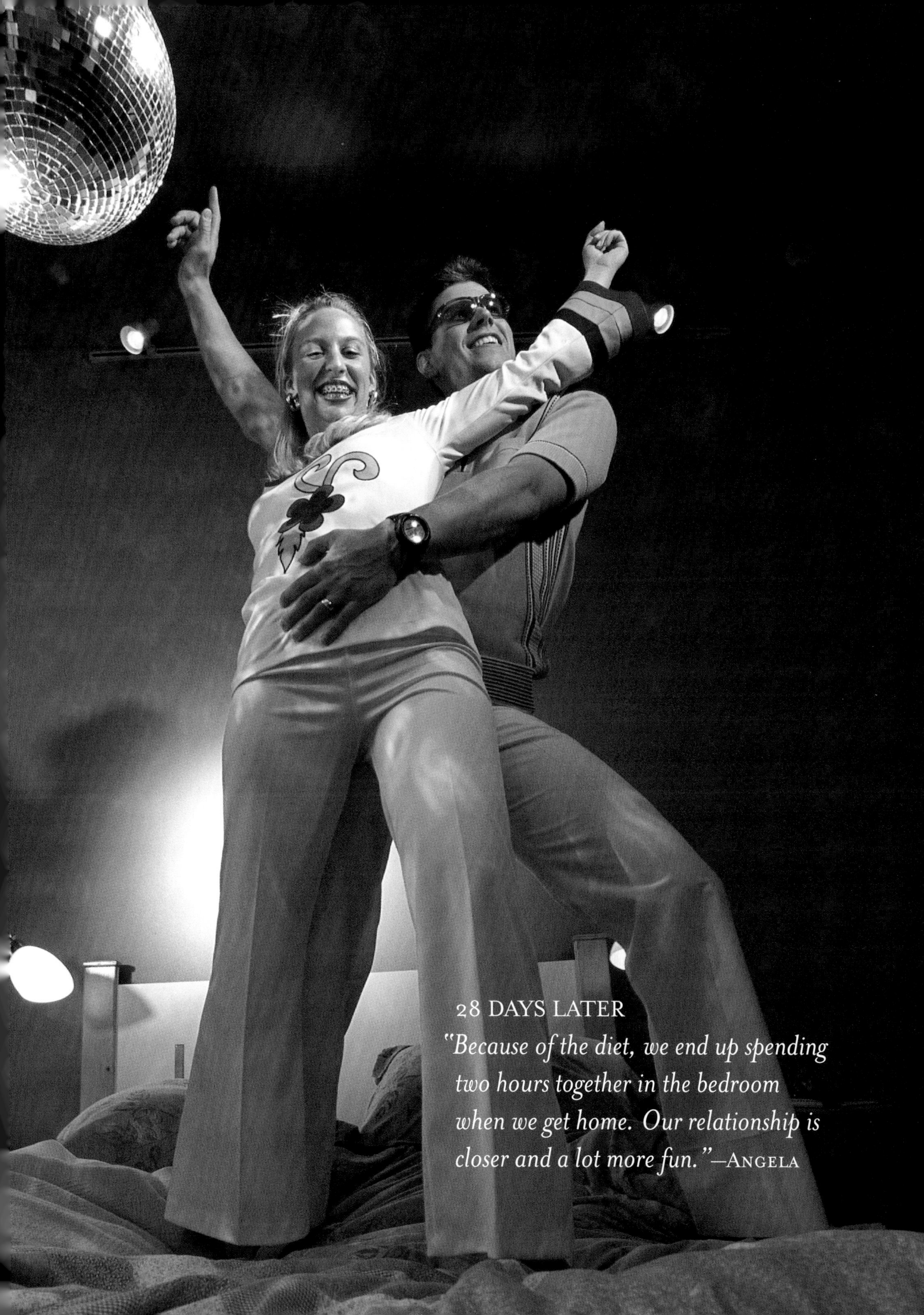

28 DAYS LATER

"Because of the diet, we end up spending two hours together in the bedroom when we get home. Our relationship is closer and a lot more fun."—Angela

actually waited to consummate their relationship until they were married. I believe this deep commitment to each other is one underlying reason for their passionate connection.

As one of the few couples to have sex virtually every night of the diet, it was clear I didn't need to prompt them to open up and have fun—they were already married to that! They're young, they're carefree, and they're always raring to go. They share an absolute passion for the outdoors, and hike, snowboard, and ski together—and it's clear that this physicality just takes over in the bedroom.

Although they used the Spice Menus to inspire some wild activities (Angela was especially creative using rose petals for lingerie), they didn't feel they needed to use the calendar. Well, that makes sense; after all, they had sex almost every night—no reminders needed!

The more experimental Angela was, the more confident she became. One day, when Jeremy opened the door after a hard day at work, he heard a voice calling from the living room. "Honey, are you alone?" Angela purred. When Jeremy said he was by himself, he went to find out what was going on. After turning the corner, he had his answer: There was Angela, leaning against the wall in a very seductive pose. His stunned gaze fell upon her five-inch pumps and traveled slowly up her body: from her sexy thigh-high fishnets, to a form-fitting purple leather miniskirt, and a black leather tank top that hugged every one of her voluptuous curves. Topping it off was a purple hair extension that dangled seductively down her shoulders. Jeremy barely had time to mutter, "Holy Moly!" before Angela demanded he take his clothes off. She was a woman in charge, and she would not be denied. After he followed her orders, she led him to the couch and did a slow, sensual striptease. But she didn't take off everything: The skirt stayed on—but what was underneath did not.

Angela had never been quite this brazen or experimental before, and her every last move

> *"Being on the diet was like starting a new workout program. And it's always exciting when you've got a new program."*
>
> —Jeremy

seared itself into Jeremy's memory. In fact, the entire next day he couldn't get the experience out of his mind, which could have been dangerous, he says, since he's in construction! He was so moved, the next night he asked Angela for an encore performance the minute he got home. And Angela happily complied.

But she wasn't the only one who had a few surprises up her sleeve. One evening, Angela arrived home to find an inflated bright red balloon resting on her pillow with something inside. "What's this?" she asked. Jeremy told her she'd have to wait until later to find out. First they had a party to prepare for. By the time they made it to bed it was after midnight and they were both exhausted. But Angela was still curious. Before they hit the sheets, Angela asked if she could pop her balloon. Jeremy flashed her a devilish grin, set the balloon next to the bed, and told her she'd have to wait until tomorrow!

"We loved the Spice Menu, but we didn't use the calendar. Instead, we took turns. I'd surprise him with a spice one night, and he'd surprise me the next."

—ANGELA

The next day at work, Angela couldn't get the balloon off her mind. *What was in it?* She was in total suspense. She arrived home before Jeremy and the temptation to pop the balloon was almost overwhelming. She shook it a few times, but fought the urge to puncture it. When Jeremy finally did get home, she made sure *nothing* came between her and that balloon! Jeremy relented and took Angela in his arms and led her to the bedroom, telling her that she could pop the balloon *after* they'd made love. Just imagine how charged their lovemaking was with anticipation! When they were done, Angela finally got her sweet reward. What was in the balloon? "I don't want to spoil it for any other women out there whose guys might do this spice for them," she says. *(What a tease!)* But she will say it was definitely worth the forty-eight-hour wait: "It's one of those things I'll save forever."

Angela and Jeremy prove that a hot couple can get even hotter when they up the frequency and get creative. Angela says she now has the confidence to be bolder in the bedroom. "It gave me that extra encouragement to do something a little bit more wild," she says. And Jeremy says they're both more playful now and feel even closer. "It added another element to our relationship that wasn't there before," he says. "It's really made a good thing better."

BEFORE THE DIET

"We have four kids, and we're living with my parents right now in a three-bedroom house. It's kind of a struggle for us to be intimate or spontaneous. What we really want is to spend more one-on-one time together."

—ROBIN

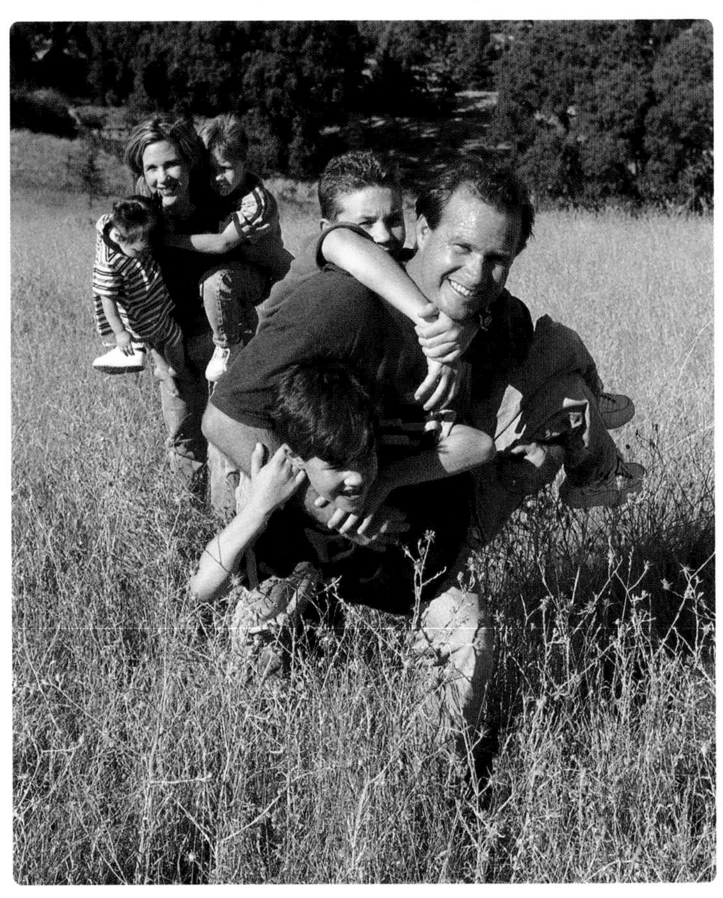

A Divine Romance

ROBIN & ERIC

SHE: 30s, home-schools her kids, counsels couples at her church, and runs a home business

HE: 30s, co-pastor at Vine Life Ministries in Lincoln, California, and stucco plasterer

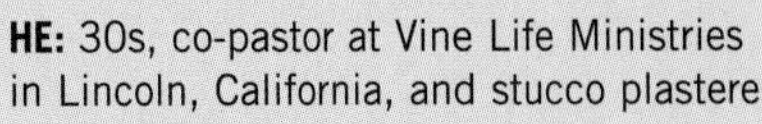

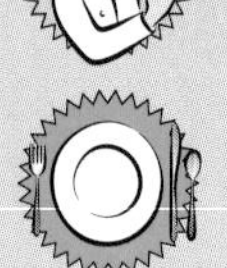

STATUS: together 15 years, married 12 years; 4 kids and they take care of Eric's teenage sister

I am simply in awe of Robin. I am blown away by her energy, passion, and gusto and how she brings that strong commitment to all of the many facets of her life.

One of the reasons Robin has become such an incredible inspiration to me is because, like me, she has a low sex drive. What I can't quite believe is how she has overcome that in

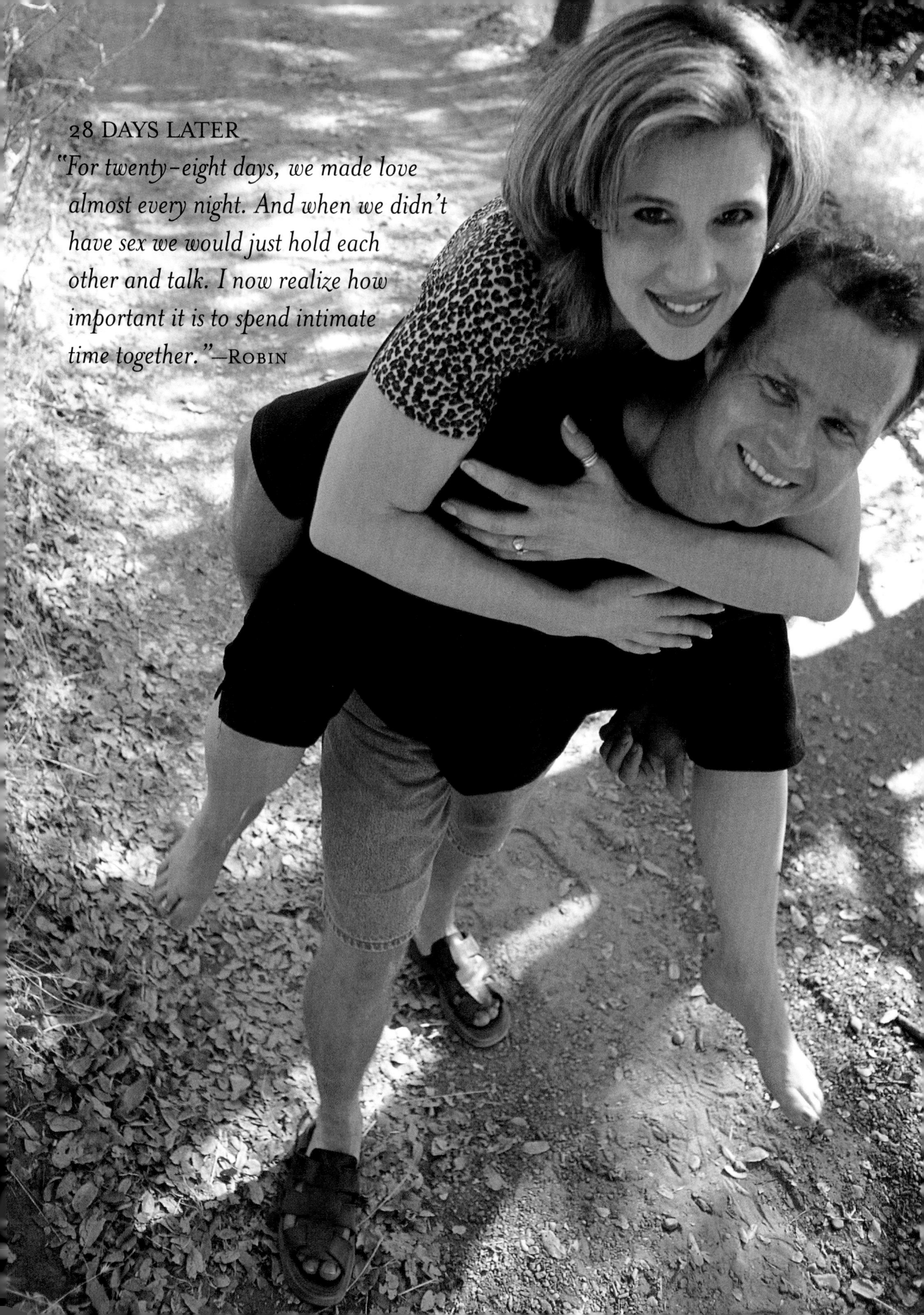

28 DAYS LATER

"For twenty-eight days, we made love almost every night. And when we didn't have sex we would just hold each other and talk. I now realize how important it is to spend intimate time together."—Robin

addition to everything else she does in her life. She has her own business, counsels couples at her church, home-schools her four kids, *and* lives in her parents' home. Yet she was able to go on this diet and have sex almost *every night*. Her amazing story illustrates how powerful it can be to make a commitment to your relationship and stick to it. Whenever I think I'm too tired for sex, I think of Robin. If *she* can find the energy, I certainly can, too.

Robin and Eric have a unique relationship that is rooted in their belief in God and love for each other. With four young children and Eric's teenage sister to raise, they moved in with Robin's parents more than a year ago when they sold their former home. They all live together in a three-bedroom house. Robin and Eric share one bathroom with their five children and their only sanctuary is their bedroom, which they still share with their youngest child, who is eighteen months old. Needless to say, their lives at the moment are very challenging.

Although Eric's passion and vocation is his work as co-pastor of their congregation, he also works ten-hour days as a stucco plasterer for a construction company. Their first priority after God is raising a strong, healthy family. Since Eric came from a dysfunctional family with an abusive father, he was especially determined to create a different family for him and Robin. With their full lives, how do they find the time for one-on-one intimacy?

Robin says spending time together and finding out about each other is of the utmost importance to them. "When I give to him, I just receive automatically," she says. "It's a blessing for me to give to him and meet his needs." Eric reciprocates Robin's feelings—in both feeling and gesture. Although they've always had a good sex life, they were finding it a lot harder to make the time to get together and that's why the diet and the idea of using the calendar and planning sex was so appealing. "It works better for me if I know that night that we're going to spend some time together," Robin says. "Then I am not caught off guard." So

"After all this intimacy, I find my husband even more attractive. I want to talk to him more. I want to sit by him more. I want to look at him more. I want to hear his voice more. I want to call him on the phone more."—Robin

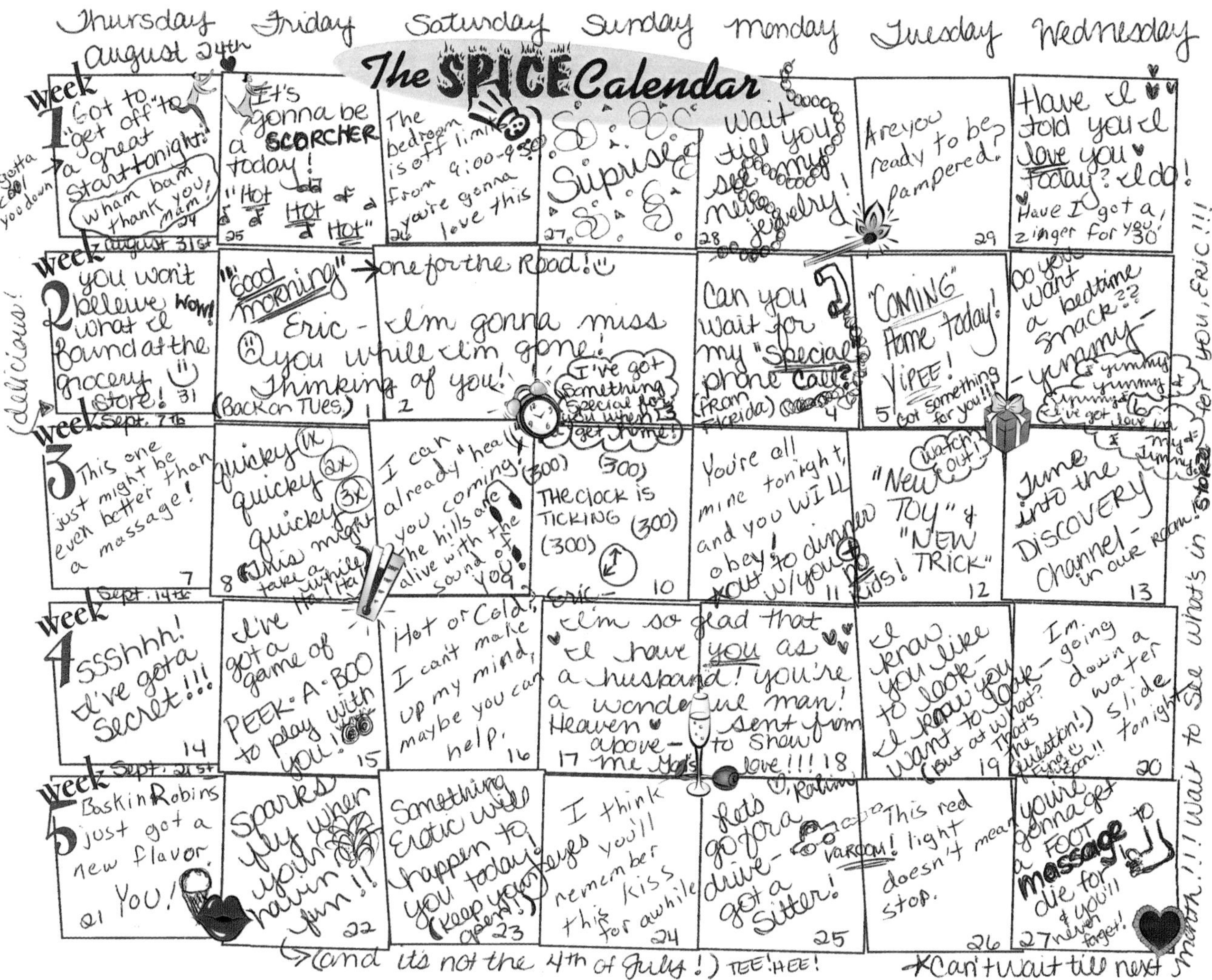

"Writing on the calendar is kind of like leaving little love notes just to help you remember you're thinking of each other and you're making the time to surprise each other."—Robin

although they weren't sure at the beginning of the diet whether they were going to be able to have sex four times a week, they wanted to try.

And try they did. Outside of a few times when one of their kids got very sick, Robin and Eric made love almost every night when they were on the diet. And this passion and commitment happened even in the presence of Robin's low desire and chronic pain with intercourse, about which she'd been consulting doctors for eighteen months. "We were still able to do it because it was important," Robin says. "Even though I had all these physical problems, I was committed to this. It was a promise we had made to each other."

And they certainly kept that promise! As Robin

points out, "As I read through the menu, I was trying to do new things, so I adapted one of the spices that you do in the bathroom. Instead of having Eric sit on a chair and watch me while I did a little performance for him, I told him to climb on the roof and watch me through the skylight! We had to be careful about the kids, you know. If one of them saw Eric on the roof, they would have climbed up after him!"

Robin continues: "I had a bathrobe on and under the bathrobe I had on lingerie. Then I took off the lingerie and did a little bit of everything. . . . By the time I got in the tub, I was calling him into the bathroom and all of a sudden I heard him climbing down off the roof and into the bathroom. It was great fun!"

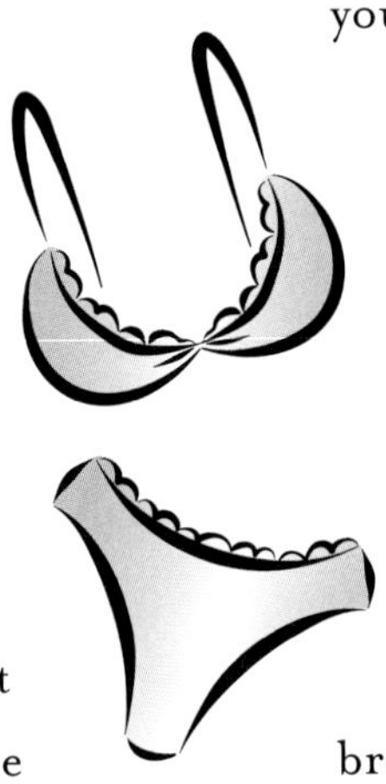

Robin and Eric became so creative and adventurous, they filled every inch of space on their calendar! Robin explains, "My problem was that I'd start writing a spice on the calendar and then I'd think, 'Oh, I want to do that one, too,' and then I'd write it in again and before you know it, I'm writing all kinds of notes all over it. There was no room for him!"

And once they were on the diet, Robin's pain miraculously subsided. Robin explains, "I think the hormonal factors have a lot to do with it. When you're more frequent and you're thinking about sex and your mate, your hormone levels are going to be higher, so you secrete more, and as a result, the pain isn't as severe. We've noticed this last month [that] the pain hasn't been there. I think it has to be the frequency. And now it's like a habit. We started making the time for each other every night."

In addition to this miraculous relief from her pain, another breakthrough moment occurred when Eric actually took off from work to stay home with Robin for the day. "If you knew my husband, you'd understand what a big deal this was. He never, ever takes off from work. Never misses a day being sick. And this last month he called in a couple of times and went to work late so he could stay in bed with me and snuggle. I mean, that's amazing."

I think *they're* amazing. Their love and commitment is an inspiration to us all.

"When we're having frequent sex, I feel security from him and I feel loved. I feel that everything is going to be taken care of. Any insecurities that you have just vanish."—Robin

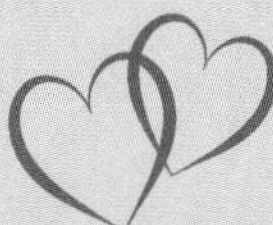

HOW TO LOVE AND BE LOVED

"The advice that I'd give to any man in a relationship—the advice that's always worked for me—is to *always put her first.* Think of her needs and the way that she needs to be loved first and, in turn, all of your own desires will be met because she will eagerly meet them.

"But you can't be doing it thinking, 'I'm going to give so I can get.' When your true attitude is to just give and to bless her—basically just give *everything* to her—then *any* woman will gladly give back. And it goes both ways. That works for both men *and* women in their relationships. If your heart is in the right place and you're just giving because of the love of giving, your partner will sense that. If you truly give out of love, then it will be returned to you.

"The first time I tried this and actually put it into practice, I thought, Well, man, she's just going to take advantage of me. That was my thought, because I had never attempted to give without expecting something in return. I thought, Well, she'll just want me to give to her all the time. But what I've learned—and this is what's so exciting—is that it doesn't work that way. What you get in return is probably *ten times* better than what you ever expected to get. It's unbelievable!

"This is something that I've always shared with anybody who's struggling with this what-about-me mentality. Because that's where a lot of people are at right now. It's a selfish thing. They're thinking, What about me?—and *everything* revolves around that. That's the root of a lot of their problems. They never learned to give of themselves and never learned to love. If they could instead give that attention to their partner, then everything in their life would be so much better."

—Eric

BEFORE THE DIET

"Since most of the kids have left the nest, we're just beginning to dive into intimacy."

—JoAnn

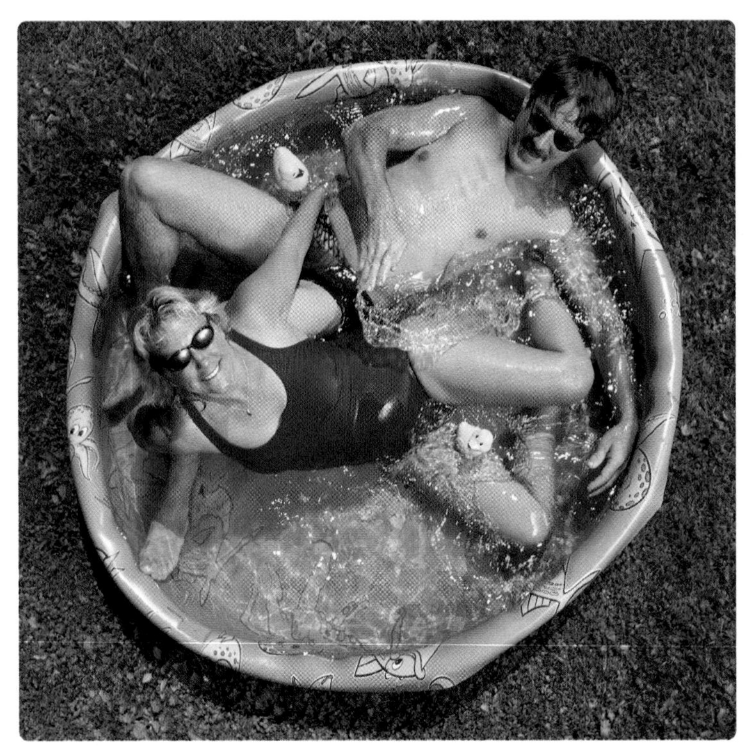

Sweeter the Second Time Around

JoAnn & Jerry

SHE: 40s, owns a cleaning service

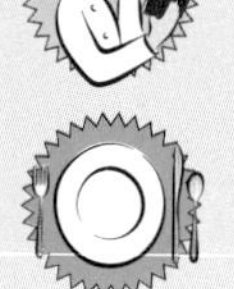

HE: 40s, tool and die maker

STATUS: together 3 years, married for 10 months; she has 3 grown children from her previous marriage, he has 2 from his previous marriage

When I first saw JoAnn and Jerry's before picture, I assumed there had to be a mistake. The photographer must have sent me their after photo instead. They looked so in love and were obviously having so much fun with each other, like kids splashing around in a pool—what could a couple like *this*

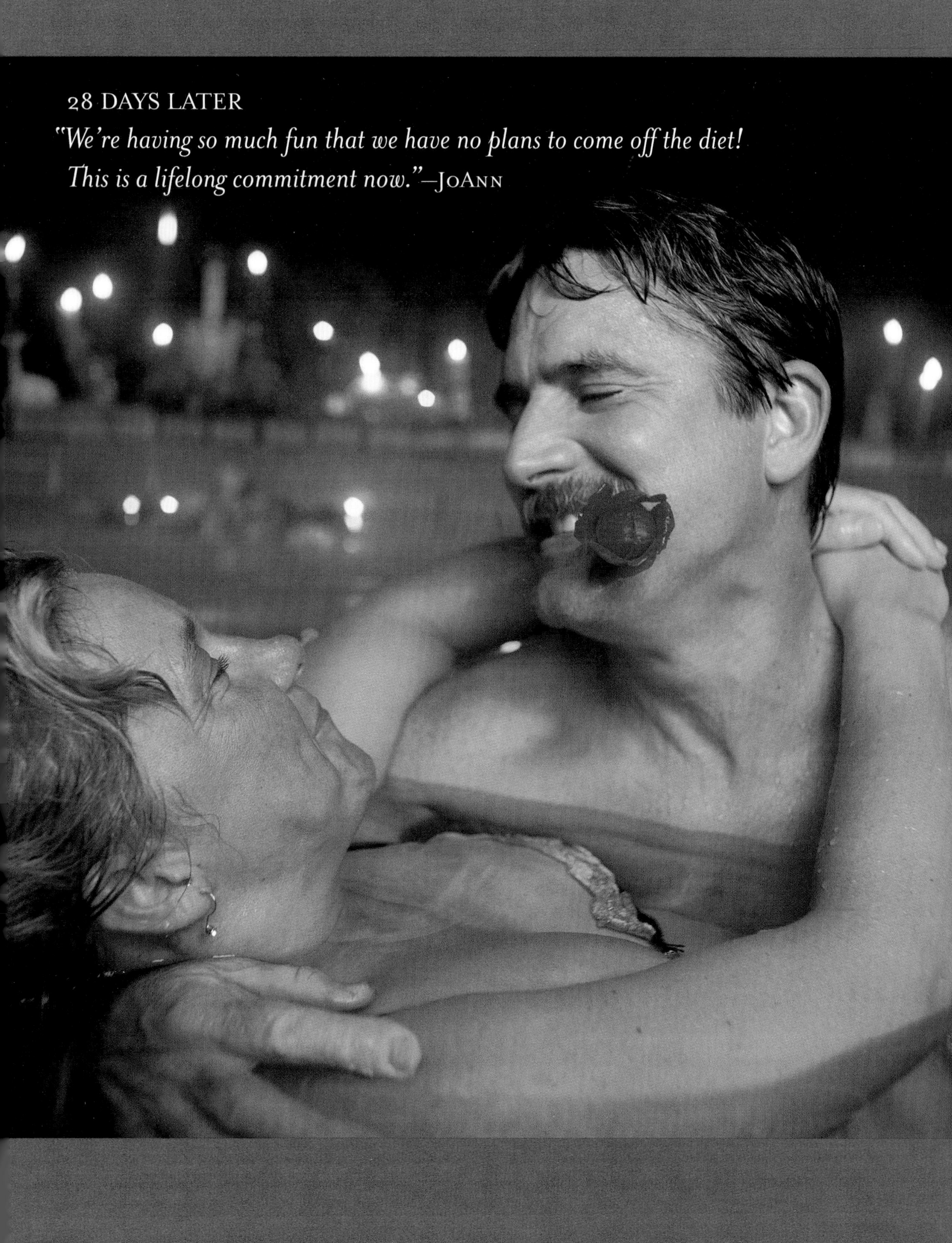
28 DAYS LATER
"We're having so much fun that we have no plans to come off the diet! This is a lifelong commitment now."—JoAnn

get out of the diet? I couldn't wait to find out!

And when I discovered where these two wonderful people came from emotionally, I found them even more remarkable. Since both of their former spouses of more than twenty years cheated during their respective marriages, trust is a major issue for Jerry and JoAnn. "When you come out of an unfaithful relationship, knowing you can always count on your partner is really important," explains JoAnn. "And that's why I was drawn to Jerry. He's very honest, and he makes me feel secure."

It's clear that Jerry is bringing JoAnn out of her shell sexually. "I've always been very conservative," she says. "Jerry is really bringing me out of that. I feel like I'm a teenager and I'm learning. He makes me want to try new things."

"I'm the more adventurous one," Jerry agrees. "I'm pretty much up for anything. But I love it when she seduces me, and I wish she'd do it more. It makes me feel good to be hunted."

So hunt Jerry she did. During the second week of the diet, JoAnn planned a surprise attack during their Vegas vacation. "Before we left, I wrote, 'Show me the money!' on our Spice Calendar," she says. "And since we were going to Las Vegas, I decided to stick with a gambling theme for the spice. I gave him a pair of boxers with dollar signs all over it, then I bet him that I could make him have an orgasm before he could make me have one. In that game, everybody was a winner!"

"One day, she surprised me by slipping her panties in my lunchbox!"

—Jerry

When they left the hotel, they swiped some Do Not Disturb signs for their bedroom door. "We have three or four hanging on our doorknob," Jerry says. "It's a fun way for us to say we need our private time."

JoAnn says one of the biggest lessons she learned on the diet was that she should protect that private time. "We still have a seventeen-year-old living at home, and I've always had a habit of putting my kids first," she says. "But this month, I didn't do that. I put *us* first."

Her newfound attitude helped Jerry give JoAnn her first oral orgasm. "She'd never experienced an orgasm that way before," he says. "The frequency and the creativity of the diet helped her relax and

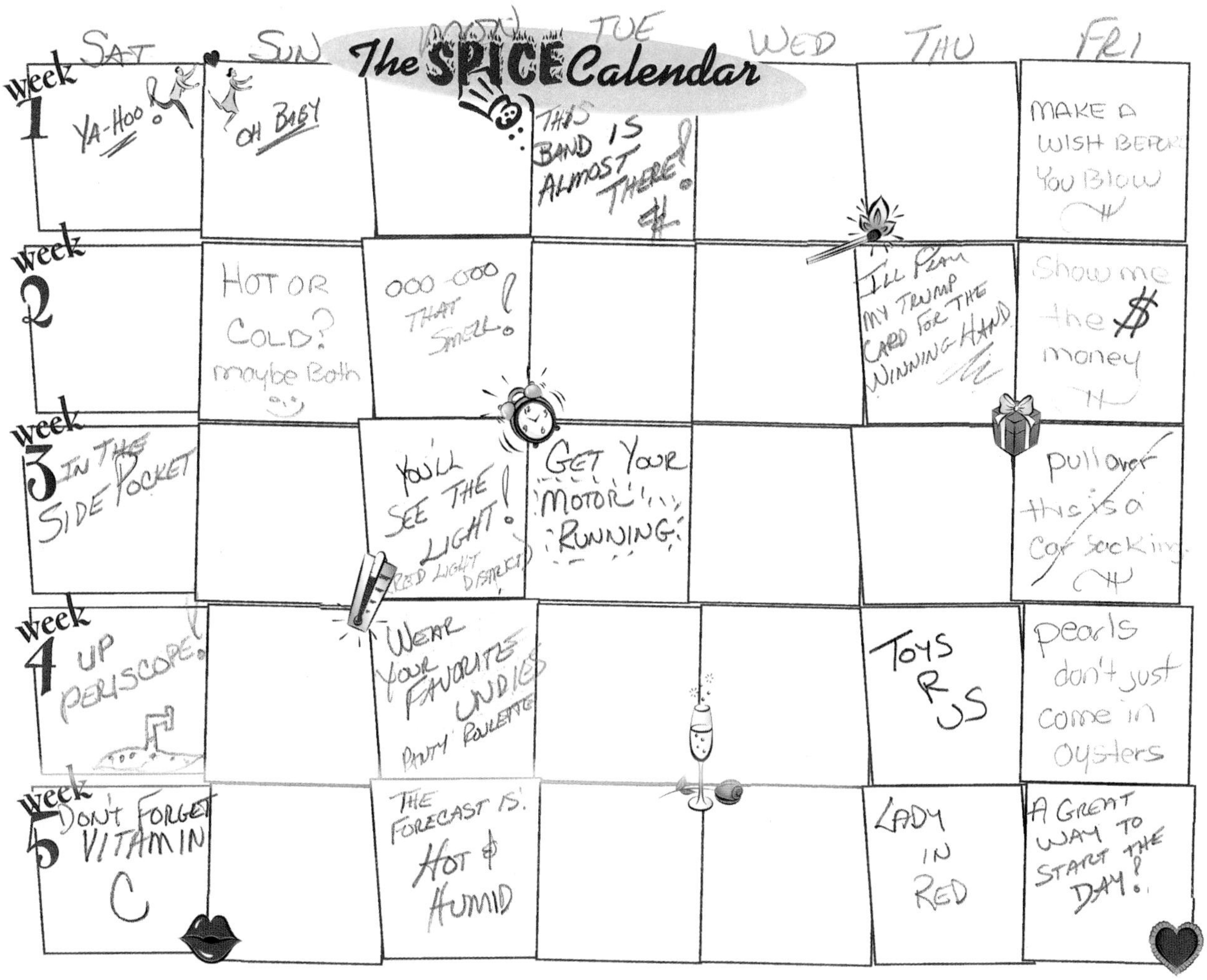

The SPICE Calendar

	SAT	SUN	MON	TUE	WED	THU	FRI
week 1	YA-HOO	OH BABY		THIS BAND IS ALMOST THERE!			MAKE A WISH BEFO YOU BLOW
week 2		HOT OR COLD? maybe Both	OOO OOO THAT SMELL!			I'LL PLAY MY TRUMP CARD FOR THE WINNING HAND	Show me the $ money
week 3	IN THE SIDE POCKET		YOU'LL SEE THE LIGHT! RED LIGHT DISTRICT	GET YOUR MOTOR RUNNING			pull over this is a car jacking
week 4	UP PERISCOPE!		WEAR YOUR FAVORITE UNDIES PANTY ROULETTE			TOYS R US	pearls don't just come in oysters
week 5	DON'T FORGET VITAMIN C		THE FORECAST IS: HOT & HUMID			LADY IN RED	A GREAT WAY TO START THE DAY!

"I wrote 'Don't Forget Your Vitamin C' on the calendar, then did a spice for him called Passion Fruit. I led him to the edge of the hot tub, so his feet could dangle in the water. Then I . . ."—JoAnn

really let go. Now I feel like I'm *the man*!"

Since they had so much success on the diet, JoAnn and Jerry say they have no plans to come off of it. "This is a lifelong commitment now," JoAnn says. "We probably won't make love four days a week, but it will be frequent. And we'll use the spices forever, because they're just too fun to give up!"

I know it was fate that JoAnn and Jerry found each other. They not only overcame deep issues, they *jumped* the hurdles in exhilaration and excitement.

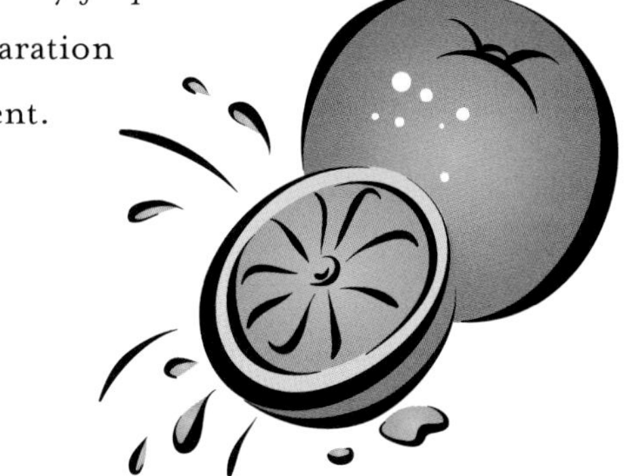

BEFORE THE DIET

"Burnie and I have good sex, and he knows the right buttons to push! But we'd like to be a little more creative and to schedule more time just for us. If your mind's on the sixteen million things that you need to be doing, then sex can really get lost in the shuffle."

—PENNI

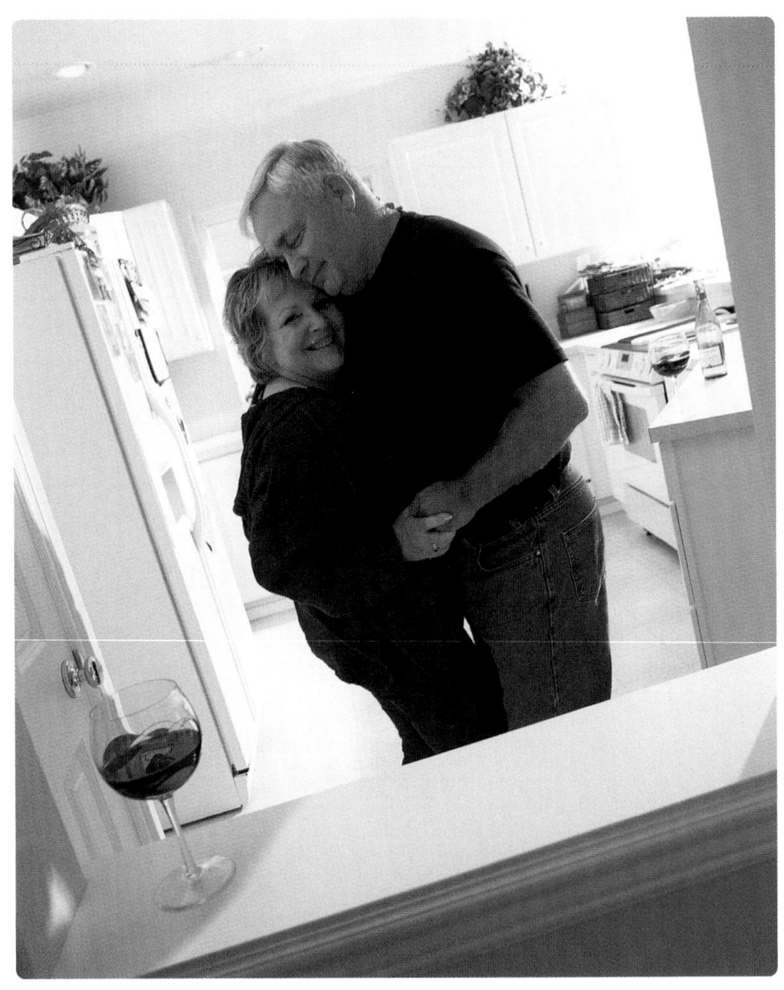

Drop-Dead Gorgeous

PENNI & BURNIE

SHE: 50s, RN and educator at a sexual assault center

HE: 50s, training manager, retired pilot instructor for the U.S. Army

STATUS: married 11 years, 3 kids from her previous marriage

The first thing anyone notices about Penni and Burnie is their unwavering sense of humor. As Burnie says, "We always laugh together. There is great communication between the two of us and we laugh our buns off all the time. We find something funny and humorous in just about everything."

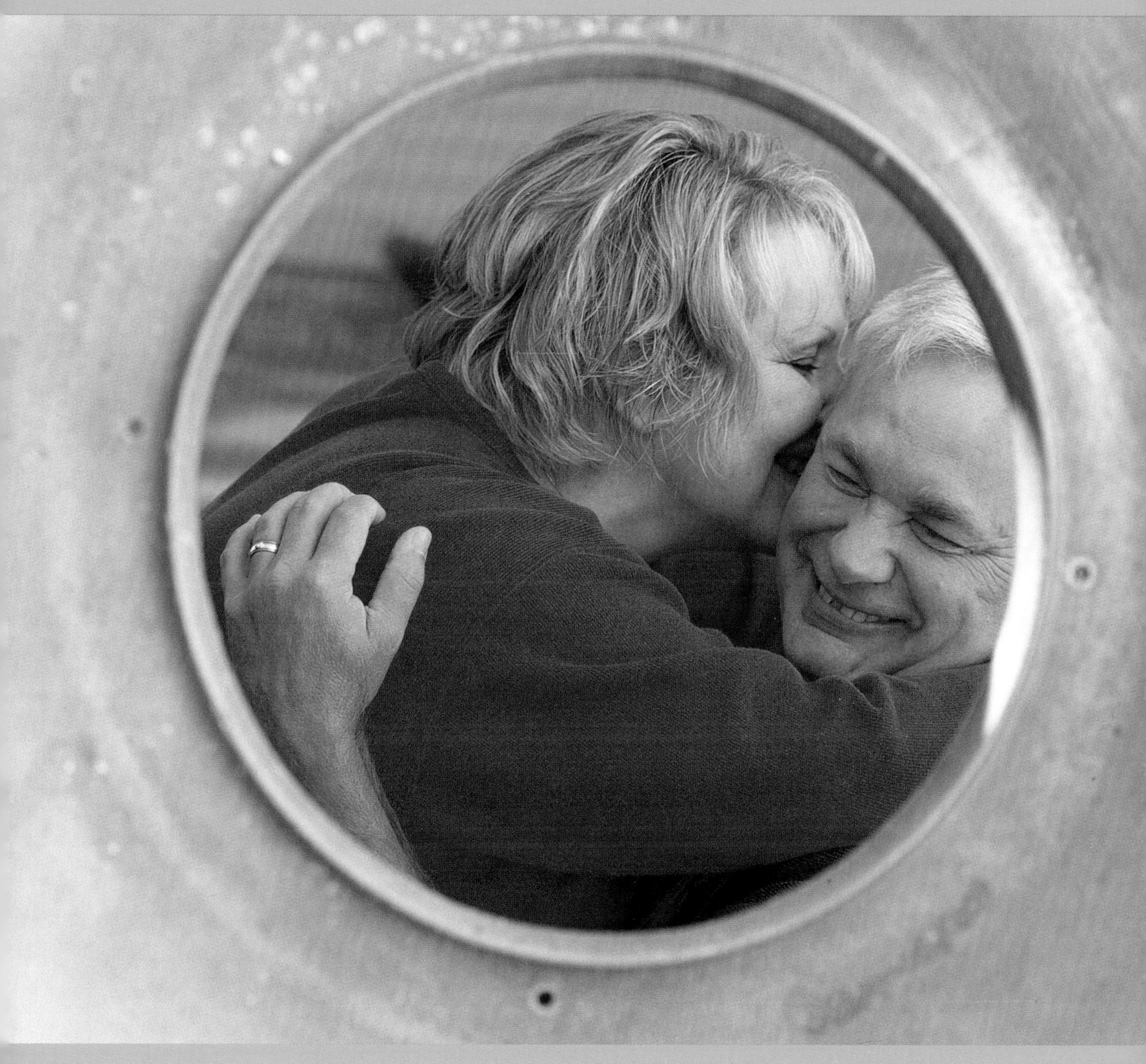

28 DAYS LATER

"The first thing that popped into my head is that we're having more fun. We aren't in a rut anymore! We're making time for ourselves. The diet just helped us put the fun back into everything."—PENNI

This proved true during the entire diet. When I called them for their after interview, Penni said to me, "You know, you interrupted us this morning." They knew I was going to call at the scheduled time, but when they called me back, they couldn't wait to tell me that I had caught them having sex! These two are just a hoot!

And Penni is not only funny, she simply oozes with sexual confidence. As she likes to say, "There's really no reason for us women to fret about our looks and age. Because when you're the only naked broad in the room, you're drop-dead gorgeous!" This great attitude and sense of playfulness were some of the reasons they were so successful on the diet. The other reasons . . . well, just keep reading. I don't want to spoil your fun!

Penni had always been in charge of the adventurous part of their relationship. As she explains, "In the beginning, I was the one who always set up all the fantasies. I was the one who picked him up in the white teddy and the raincoat. I was the one who got into the tub with him with just lingerie on. I was the one who picked him up from the airport in crotchless panties. But when you don't get any of that back, pretty soon it's like, why bother?"

Penni was very aware of the reasons behind Burnie's hesitancy to surprise her. "Because of his past experiences," she explains, "he would never really reciprocate because of his feelings of rejection." His ex-wives often used sex as a weapon or tool to manipulate him and Penni wanted to avoid that at all costs. It has been very important for her to make him feel comfortable, make him feel loved. But she also wanted him to be more creative. Before the diet, Burnie says, he would back off quickly any time he *thought* Penni was unsure or hesitant about sex. In his former relationships, he felt he had to earn sex. "I had to do the laundry or go to the grocery store or buy her something. I had to perform, and it demotivated me, made me more on edge." Burnie

"The most exciting thing about the diet was the anticipation. You know something is going to happen when you get home, but you don't know what it is. It's like you're a kid in a candy store— 'I can't wait, I can't wait!' I was close to getting speeding tickets on the way home!"—Burnie

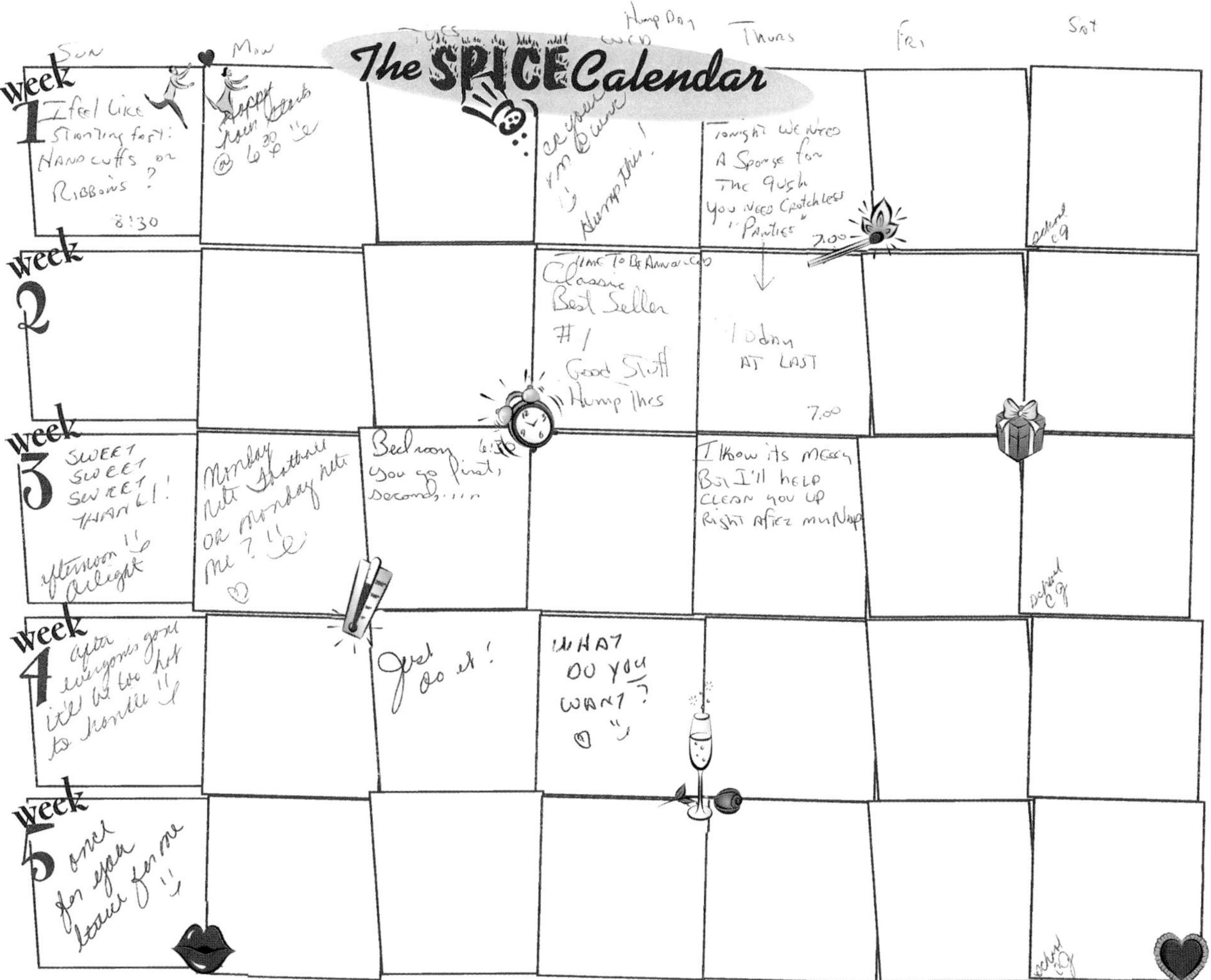

"People schedule going to the gym, going to work, going to their kids' softball and soccer practices. They schedule the car going to the shop. They schedule dinners. They schedule everything else. So why the hell not schedule sex?"—Burnie

also admits that as a retired military man, "I'm a tight-ass in some situations."

Now don't get me wrong. Before the diet, they didn't have a bad sex life. In fact, they were both pretty satisfied with it. "It's fine," says Burnie, "but in a perfect world, it would be fantasy week all the time." Basically, they both wanted a jump-start!

This relationship is the third one for each of them. With that kind of history, it makes sense that they would be a bit reticent about making themselves emotionally vulnerable. But the calendar got them to the point where they put themselves first and ricocheted them out of the past and into the future! Penni would think about their romantic plans for that evening all day long. "When it was on the calendar, I knew what was happening when he got home from work. Whatever was going on, I knew that it was going to happen, so I could think about it and be excited about it."

The anticipation also worked wonders for Burnie. He loved how the calendar created the anticipation. "I loved being surprised. The most exciting thing about the diet was the anticipation. . . . It's like you're a kid in a candy store—'I can't wait, I can't wait!' I was close to getting speeding tickets on the way home!"

Clearly the diet enabled them to put the fun back into their relationship. As Penni says, "Now he is actually doing things more creatively and taking the time to put something together that he thinks will please me. The fact that he put some thought into it probably turned me on more than anything. It wasn't just 'Let's go to bed and f—!'"

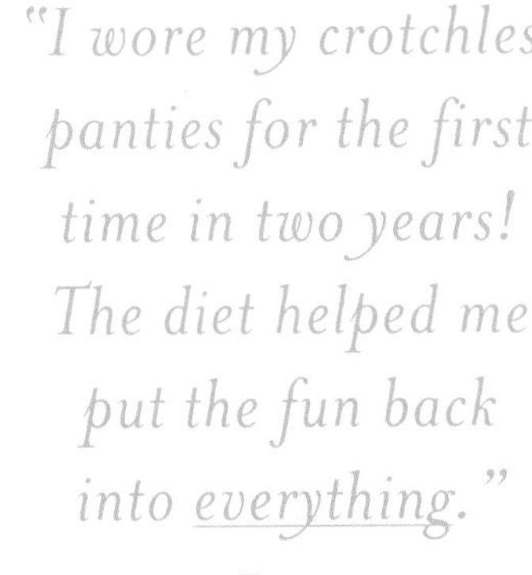

"*I wore my crotchless panties for the first time in two years! The diet helped me put the fun back into everything.*"

—PENNI

And Burnie feels freer to experiment. "The diet allowed Penni and me to get past those original boundaries and find out that there's a whole world of experimentation that we haven't tried before." He not only surprised Penni by donning a pair of boxers that said "Sweet Thang" on them (a reference to an old license plate), he also treated Penni to a wild spice called Thighs and Whispers. "It was something. It was very unique," Burnie says. "I definitely got the reaction I was looking for. I teased her a lot longer than I normally would have. Then I did the Gee! Stroke and I started doing something a little bit different with my fingers, and that got a pretty good reaction out of her, too."

And Burnie certainly was treated to a few scintillating surprises! Penni says that after she did the I'm Famous for This spice on Burnie, he said, "I've been screwed, blewed, and tattooed!" And Penni recalls, "He's already put in a request for it again tonight! I'm going to combine it with the Finger Zinger and another spice, so basically we're going to have a flippin' smorgasbord!"

Penni and Burnie's energy is on fire! I hope all couples can find as much sweetness and pleasure in the anticipation and variety of the diet and take it to such wonderful, hair-raising extremes.

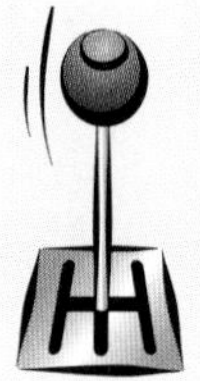

I'M A NINETEEN-YEAR-OLD MAN TRAPPED IN A FIFTY-ONE-YEAR-OLD BODY!

"I kind of look at it this way: I'm a nineteen-year-old man trapped in a fifty-one-year-old body! Things still work, but they don't work as well as they used to. I'm having fun with the equipment I have. And if those people in Hollywood and on Madison Avenue think that just because somebody's got gray hair they don't think about the finer things in life, those people need to get off the truck and get on the street. I mean, this over-the-hill generation has put more stuff in your garage, more stuff on the highway, more stuff on your computer than anybody else around. And then the younger generations come along and tell us that we don't know how to live. And that's wrong. We're still living. I'm still nineteen in my brain. I'm just a little more experienced, a little more educated, and a little bit slower. There's just a lack of understanding that people are still alive after thirty. I mean, too many people are looking at the television and seeing all the sexy models. I love to look at them, too, just as much as any other man. But that's not reality. I mean, the person who's in the body may not have the personality to go with it. You fall in love with someone because of who they are on the inside. And if you're just looking at them for what's on the outside, you're setting yourself up for a fall. Luckily, my wife is one of the most beautiful women I have ever met—inside *and* out."

—BURNIE

BEFORE THE DIET

"We have issues with the kids all the time. We aren't connecting and our bond is chipping away. We have no time. It seems like we're mad at each other more of the time than we ever spend holding hands or cuddling."

—CHRISTINE

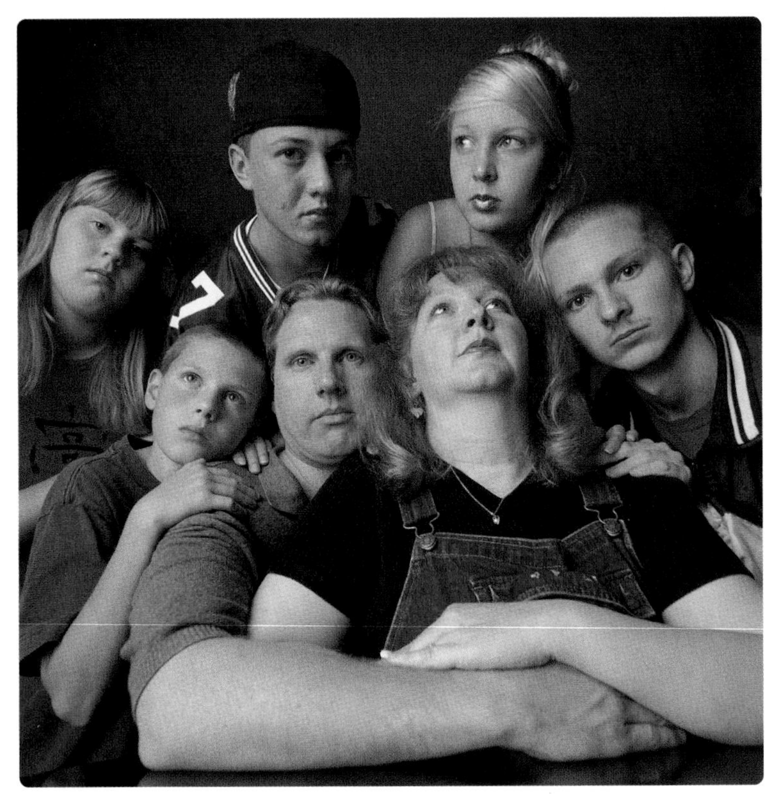

From Sad Eyes to Bright Eyes

CHRISTINE & KEVIN

	**SHE:** 30s, office coordinator
	**HE:** 30s, computer consultant
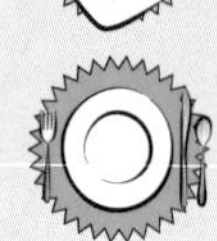	**STATUS:** together 5 years, married 4 years; she has 3 kids from previous marriage, he has 3 kids from a previous marriage

When I talk to people about going on the diet, one of their first reactions is "Well, we have kids. I couldn't possibly find the time." That's when I tell them the story about Kevin and Christine.

Their blended family is made up of his three kids and her three kids—all teenagers. They like

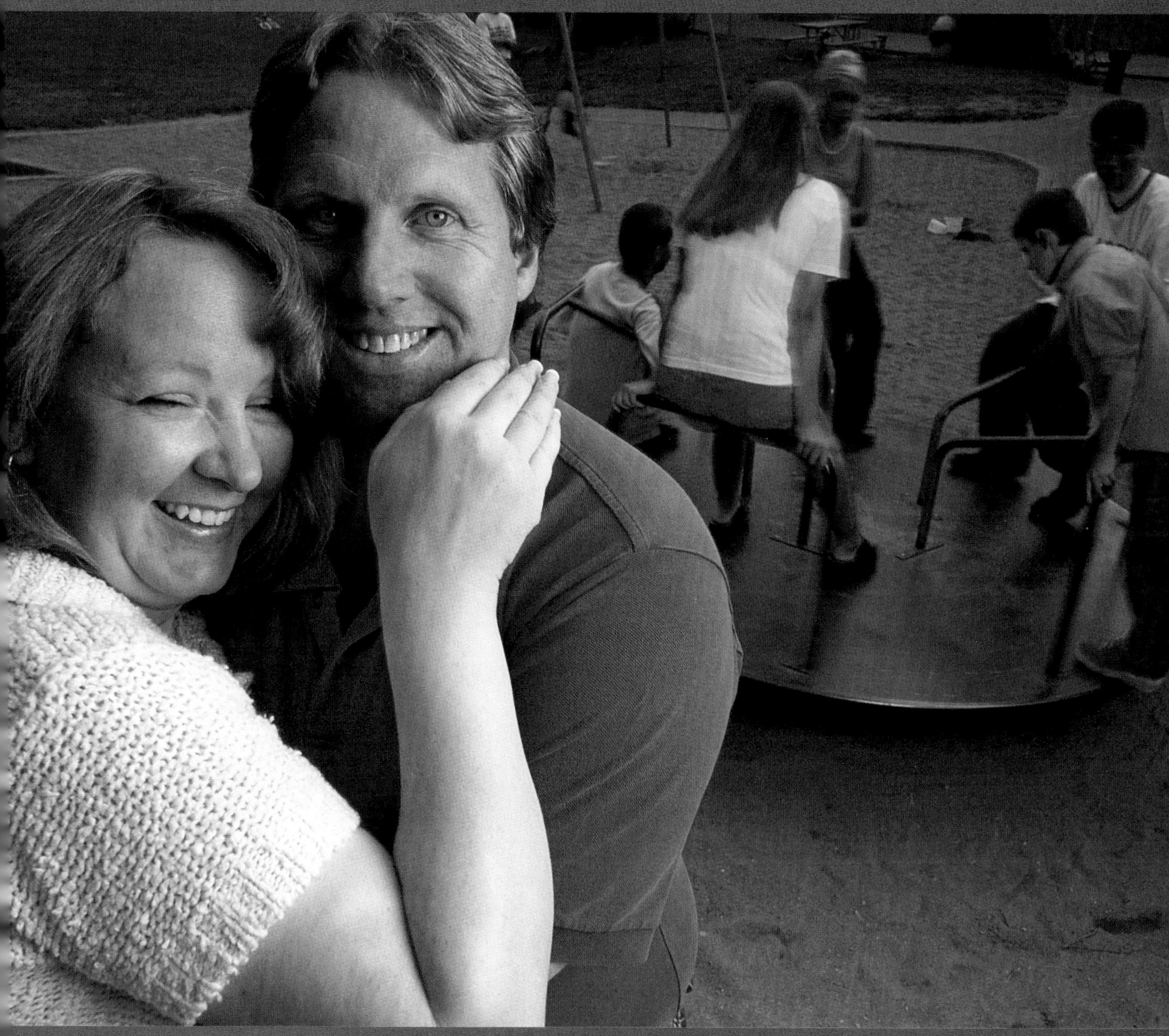

28 DAYS LATER

"The kids have been just as wild as they've ever been, but we still made time for each other. We started talking and communicating. And we were being sensitive, touching and listening to one another. We saw rewards in our family, our relationship, our bond. We saw ***everything*** *change."*—KEVIN

to call themselves "The Crazy Bunch." Ten months before the diet, they were living in separate homes but had moved back in together. Then just two days before the diet Christine and Kevin were again talking about divorce. They felt they were at the end of the road.

Both Kevin and Christine agree that part of the reason for all the tension were the conflicts brought on by the blendedness of their family. The children all vied for the attention of their parents. Yet Kevin and Christine both knew the real changes had to come from within themselves. And to a large degree this internal change had to happen within Kevin. As he admits, "It was mainly because I wasn't hearing what Christine needed. I wasn't loving her the way that a husband should."

As an independent computer consultant, Kevin feels a lot of pressure to keep his business up and running. "I am quite dedicated to my work," he explains, "and sometimes I don't think about what Christine really needs. That she needs my loving her and supporting her and being there for her with the kids. She tends to take up most of the responsibility for them."

Though they've always had a strong sexual bond, they began the diet because their connection had weakened and they wanted to make more time for each other. "We used to be a lot more playful. We used to tease each other and make each other hot, so that by the time we'd get in bed, it'd all be over. But it's been really tough to do that with all the stress," explains Kevin. Christine says, "We aren't connecting and our bond was chipping away. We have no time. It seems like we're mad at each other more of the time than we ever spend holding hands or cuddling."

It was up to Kevin to make the first move and break the ice. "I was taking Christine for granted and the diet became the focal point for us to reconnect and for me to begin to see her as a woman and as my lover and partner again. I definitely started to appreciate and value what Christine brings to my life and because of that realization our love has

"Before I started this diet, I had a very low sex drive. But now I'm much more excited because of the bond and the intimacy. I didn't feel it was there before. If I'm not emotionally connected, then I don't want to make love. But now I'm really in the mood."—CHRISTINE

amplified," says Kevin. "The lovemaking just catalyzed everything. The real words for what we've accomplished in the last four weeks are reconnection, appreciation, and tenderness. Those three words are the key to my experience on the Great American Sex Diet."

And what did he do after such an incredible epiphany? Kevin wanted to show Christine just how much he appreciated her, so he "went out and got her a bouquet of flowers and a card. The card says, 'It's easy to love you for what you are because what you are is wonderful, Bright Eyes'—because that's what I call her." But Kevin didn't stop there. After reading over the Secret Spice Menu, he became inspired and wrote all sorts of anticipation teasers on the greeting card, which he called "Coming Attractions." Check out some of what Kevin wrote to Christine:

- ♥ Back rub and special attention.
- ♥ Set up the computer: you've got M-A-L-E.
- ♥ I'll clean the bedroom and change the sheets.
- ♥ Hide and seek, ready or not, here you come!
- ♥ Wet kitty—I'll leave that one to your imagination.
- ♥ Blind man's buff.
- ♥ Dinner and dancing with dessert at home.
- ♥ Shopping spree!! My pleasure, your treat.
- ♥ Hot stuff! This will warm more than your heart.
- ♥ Surprises! Surprises! And more surprises!

"They're all over the card," Kevin explains. "And then I gave her the card and the bouquet of flowers. It was on a day when she was really tired from working hard all week. And when Christine opened the card, her eyes just lit up! For the next twenty-eight days I did everything on the card and more."

Besides being swept off her feet by this change in Kevin, Christine also noticed "a stronger bond between us." She explains, "And it's everywhere. We try not to make it really obvious in front of the kids, because they're teenagers. But we do know that it's healthy and okay for two adults in a committed relationship to be sexual." And the kids definitely notice a difference. Christine says that the kids were always aware when there was stress between her and Kevin. "They'd ask questions like 'Are you mad at Daddy?' That kind of thing." During and after the diet, the questions became more like Who loves each other more? "It's really a kind of shock," admits Christine. "But now the outside pressures don't have as much power because our bond is stronger."

Kevin sums up the impact of the diet this way: "I feel so much better about myself and our relationship because of the love that we are giving to each other. We brought back the romance and tenderness that had been missing. And I think if other couples would use the diet as a catalyst, it can't help but transform their relationships, too."

BEFORE THE DIET

"We have a little one on the way, so I'm trying to get close to Julie and the baby. I'm really listening and trying to see what she's going through."

—Jay

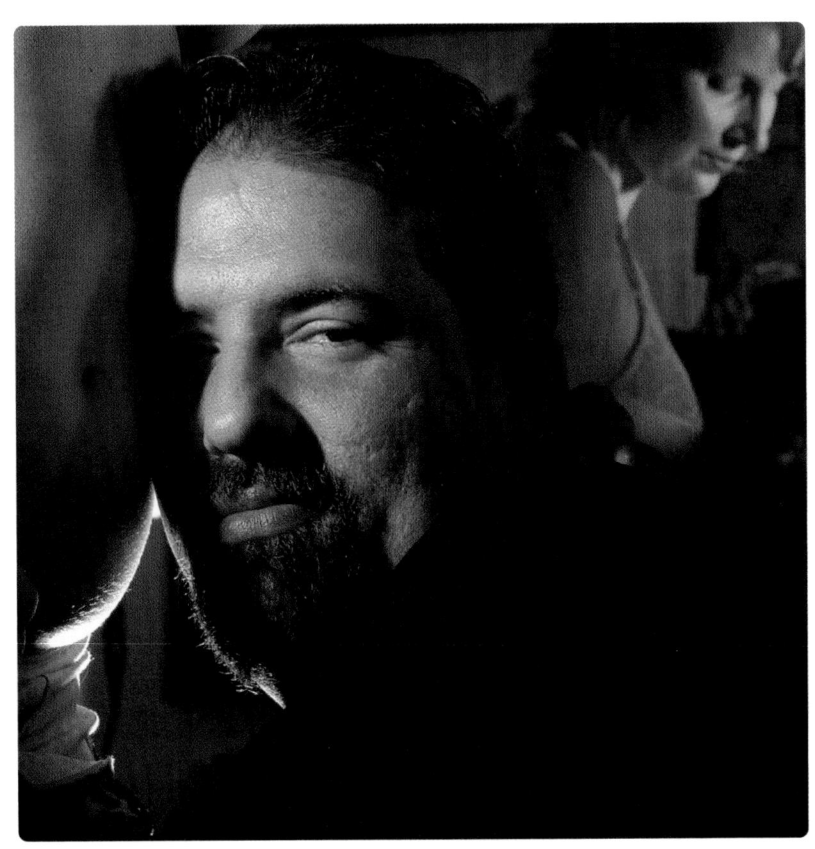

A Blessing in Disguise

Julie & Jay

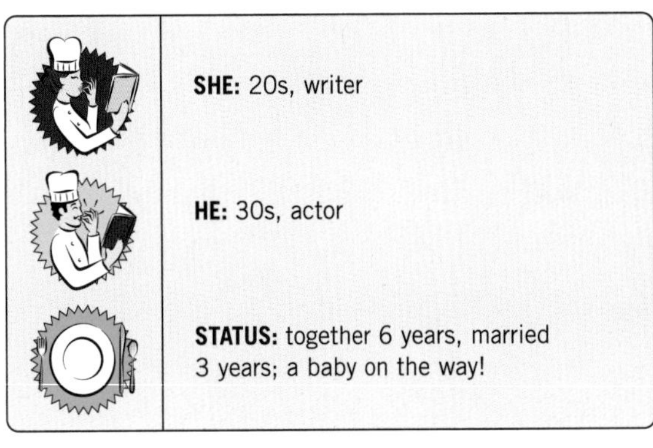

SHE: 20s, writer

HE: 30s, actor

STATUS: together 6 years, married 3 years; a baby on the way!

Check out Julie and Jay's after picture. Would you believe the girl in the pink fur cowboy hat holding a sex toy is five months pregnant? While some women totally lose their sex drive during pregnancy, Julie's went into overdrive on the diet! *Vrrroom, vrrroom!*

But in most ways Julie and Jay had always had a terrific sex life. Julie says of Jay that "he makes me feel like I am a total princess, and the best thing that's ever happened to him."

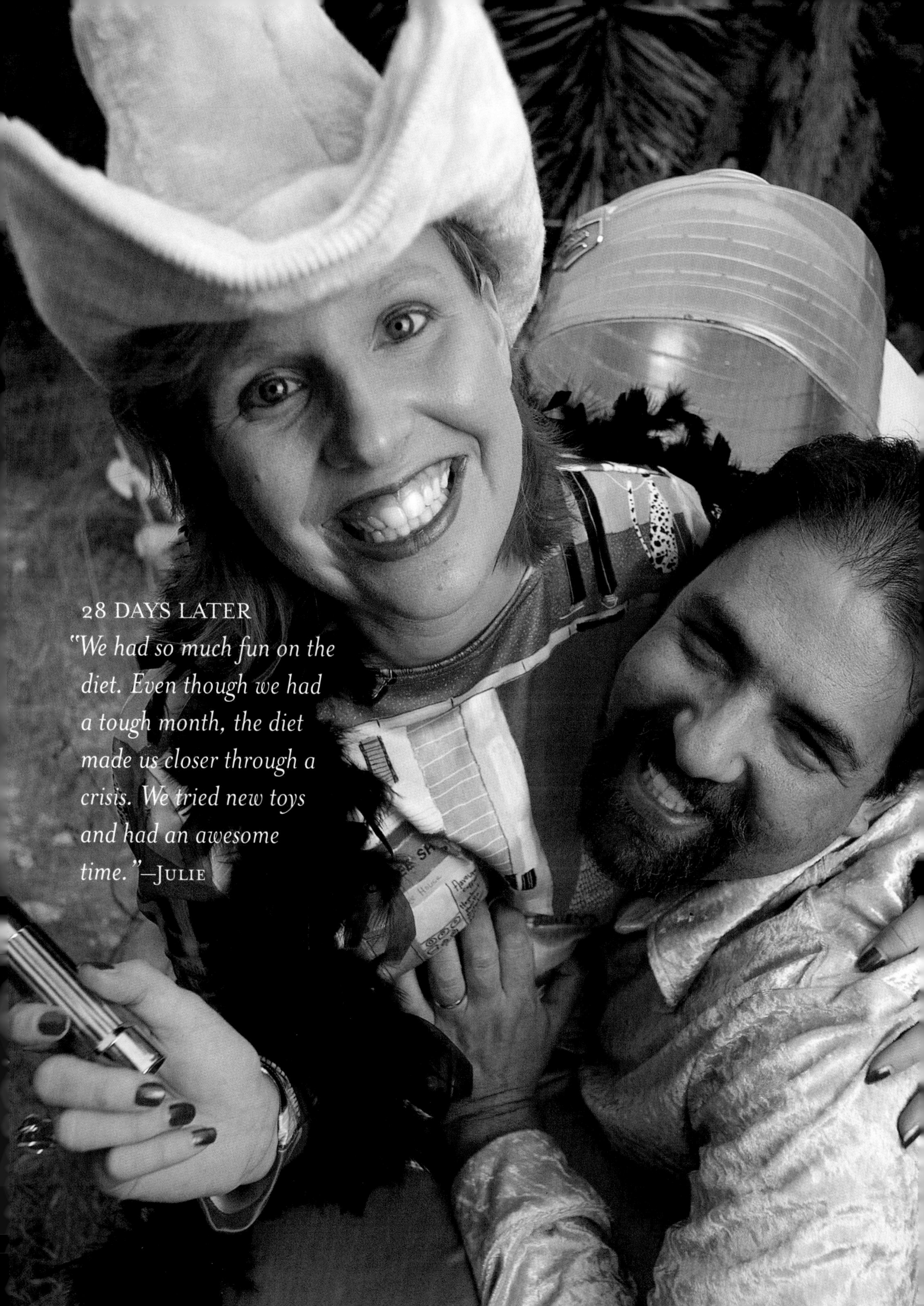

28 DAYS LATER

"We had so much fun on the diet. Even though we had a tough month, the diet made us closer through a crisis. We tried new toys and had an awesome time."—JULIE

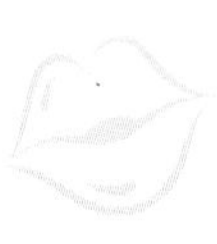

And Jay feels the same way: "Nobody has ever made me feel as special as Julie makes me feel. I've certainly learned to like myself a whole lot more since we got together." But they wanted to try the diet to see if it could get even better. And I say, why not turn great into greater!

Unlike some women who lose their self-confidence when they are pregnant and begin to question their attractiveness, Julie saw only the positive. "I don't have a perfect body but I've always had a pretty good body image," she explains. "And being pregnant hasn't changed that. I mean, I'm carrying Jay's child. What could be more beautiful than that?"

And both Julie and Jay believe sex should be fun. "We always try to play a little," Julie says. "I bought a Girl Scout uniform at a thrift store and now I use it as a great sex prop. A little role-playing is always fun for us."

But Julie and Jay experienced a derailment two weeks into the diet. One day Julie had severe cramping and went to the doctor. She was told by her Ob/Gyn that because of her short cervix, she was at risk for going into premature labor. She was ordered to take it easy and refrain from sexual intercourse for two weeks.

Since they wanted to obey the doctor's orders, they began to explore each other sexually in ways they hadn't since their early dating days. "When Julie and I first started to go together, we didn't have sex for about five months and we were very creative without having intercourse," Jay explains. "It was good to see that we haven't lost that." Remember what it felt like to try and have sex without having intercourse?

There was a teasing element about kissing, touching, licking—doing everything but intercourse. In fact, Julie gave Jay the best oral sex of his life when she tried the Sensory Overload spice. He says it was one of the top three sexual experiences of his life—and he can't even remember the other two! "I felt like the king of the world; nothing could hurt me at that moment," Jay recalls. "So many things were going through my mind while I was being serviced, so to speak. You know, it was like I'm the luckiest guy in the world. Everybody should feel as I feel right now and the world would be a better place."

And Jay took Julie to a *much* better place when he tried the Heat Is On spice on her. "It was such a little spice, but it totally got the biggest reaction from me," she says. "It's something a little different, and one I'd love to do again and again!"

Remarkably, despite all the stress and restrictions, Julie and Jay had found their own slice of paradise. As Julie says, "Even though I'm pregnant, it still got pretty crazy."

Getting a bit more serious, Jay remarks how the diet "gives you a chance to be in sync with

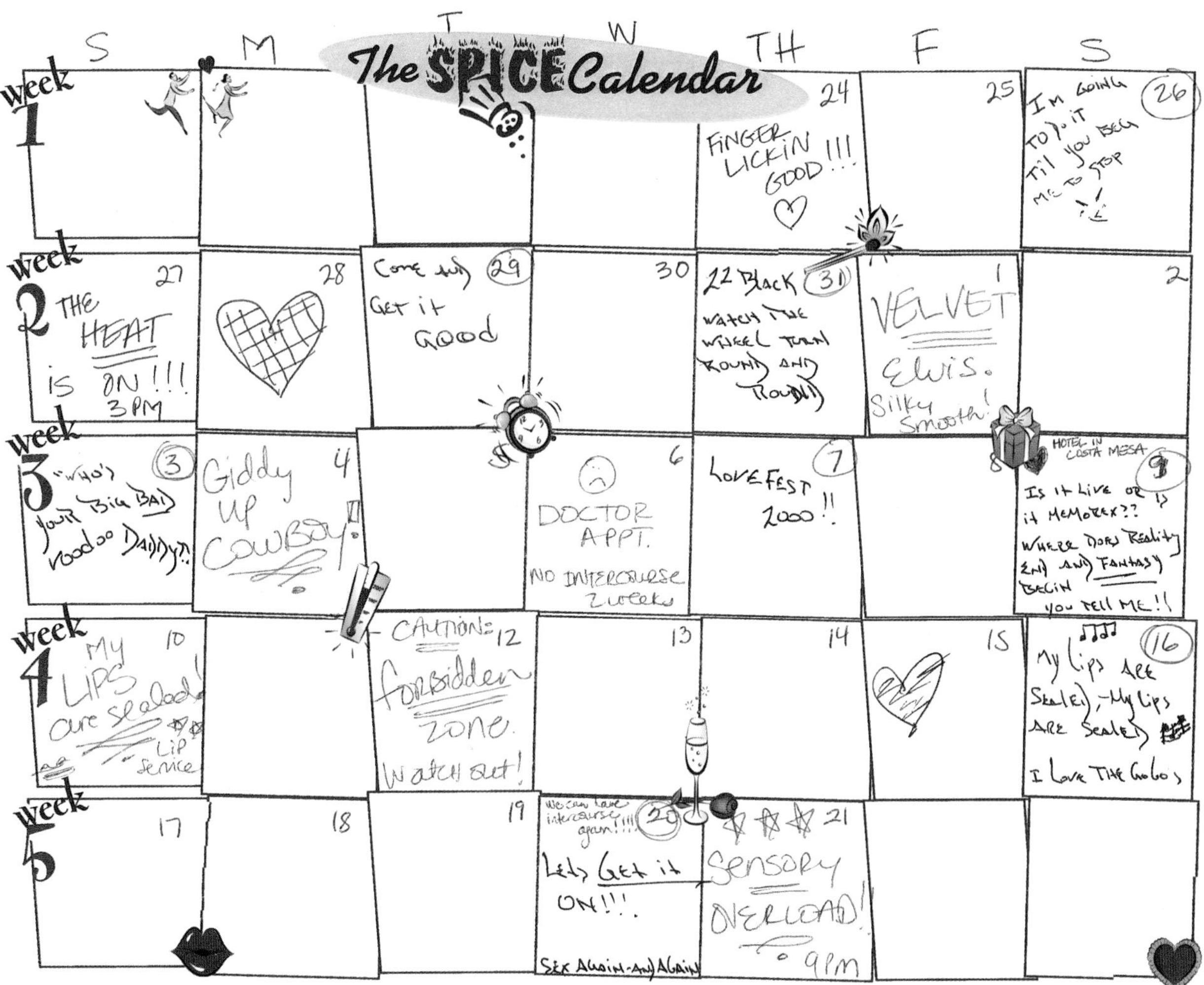

"Julie did a spice on me called Sensory Overload. When she was finished, I said, 'That was one of the top three sexual experiences of my life. And I can't remember the other two!'"—Jay

your partner in a way that creates a huge bond. Let's call it the glue." Julie agrees and says, "It's important for couples to always make the effort. We had two very tense weeks and thank God the doctor said that everything is going to be okay. But having to be creative sexually really brought us a lot closer together through a crisis."

I think that Julie and Jay's story shows how certain circumstances can help us look at sex from a different point of view. If they hadn't needed to stay away from intercourse, would they have discovered all those other avenues of pleasure? When you take time to be intimate with each other—whether it's giving him oral sex or pleasing her with a toy—you're still connecting sexually and sometimes this leads to an even stronger, more satisfying bond.

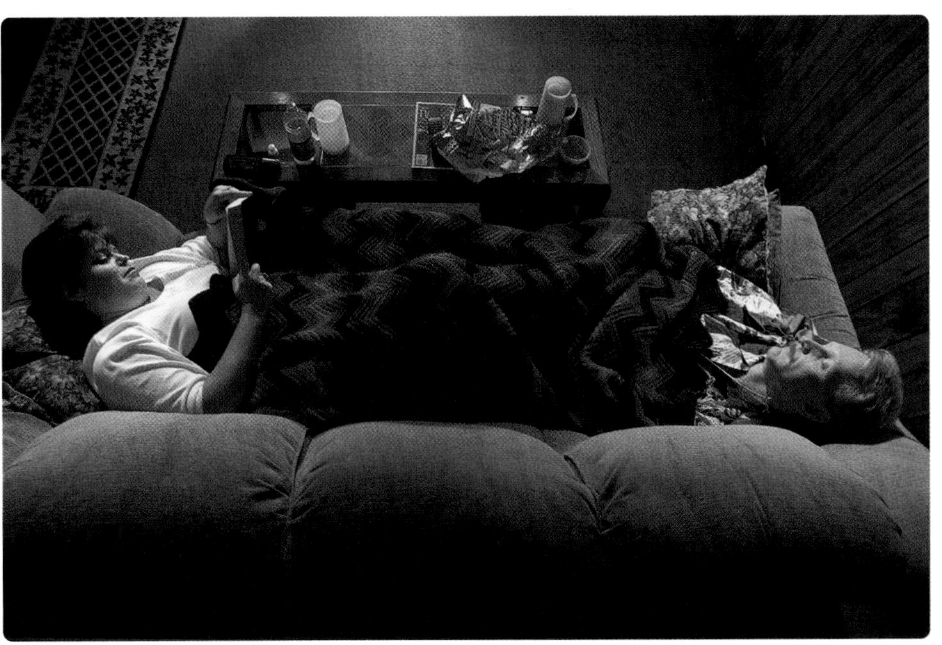

BEFORE THE DIET

"I'd like to get that spark and spontaneity back into our relationship. Right now, we're letting life get between us and we're always at separate ends of the couch."—ELIZABETH

Romancing the Toes

JEFF & ELIZABETH

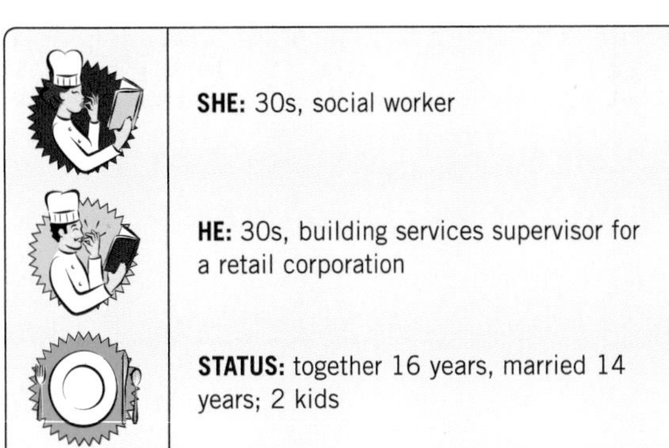

From the moment I met them, I could tell that Jeff and Elizabeth are a very caring, nurturing couple who are used to working on their relationship in a serious, committed way. They even belong to a couples group that meets every Saturday night to discuss and process issues that affect their respective relationships.

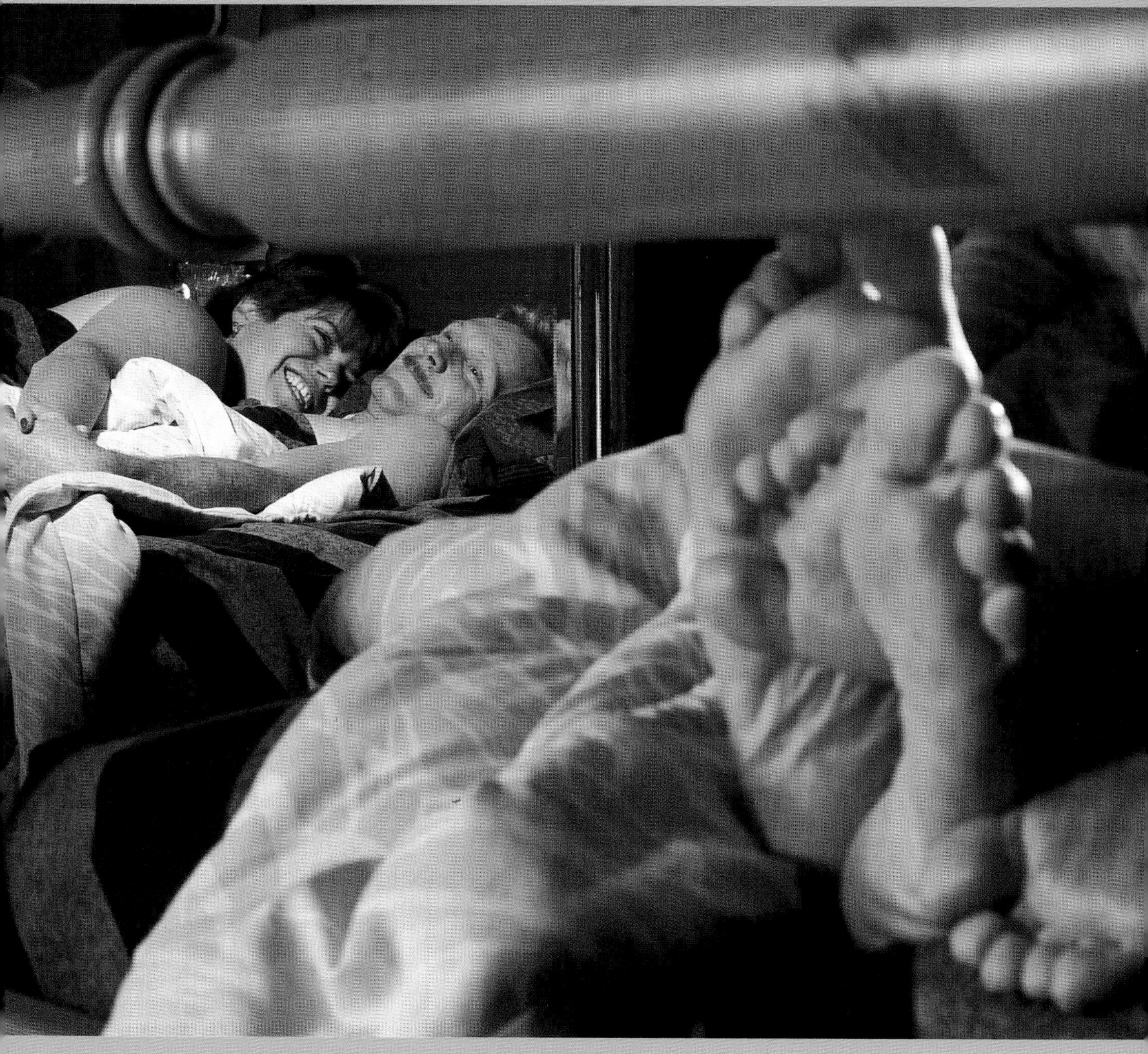

28 DAYS LATER

"We've always said we know we're connected as long as our toes are touching at night in bed. And now we're touching toes again. Our connection is just so much stronger."—Elizabeth

But even though they had all this knowledge and insight into their relationship, they still couldn't find a way to address their flagging sex life. They needed a plan of action, and that's where the Great American Sex Diet came in.

Like many couples, they are busy with work and kids. In addition, a few months before the diet, Elizabeth had hurt her back and as a result sex had become painful. "We would compensate with a lot of cuddling, but I felt guilty," said Elizabeth. But the lack of sex was definitely affecting their relationship. When they are having sex a lot, "there is more of a gentleness in our tone, our word choices," Elizabeth says. "When we sit at dinner, we hold hands under the table, which we are not doing right now."

"One of the greatest things about the diet was that Elizabeth surprised me as much as I surprised her. There was a lot of anticipation and excitement. She was leaving me sexy voice mails at work and doing things she'd never done before."

—Jeff

In addition to trying to balance the responsibilities of kids with their relationship, Elizabeth also struggled with low desire that was clearly linked to her feeling unattractive and undesirable. Like so many women, Elizabeth doesn't think she is as attractive now as when she and Jeff got married. "I was thin and really athletic when we met. Then after having the kids, I gained weight and I personally don't feel that I'm as beautiful. Jeff doesn't have an issue with that; it's my hang-up." So even though Jeff thinks, believes, and tells her she is beautiful, Elizabeth holds back. Their sexual tension also affects their children. "When Jeff and I are clicking and intimate and sharing, the atmosphere in the house is different, too. The kids even notice when we don't kiss or ask each other how our day was."

Elizabeth turned to the diet to put spontaneity and energy back into their sex life and relationship. Jeff was more practical. He simply wanted her to initiate more. "For the past few years, it seems like I'm the one doing all the foreplay and all the seducing. If I don't, then it won't happen at all."

The SPICE Calendar

"When I would pass by and see something new written on the calendar, it would just make me tingly. And if he wrote a specific time down and I had to wait, I was like a little kid. My curiosity was overflowing."—Elizabeth

But, boy, did that ever change on the diet! "I did a spice for Jeff where I had to wear lingerie, and I'd never worn garters and stockings before," Elizabeth explains. "I was telling the lady at Victoria's Secret I have less of a problem walking around naked then I do walking around in lingerie. It took me an hour and a half to pick out the perfect outfit! But I have to tell you, I got so excited putting this on. I kept spraying myself with body splash to calm down. When I finally got dressed, I looked at myself in the mirror and I said, you know, I spend so much time being critical of myself for being overweight. It doesn't bother Jeff, so why does it bother me? And he was so excited when he saw me, I realized I need to let go of that stuff."

And did she ever succeed in turning Jeff on. "She was hot looking," he says. "She kind of peeked around the corner and put a leg out so I could see the stocking." Elizabeth remembers, "His eyes nearly popped out of his head. And then I stepped around the corner so he could get the sense of the whole outfit." Jeff continues, "One of the greatest things about the diet was that she surprised me as much as I surprised her." One night, after Elizabeth had had a particularly grueling day of work, Jeff knocked on the front door and, dressed in a robe, handed her a towel and said, "I'm Sven, your out-call masseur, are you ready?" Elizabeth remembers, "I'm just thinking, ohmigosh, if any of our neighbors saw him! And I started giggling. It was the first time I had laughed all day, so I let him in the door and he led me into the bedroom. There were lit candles everywhere!

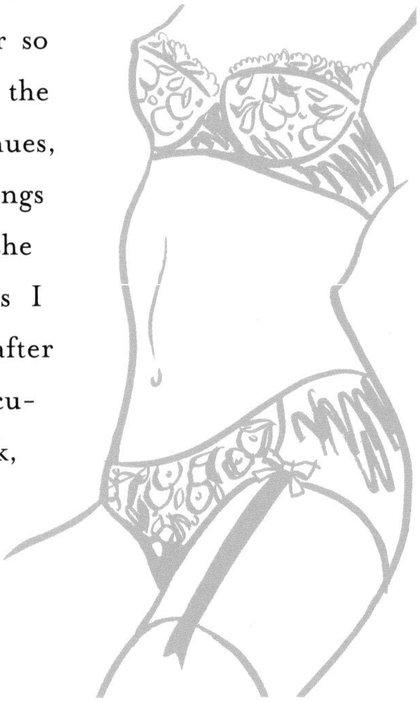

"He told me to get comfortable, then he started rubbing my feet. A couple of minutes after, he handed me a poem. He knew I'd had a really bad day at work. It was so romantic and so touching. I started crying. It just made my whole bad day wash away and made me really get into the night!"

Elizabeth and Jeff reconnected on the diet. I'm always surprised at the impact doing something as simple as wearing sexy lingerie can have on a relationship and a woman's self-confidence. After talking to Elizabeth, I was inspired to wear garters for my boyfriend Jeff for the first time in ages! He was blown away, too. Afterward, he even called me from the freeway to say what a lucky man he was. *Wow*. Thanks, Elizabeth, for the inspiration!

"Our kids definitely noticed a difference during the diet. I think it's very important for kids, especially boys, to see their parents showing love and affection and all the little romantic things that we do." —Elizabeth

Can We Get Back on Track?
Or are we all Washed up?
I'll Take Tue/Wed.
Can You do Thurs/Fri?
Let's make like Bunnies
And Hop, Hop, Hop. Jump, Ju
Funny, Funny, Funny (Fa
Love Ya Lots

Elizabeth:
My Sweet Love
Caress your Body
Sooth thy Soul
Your Tensions Arrested
This nights Goal!
While rubbing your Feet
I'll tickle your Toes!
Feelings are High
No more Lows
My touch is the Cure
For all your Woes
Nothing so Pure
As my Love for you
And just for Tonight
You'll know for Sure
Our Loves all Right
For me and You Too!
Jeff
xoxoxo

"The poem Jeff surprised me with during the diet made me feel all of the things that you want to feel in your relationship—love, support, and nurturing. And it reminded me again that the most important thing was our togetherness."—Elizabeth

BEFORE THE DIET

"Melanie and I are best friends. We communicate, we talk, we laugh. We're open to each other. There isn't a wall between us. We've made the commitment to grow together and that's why we want to do the diet."

—Mo

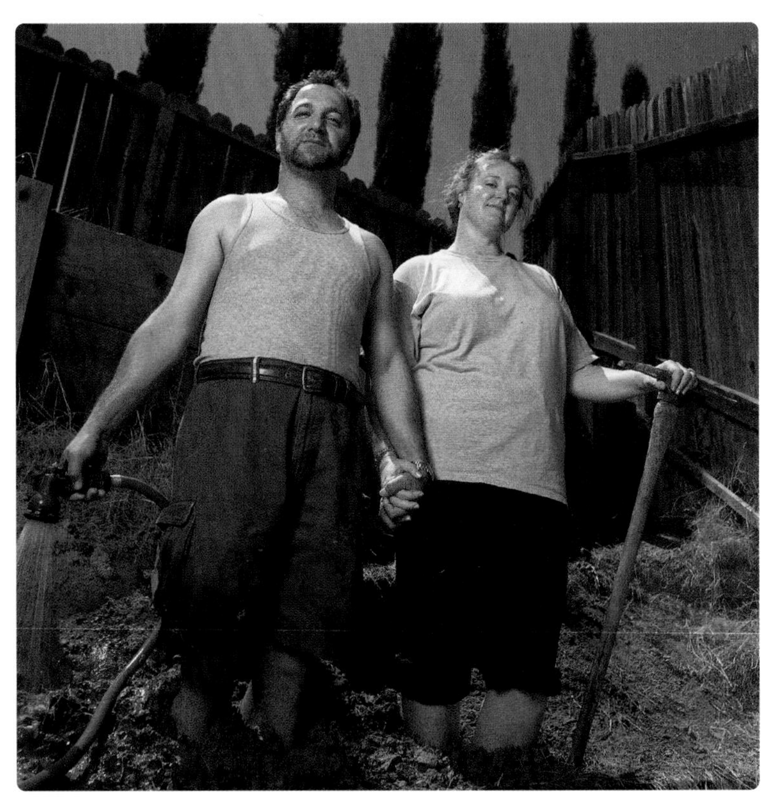

And the Walls Come Tumbling Down

MELANIE & MO

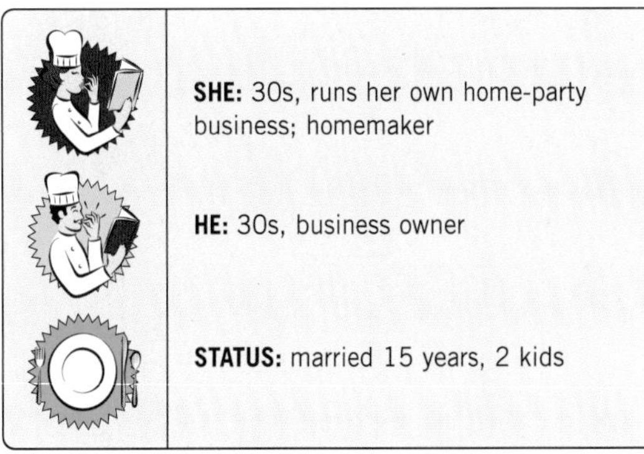

SHE: 30s, runs her own home-party business; homemaker

HE: 30s, business owner

STATUS: married 15 years, 2 kids

You may remember Melanie and Mo if you read Melanie's astounding intimate diary that recorded the couple's experience on the diet. This real-life account captures not only the emotional intensity of the diet but also its sexual power.

Melanie and Mo dated only five months

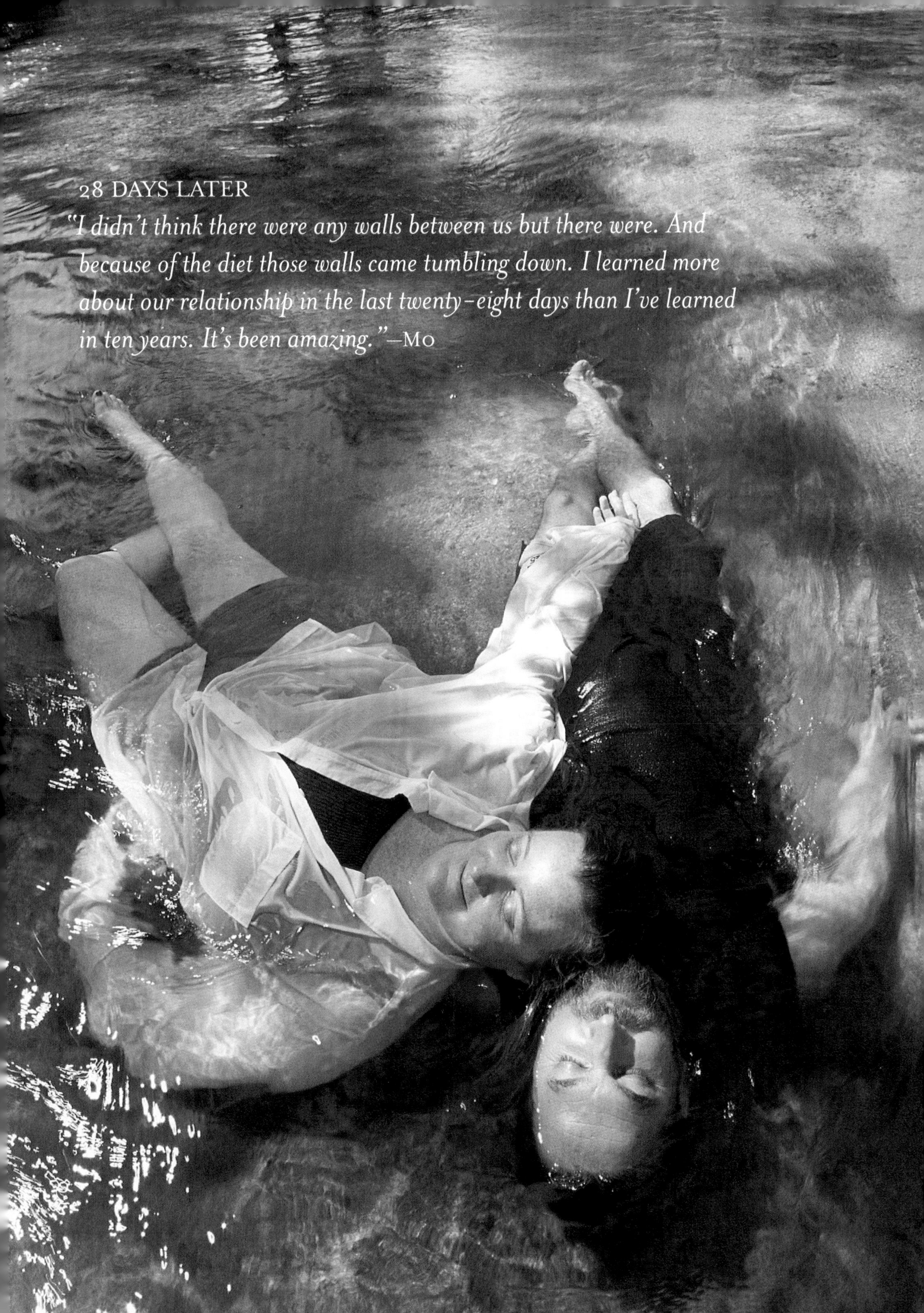

28 DAYS LATER

"I didn't think there were any walls between us but there were. And because of the diet those walls came tumbling down. I learned more about our relationship in the last twenty-eight days than I've learned in ten years. It's been amazing." —Mo

before deciding to get married. As Melanie admits, "I totally took a chance and it worked out." She went into the marriage thinking "this is a guy I could have an adventure with." At the time, Mo, who had recently moved from Iran, barely spoke English. "I like to think of him as Aladdin—like a prince on the inside, but like a street rat on the outside," she says. "At first my parents wanted to disown me for marrying him, but now, after fifteen years, they would trade me for him in a minute!"

Melanie and Mo laugh a lot together and it's obvious to an observer how actively committed they are to growing their relationship. They are very conscious about this—hence their photo in their garden, which shows how they like to grow—both as a couple and as individuals. "Mo taught me that I'm beautiful and I should believe I'm beautiful," Melanie says. "I was always kind of afraid of things and thought maybe I wasn't good enough. I have a BA in English from UC Berkeley and I'm a member of MENSA [the high IQ society]. What's ironic is that you can be educated, you can be smart, you can be everything, but if you don't have that confidence, you can't get very far. Mo gave me that confidence."

From Mo's point of view, he feels they are best friends: "There isn't a wall between us," he says. When Mo told me how close they are, I wondered what such a couple would learn on the diet. But was I in for a surprise. I never knew their revelation would be so big!

During much of the diet, they had a lot of extended family around. Melanie's stepfather had just passed away, so her mother was staying with them, and Mo's parents were also visiting for a while. As you might imagine, there was a lot of grief in the house, and as a result a lot of tension with all the intense feelings. "You can't even think about sex with your parents in the house!" Mo says jokingly. But this didn't stop them from sticking to the diet.

Again, it was their commitment to growing and learning that shined through. They were determined to break the monotony of their sexual relationship. Melanie says, "It's like this bed is looking very boring and unspontaneous after all these years." *Not anymore!*

One night, Mo surprised Melanie with the Foreplay Gourmet spice. "I was in the

"Knowing ahead of time how many days a week we're going to have sex has taken the edge off completely. It helps in two ways: helps me get psyched for sex and helps him to relax because he knows it's gonna happen. I thought that was awesome."—Melanie

The SPICE Calendar

week 1	Wed 8/23 (Mo) (impromptu) TRANSITION NOW!	Th 8/24	Fri. 8/25 (Mel) "Yee-Haw" at 9pm!	Sat. 8/26	Sun 8/27 (Mo) "Cleaning the Fan" 7:45pm	Mon. 8/28 (Mel) "ICY-HOT FOOT FREAK MASSAGE PLUS" 8:30pm	Tues. 8/29 DO "ICY-HOT" TONIGHT. (SWITCHED TO THE COOKIE JAR)
week 2	Wed 8/30 (MO) "The Gentleman" 9pm MOVED TO THURS.	Th 8/31 DID NOT HAPPEN: BAD NEWS CALL	Fri 9/01 (Mo) Did not happen "Going Fishing" 5:30pm	Sat 9/02	Sun 9/03 (Mel) ~~Attack~~ at 9PM, Wear an old t-shirt, shorts + NO undies! Did not happen	Mon 9/04 (Mel) Kissing 101 9pm Did not happen	Tues 9/05
week 3	Wed 9/6	Thurs 9/7 (Mel) Sweet, Lazy Love: ready or not. Time: whenever we can	Fri. 9/8 (Mel) Liquid Ecstasy 8:30pm	Sat 9/9	Sun. 9/10 (Mo) surprised me with bath	Mon. 9/11	Tues 9/12 (Mo) Birthday Balloons
week 4	Wed. 9/13 (Mel) DO NOT EAT dessert... unless you want it in your LAP! tonight	Thurs. 9/14 (Mel) FLASH FRIDAY	Fri 9/15	Sat. 9/16	Sun. 9/17 (Mo) Party Raid!	Mon. 9/18	Tues. 9/19 (Mo) The Iceman Cometh: let's celebrate!
week 5							

"One thing I learned using the calendar was that if you fail to plan, you plan to fail!"—Melanie

bedroom, and Mo walked in with his painting clothes, carrying a ladder," she recalls. "He even had a tool belt on. I asked what he was doing, and he said he was going to clean the ceiling fan before we got started on our spice. And I thought, Ooooookay. He was so cute. After he set up the ladder, he took off his shirt. Then he climbed up a couple steps and undid his belt. He was doing this striptease up the ladder, pretending I wasn't even there. It was the cutest! I kept going from cracking up to being really excited."

After he got to the top of the ladder, Mo dropped his pants . . . and his inhibitions. "His groin area was eye level to me, and he was trying not to let me touch him," Melanie continues. "That really drove me crazy, because that zeroed in

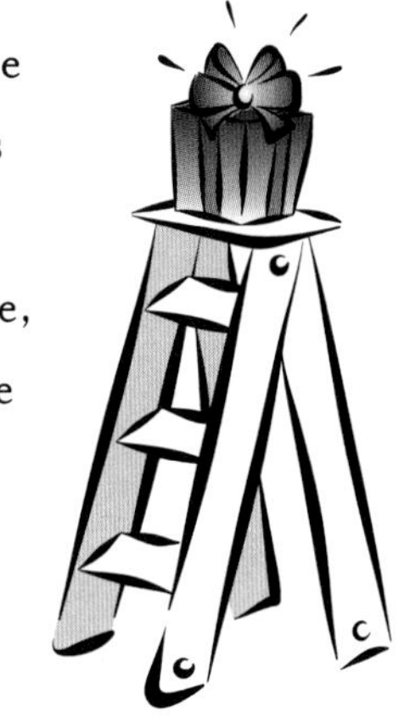

on what I really need—the tease. And after a few more minutes of driving me wild, he finally let me pull him down off the ladder." But that wasn't the end of the sensual surprise. In fact, it was only the beginning. "Things got pretty crazy from there, because out of nowhere he mixed in another spice," Melanie explains. "He really kept me on my toes because I didn't know what to expect next. I was really getting into it."

But even though they added spice and variety, some of their old issues lingered. One of their issues as a couple was Melanie's need to control things, especially Mo. "I'd say the hardest thing about keeping the relationship on track is remembering not to consume him," she says. "I struggle to let him be him, to laugh with him and enjoy him and to help make his dreams come true. It's a struggle to let go and not to try to control him—it doesn't come naturally." Interestingly, this particular issue actually played itself out sexually on the diet and led to one of their biggest breakthroughs.

The breakthrough occurred one Sunday morning. Instead of joining their family downstairs, Melanie made a move on Mo. She recalls, "I was feeling good because I had initiated, but he was just not into it and that sent me into a tizzy. Then we got into a big argument and he told me that he was really angry at me. He said that because he has come to me wanting sex and been rejected so many times in the past, he was bothered by my reaction to his not wanting sex right at that moment."

Melanie continues, "It was then that I finally realized how hurtful I had been being so flippant when I've rejected him. I always used the excuse of my low sex drive. I didn't realize how much pain was inside of him. For him, sexual rejection was like a failure. That's how we came up with a new rule: We just can't reject each other anymore."

But making a new rule doesn't mean the behaviors all go away instantly. As Melanie remembers, "Then we began having very passionate sex on the bathroom floor—our bathroom is an extension of our bedroom and it's carpeted—and he started doing something funky to me and I moved away from him. And I realized that I had done

"I feel I really know her now. I really truly know her. And her enjoyment is really my enjoyment. To see her face happy, it makes my life fulfilled. We had such a good time and it was so wild that you don't want to know. You don't want to go there!"—Mo

it again! So I apologized to Mo and said, 'Let's start over.'"

And they ended up having the most passionate sex ever. Melanie says, "It was just totally enjoying each other, throwing the rules out the window, wanting to completely love and not reject, and I swear to God it was the best sex I can ever remember with him in fifteen years," Melanie says. "It was just wild. I would honestly have to say that the sex that Sunday morning topped anything we'd ever had." Clearly, the emotional intensity and the resolution of that issue surrounding Mo's hurt feelings fueled their passion.

Yet their insight and change didn't end there. Melanie and Mo also came to the realization that, as with any aspect of their relationship, their sexual connection requires work. "You work at so many things, but we hadn't really worked at our sex life," Melanie says. "But now we were. Here we were scheduling sex, reading, and planning. And it was that extra effort that let us grow. That's what made us have our breakthrough."

I was struck deeply by Melanie and Mo because here was a couple that really understood the connection between working on a relationship and seeing it blossom. For any relationship to thrive, you need to accept that there is always more to learn. Even the happiest of couples can make progress and keep growing and growing.

THE WILD HORSE

That time I lived across the oceans
Not knowing what the future held for me
There I was on the other side of the world
Looking for love
Destitute, the ultimate seeming like nothing
Enemies outnumbered my friends
I left, taking nothing but wishes
Only the memories remained

Now here I am
Many many years after
Found the one I love
That time I never thought
Having a dream of her would be allowed
But now I live my dream next to her
It was not easy and it will not always be
To my best friend and my wife
Melanie

As I see her beautiful eyes
Glowing in the darkness of night
And the waves of her hair brush to the wind
And the sweetness of her lips fills the air like magic
And her free spirit
Like a wild horse
In search of my heart

Gently I run my fingers in her hair
Try to reach her lips to my own
Whispering my songs in her ear
Holding her hand so strong
Making sure
Nothing's wrong
Now I can reach to the sky
There is no limit to the high

Wonderful things I watch her do
Makes me happy and her too
There are a million ways to describe
Why I chose her as my bride

Love, Morteza

BEFORE THE DIET

"We're really happy together, but I'd like to have a higher sex drive and for Dwayne to be more fulfilled."

—MELANIE

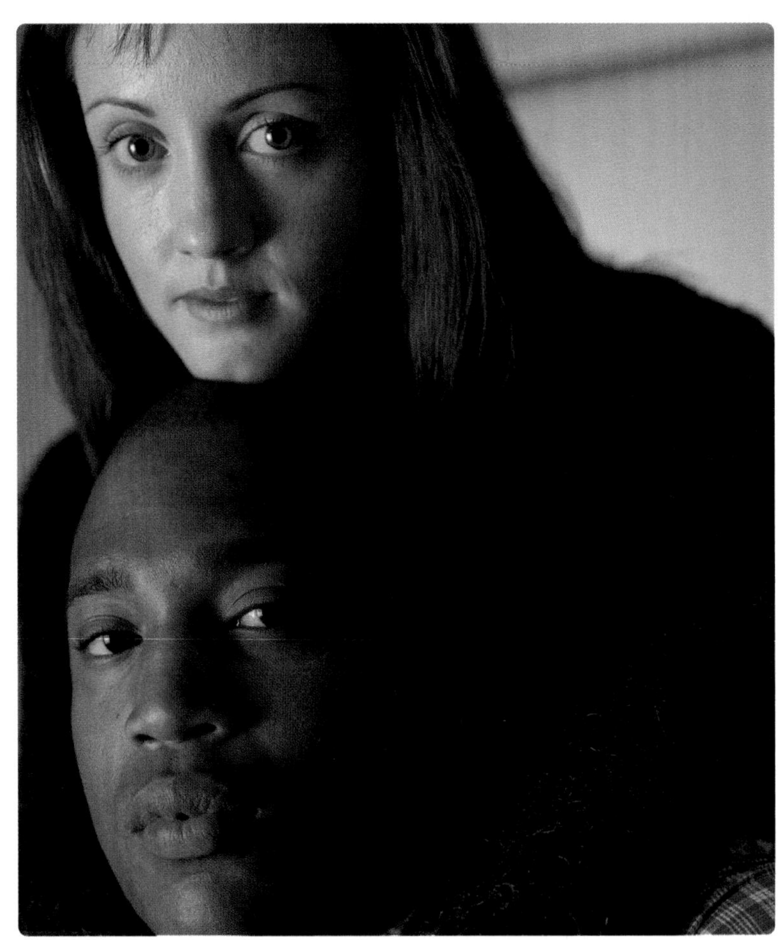

They Just Sizzle

MELANIE & DWAYNE

SHE: 20s, dental assistant

HE: 20s, child-care professional

STATUS: 3 years together, 1 daughter from her previous relationship

I just love the story of how Melanie and Dwayne got together. Melanie recalls, "One day, I visited my daughter's school and I see this really cute, young guy. My daughter's been at the school for at least a year. Well, that afternoon, when she got home, she asked if Dwayne could come over and spend the night. And I said, 'Well, let's start with dinner.'"

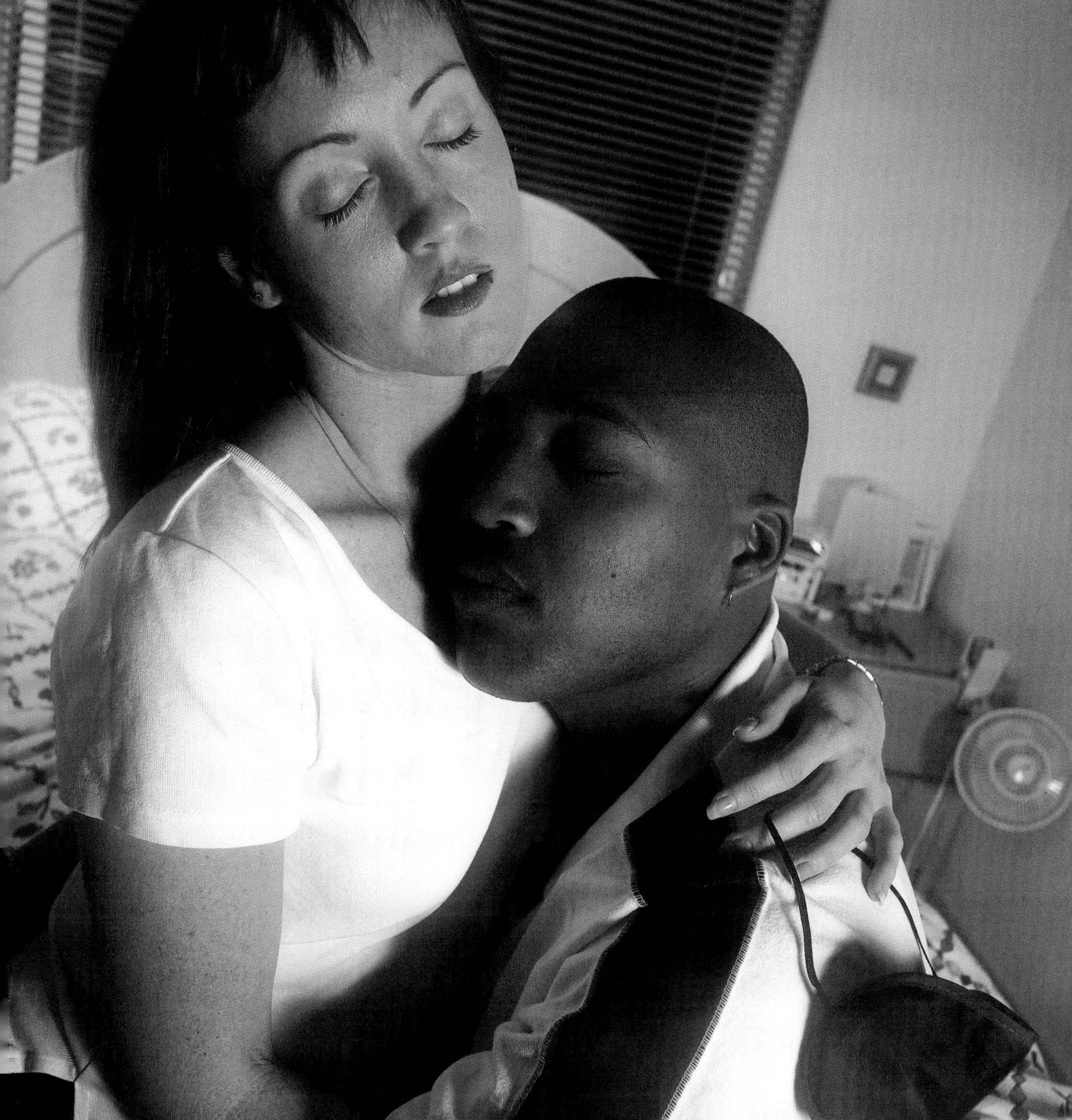

28 DAYS LATER

"Because we made love four times a week on the diet, I'm able to climax easier and my sex drive has gone way up. I feel energetic. I feel closer. I feel fulfilled. Dwayne and I have never felt happier and more connected!"—MELANIE

Melanie's daughter was only two then! Time passed and Melanie got to know Dwayne as she dropped off and picked up her daughter. Then she finally gathered the courage to ask him out. "He's pretty quiet," Melanie explains. "So I had to initiate." It's clear from how she tells the story that the fact that her daughter felt so instantly trusting and comfortable with Dwayne made it easier for *her* to trust in Dwayne, too. "My daughter really enjoyed him being around, which made it a lot easier for me to open up," Melanie says. "I didn't have to worry about her liking him."

Dwayne and Melanie were always an affectionate couple that made time for intimacy. Because they were both sensitive to Melanie's daughter's presence, they would kiss and cuddle if they didn't have the privacy to make love. Yet when I asked them what they wanted to get from the diet, Melanie spoke about wanting to boost their sex life. Dwayne could make love every day, but Melanie often turns him down, which Dwayne takes personally. Dwayne says, "I want her to be happy all the time and when she's not, that makes me feel like I'm doing something wrong." Now here's a sensitive man.

> *"This diet taught me that I had the time for sex when I made the time. It was unreal to me to find out I had that time all along."*
>
> —Melanie

Without a shadow of a doubt, Melanie was able to turn around her low libido. As she says, "One of the things that contributed to me having a low libido is the fact that I'm a mom. But once we made love four times a week, it wasn't as difficult as I thought. I'm able to climax easier and my sex drive has gone way up." Before the diet, Melanie says, "It seemed so much more important to do the laundry and make sure the dishes were done. But now I've learned that having sex is a lot more fun. After all, what do I have to show for those years of cleaning besides a sparkling kitchen and dishwater hands?"

She not only climaxed more easily, but she and Dwayne also were able to come together, something they'd been trying to do for three years. "It was wonderful," says Dwayne. "When we came together for the first time, I felt her explode. She was hugging me and holding me." Learning how to come together also improved Dwayne's performance. "I

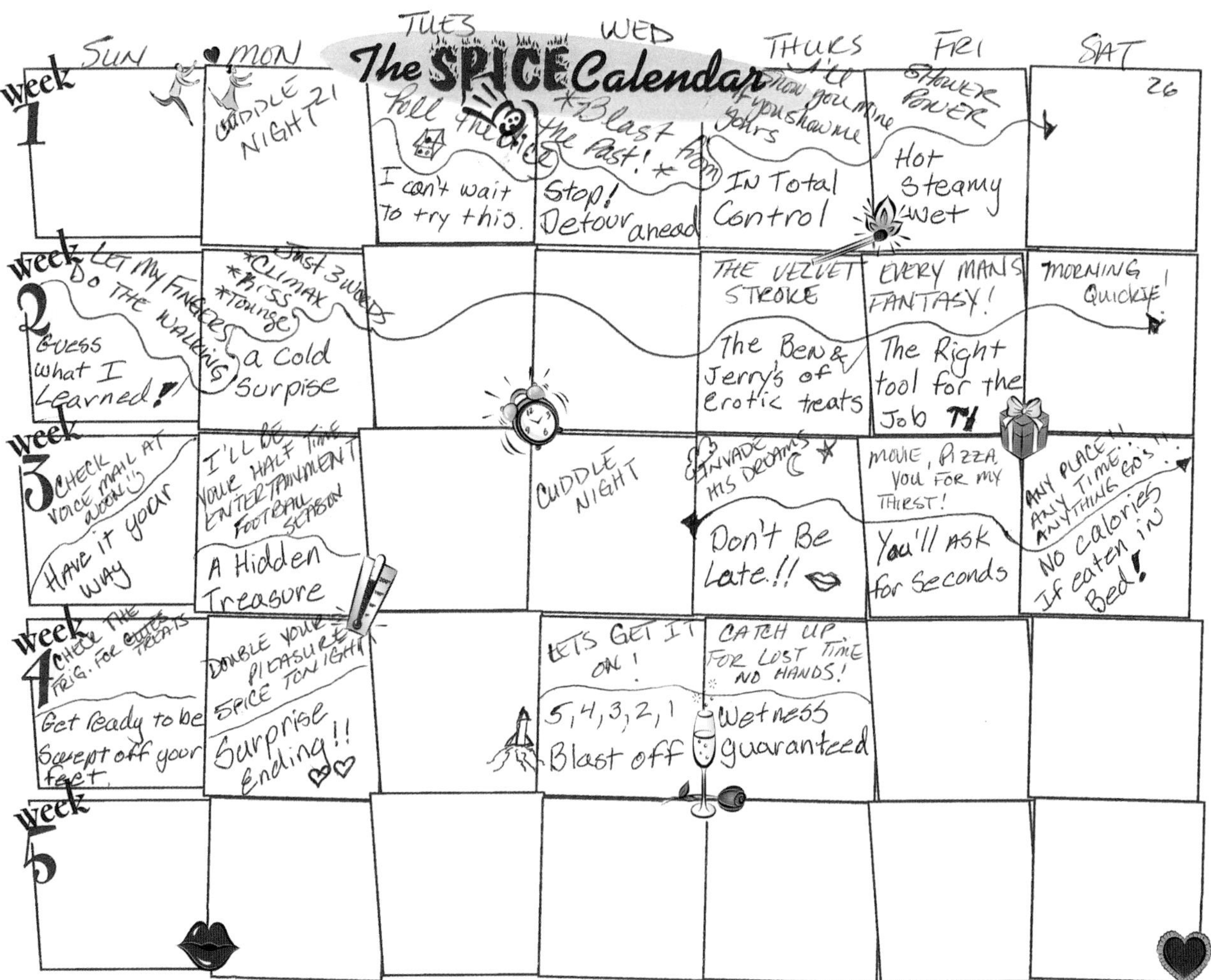

"On the first day of football season, I wrote down 'I'll be your halftime entertainment.' That really got his attention!"—Melanie

always want to last as long as I can," he explains, "and seeing the excitement on her face made me last longer."

Their adventurous spirit fueled them to try out new positions and experiment with toys. While giving Dwayne oral sex, Melanie pleasured him with a pocket-size vibrator in a couple of places, awakening erogenous zones he didn't even know he had.

There's a powerful connection between Dwayne and Melanie and it's quite visible to any observer. They're simply infused with erotic energy. Can't you just feel the heat from their after photo? They just *sizzle*.

BEFORE THE DIET

"We make the time to have cocoa together every evening, but lovemaking has moved down to the bottom of the list. We've gotten kind of mellow. We need something to get us excited again—we've run out of ideas."

—DOREEN

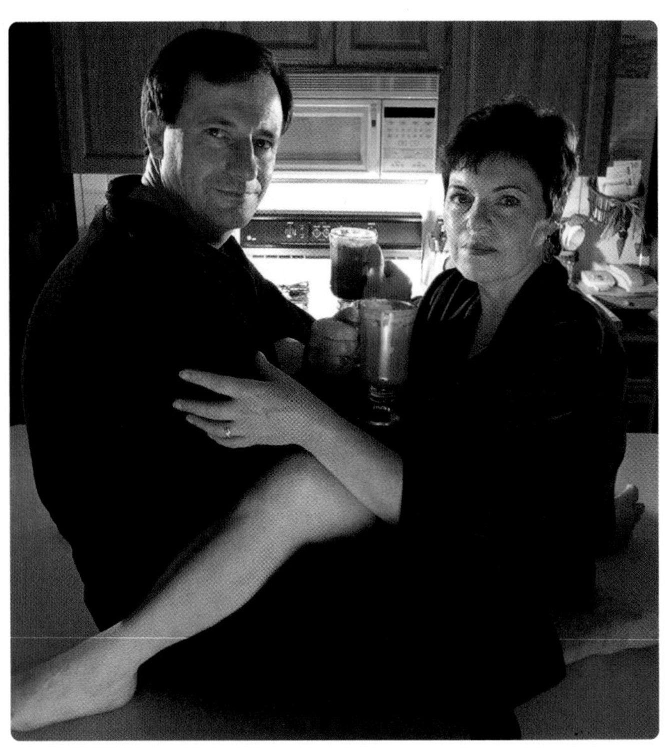

How to Turn a Good Girl Bad

DOREEN & RALPH

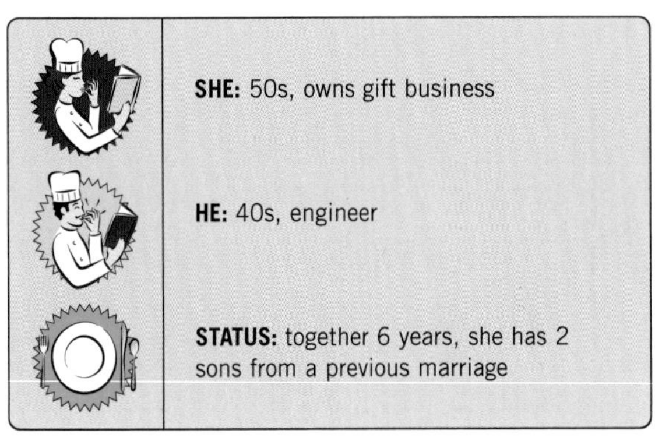

SHE: 50s, owns gift business

HE: 40s, engineer

STATUS: together 6 years, she has 2 sons from a previous marriage

I'd like you to meet Amber Rose, Doreen's sexy alter ego, someone Ralph hadn't seen in more than two years before they started the Great American Sex Diet. "When we first got together, Amber Rose was the alias I used during our fun times," Doreen explains. "She's my adventurous persona, but I haven't let her loose in quite some time."

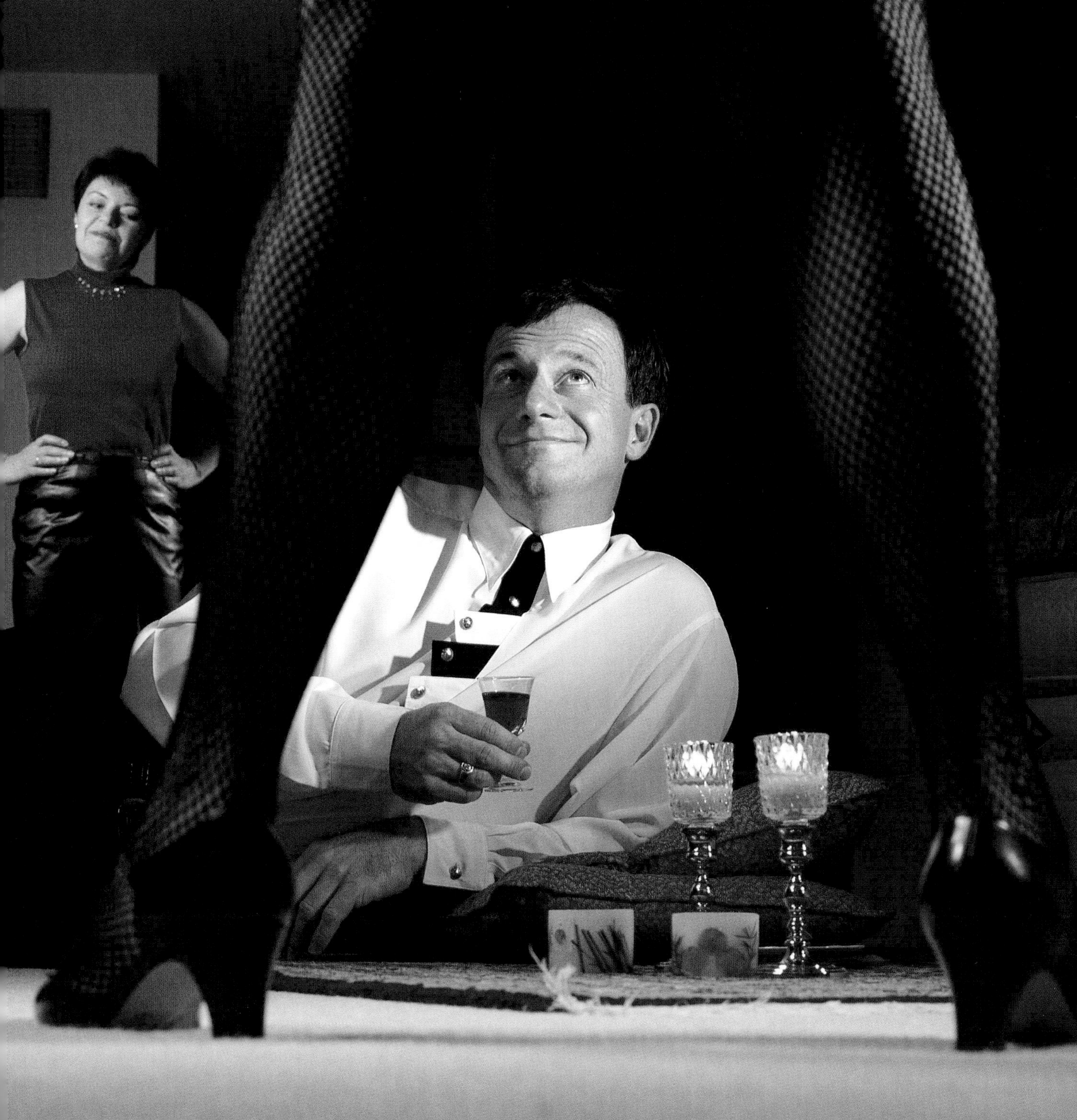

28 DAYS LATER

"When we started dating, I had an alter ego named Amber Rose—a wild, adventurous fantasy girl. And this diet brought Amber Rose out of hiding for the first time in two years." —Doreen

Speaking with this mature, thoughtful couple, I can hear the years of experience as well as their desire to not give in to a sex relationship that is dissatisfying. They want to not only make their sex life work, but make it *sizzle*.

"We always have good intentions about making time for each other," says Doreen, "but by evening we're pooped, so a lot of times our plans fall through."

Ralph says that when they have less sex, he slips back into behavior from his former marriage—specifically, he withdraws. "I think it's very important that both people have an open and willing attitude toward sex," he says. "But if one person is starting to reject the other, that can be devastating. I speak from experience."

> *"When we have frequent sex, I flirt and tease more, and I'm more playful. I feel better about myself as a person. I'm just so much more confident."*
>
> —Doreen

Early in the diet, Ralph was supposed to meet Doreen at a local restaurant for dinner. Looking around the restaurant, he didn't see her. Then a woman dressed in a tight, sleeveless red sweater and body-hugging black pants approached him. "I almost couldn't believe my eyes," remembers Ralph. "It was Doreen!" And he was even *more* surprised after dinner when she gave him this note:

Dearest Love, Don't let the innocent face fool you. You're in for a big surprise—tonight I'm gonna be a bad, bad girl! Come join me for some dirty dancing and fun and games. Wait for my call. Kisses, Amber Rose.

When they got home that night, Amber Rose told Ralph to wait in the garage with the cell phone while she got the house ready for romance. "I changed into my garters and stockings and a tight leather skirt, but left the red sweater on," Doreen says. "Then I put on some music and lit a few candles and took out a bottle of sherry and two glasses and some chocolate treats."

When the cell phone rang, Ralph ran to the front door. "We sat down and talked for a while, then my hands began to roam under her skirt," Ralph recalls. "When I discovered she had garters on, I almost went out of my mind! Then we started dancing and she began undressing me. It was like slow, sweet torture. She really outdid herself in the anticipation department."

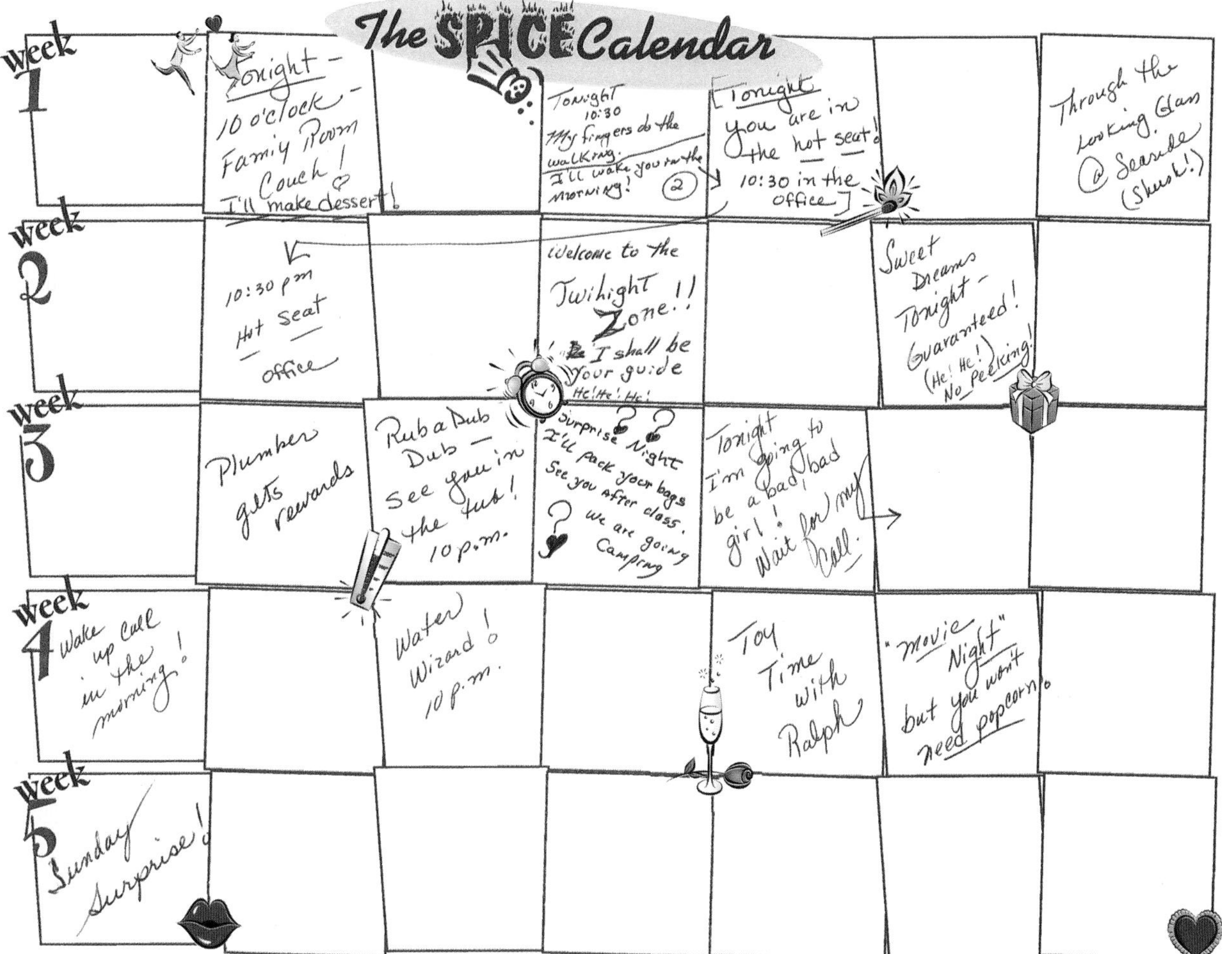

"We're putting together a scrapbook of our entire twenty-eight-day journey with the calendar, menus, pictures, and cards. It's been so amazing, we want to remember this forever."—Doreen

And Ralph had a few surprises for Doreen as well. "One morning on the calendar, he wrote, 'Surprise night! See you after class,'" Doreen says. "All through class, I was thinking, 'I want to get out of here.'" Later that evening, she returned to find the living room transformed into a campsite, complete with sleeping bags and a "campfire." "It was like we were out in the woods," Doreen recalls. "It was so romantic sitting by the fire and then crawling into our sleeping bags. It meant so much to me that he cared enough to plan something like this for me."

After twenty-eight days, Doreen and Ralph have no intentions of ever coming off the diet. "Now that we're at the end, it just keeps on getting better and better. It's one of those things you never want to end."

BEFORE THE DIET

"When you have kids, you run your life by the clock. From six in the morning until bedtime, we're running and running. And by the time we get home and get the kids in bed, we're exhausted and we're out of time for each other."

—DONNA

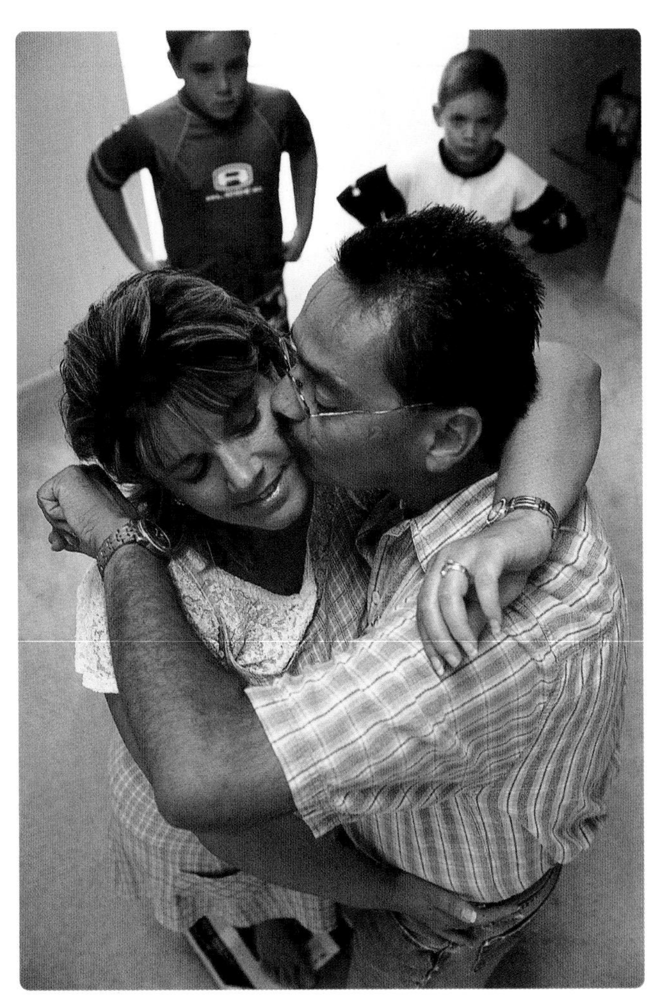

Countdown Fever

DONNA & CASEY

SHE: 30s, in sales

HE: 30s, in construction

STATUS: together 20 years, married 11; 2 kids

Donna and Casey may have two kids, but that didn't stop them from going to town on the spices! Their kids seemed to take all their free time, leaving Donna and Casey with little or no down time and certainly no time to relax and have sex. I've heard from so many parents that there is never enough time. Kids'

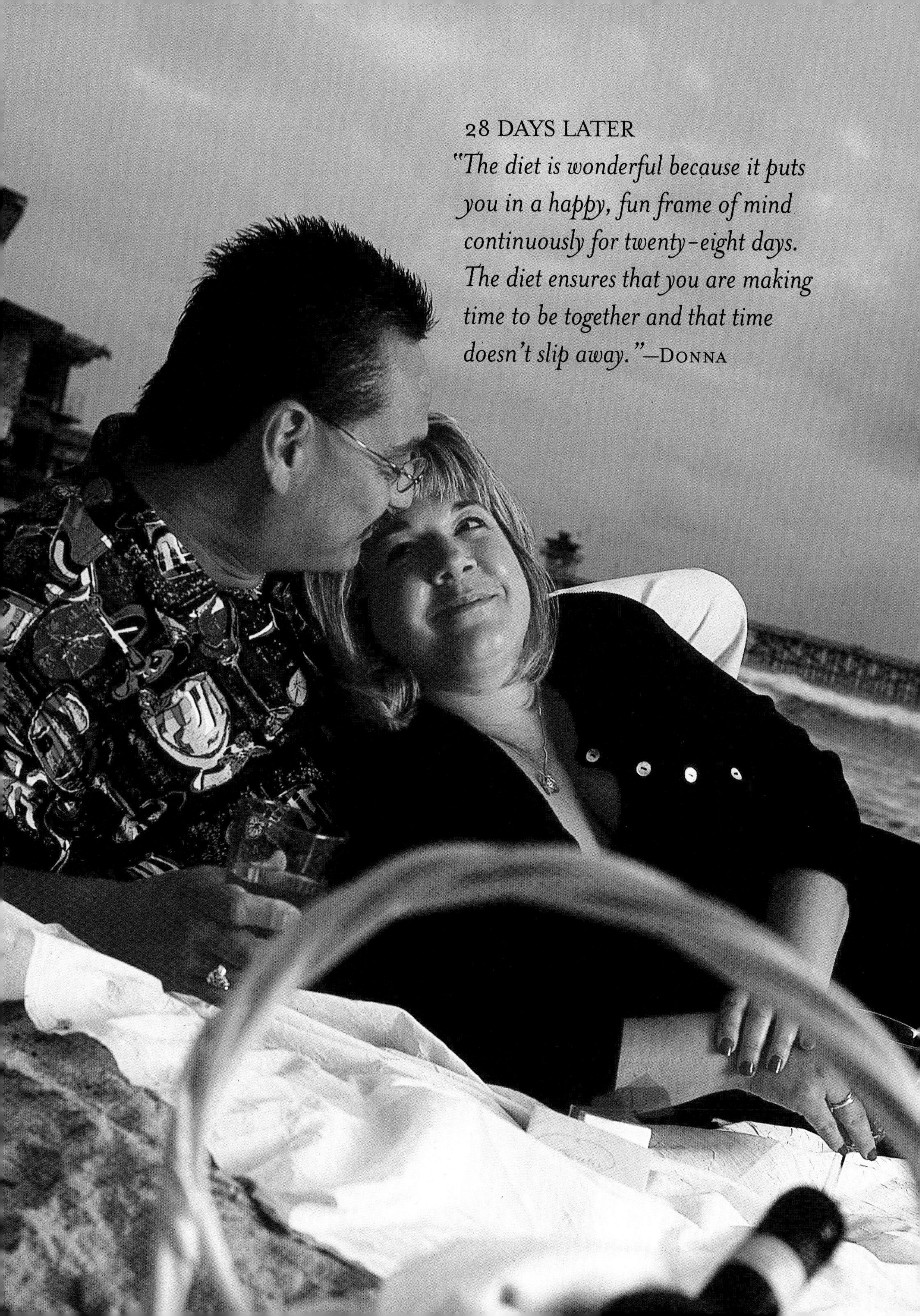

28 DAYS LATER

"The diet is wonderful because it puts you in a happy, fun frame of mind continuously for twenty-eight days. The diet ensures that you are making time to be together and that time doesn't slip away."—DONNA

lives today are so busy and structured, that parents pay a heavy price in their own personal lives. Parents are constantly running around, driving their kids from school, to play dates, to ballet lessons and soccer practice. They often start feeling like a frenzied chauffeur who never gets a day off.

When Donna and Casey decided to commit to the diet, they made their time together a priority. And guess what? They found the time! Scheduling sex on the calendar really worked. As Donna points out, "It guarantees you'll do it." She explains further, "Most of the time the day just goes by and it's later and you're saying good night, see you tomorrow. But if you plan on the calendar that you're going to be together tonight, then you make the arrangements to do that. And it just doesn't get by without happening."

But "because of the calendar," Donna explains, "we put our kids to bed on time instead of a half hour later. We made sure everything was done—dinner, the kitchen, and the kids, so that we had time together. We even finished dinner sooner and cleaned up sooner. The whole later part of the day revolved around our appointment."

The calendar also helped to create anticipation. "Looking at the calendar and not knowing what we are going to do that night," says Casey, "pretty much leaves the imagination to run wild. Just knowing the thought is being put into something for both of you is great." Casey also liked feeling desired: "It's not a question of being wanted, but knowing that you're wanted in that way, in a *sensual* way." They put the calendar on the back of their bedroom closet door and every once in a while one of them would sneak a peak. "Every time he wrote on the calendar, he'd go in the closet and shut the door. It was funny. So every time either of us saw the other in the closet, we'd run in there and read it. It kept the anticipation and excitement level really high."

Casey and Donna were so into the spices that they even rated them on a scale of one to ten, with one spice even rating a fifteen! (It was Total Control on the For His Eyes Only menu for those of you brave enough to try!) One night, Casey combined two spices and really rocked Donna's world. Using a red light for atmosphere, he then surprised her with a special kind of vibrator. "It has different sen-

"Everything that you do on the diet—the calendar, the menu, the planning—is for both of you, not just for one. You're just so happy because you both feel special." —Casey

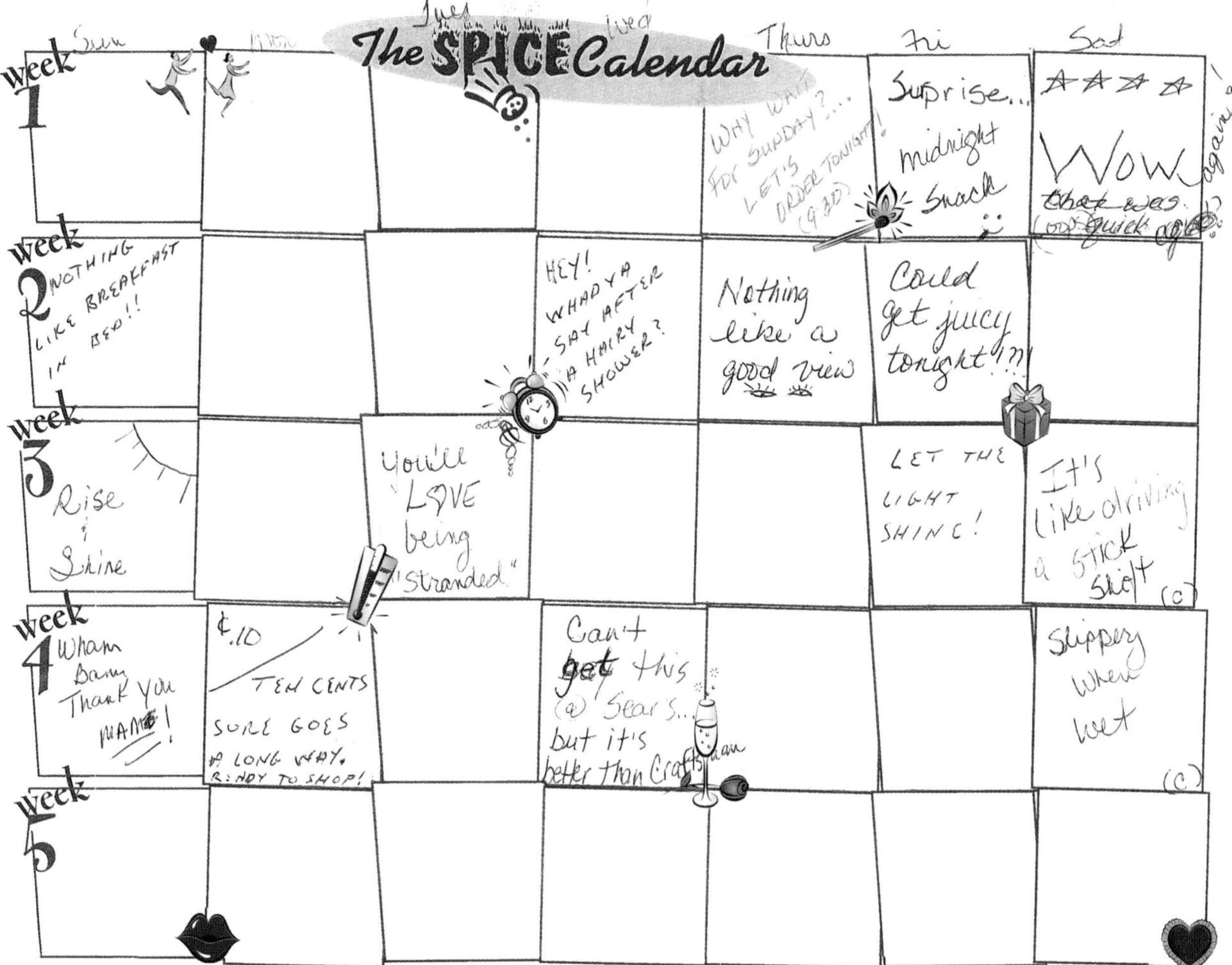

"We kept the calendar taped to the inside of our bedroom closet. Every time he wrote on the calendar, he'd go in the closet and shut the door. It was funny. So every time either of us saw the other in the closet, we'd run in there and read it. It kept the anticipation and excitement level really high."—Donna

sations," Donna describes, "it wasn't just one. It was very, very exciting." Guys, you'll have to check out the Secret Spice Menu for more info, and girls, you'll just have to wait!

Donna also surprised Casey with eighteen different spices! One of his absolute favorites was Pearl-Lingus and another was Lady Fingers. As Donna says, "That one really turns on guys. It's erotic—a real *bad girl* thing and he loved it. So I did it again!"

When I spoke to Casey and Donna after they'd completed the diet, Donna described the whole experience as "wonderful because it puts you in a happy frame of mind *all the time.*" Now that they're scheduling sex and trying new spices, Donna says she's always in the mood. And that's where we all want to be.

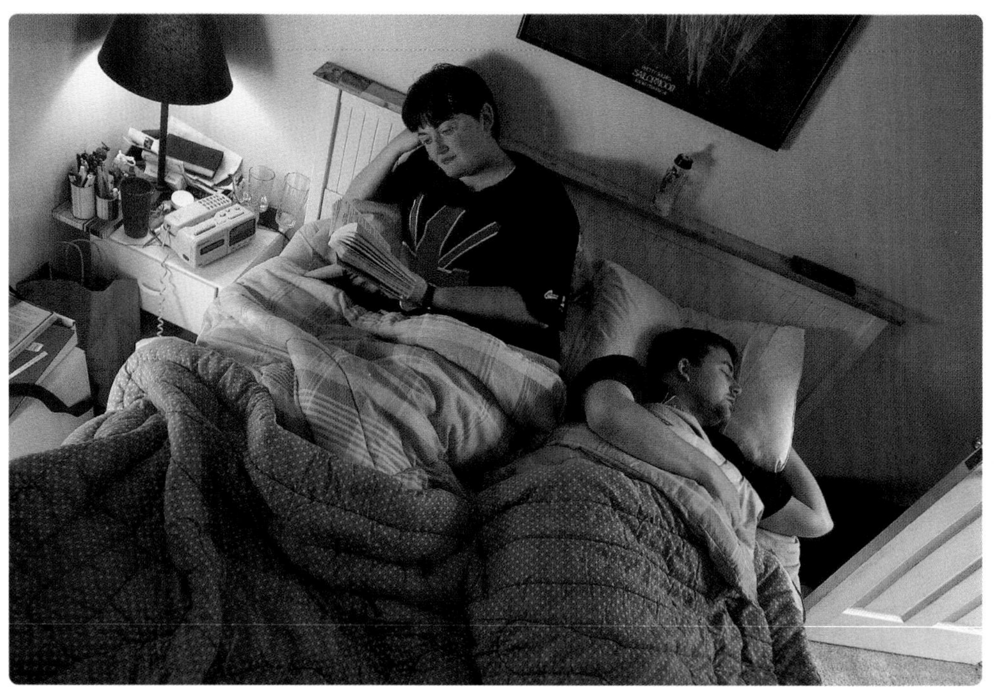

BEFORE THE DIET

"I seem to want sex more than Brian does. I have the higher sex drive. We probably make love about three times a month and it's just because he's tired. I would love it more."—AMY

Tickled Pink

AMY & BRIAN

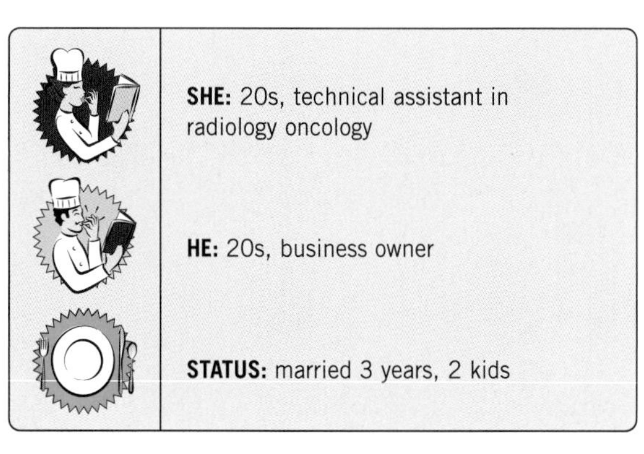

SHE: 20s, technical assistant in radiology oncology

HE: 20s, business owner

STATUS: married 3 years, 2 kids

Amy and Brian were one of the most innovative couples on the diet and are an example of how two people can learn to get mismatched desire back on track and get in synch with each other, so they simply hum with sexual energy.

Before the diet, Amy had become increasingly uncomfortable with and frustrated by her sex drive being higher than Brian's. She

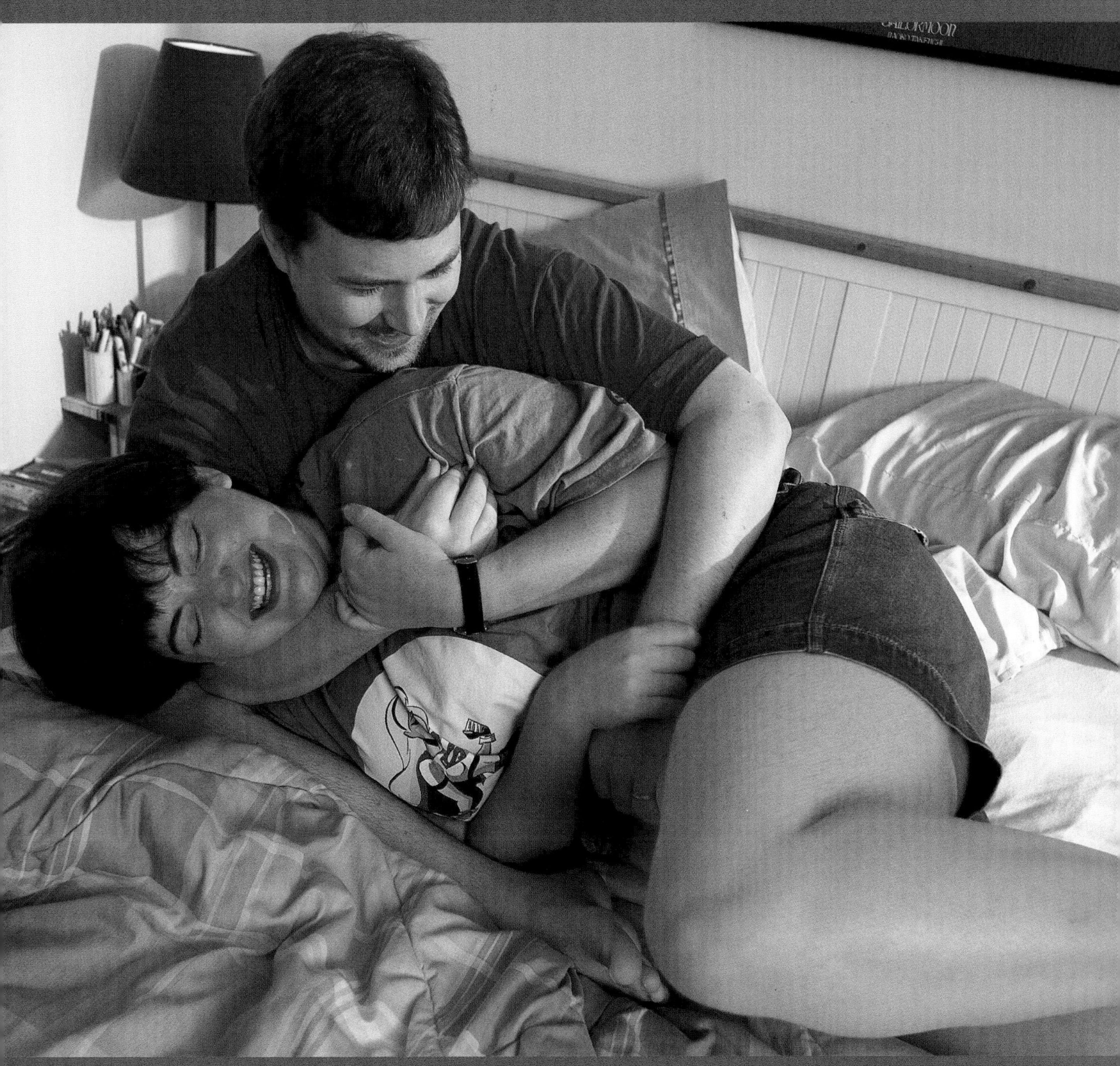

28 DAYS LATER

"This diet helped us recharge our relationship. We had so much fun! We learned that frequent sex should be part of your diet. It keeps a couple healthy and running strong."—Amy

Dear Amy,
I love you for putting up with me, my eccentricities, habits, and unusual thinking process. Only you could see through my facades to find the real me. And you're still here. Love
Brian

says that they've struggled with this issue since the beginning of their relationship. "The longest we've gone without having sex was six months. Brian was having a hard time with the relationship, and he was withdrawing into himself. I pointed out to him how long it had been. He was like, 'No, it hasn't been that long.' I said, 'Trust me, it's been that long.'"

Things got even worse. Amy says, "There was just so much more tension. I was considering ending the relationship because the closeness wasn't there. He was real closed off. And every time I tried to get close to him, he just kind of withdrew a little more. I finally told him I wanted to break up with him. And he took a look at the relationship and realized that he really cared about me more than he thought he did. And that pretty much changed it. He realized he actually needed me."

When I asked Brian whether he missed having sex during that period or whether that affected him negatively, he said something I've heard again and again in my interviews with people: "The longer you go without it, the more you think you don't need it."

But once they were on the diet, all of this turned around. Amy says enthusiastically, "We had so much fun on the diet! We joke around a lot more than we did last month. It was great having the spices. When I surprised Brian with the Now *This* Is a Massage! spice, he had a hard time moving afterward. All of his daily stresses were completely gone. It took him a while to come back to earth!"

Brian was very inventive when it came to using the spices to surprise and seduce Amy. "The first spice I did for Amy was one where you surprise her in the shower. You soap her up, rub her down, and go from there. That was a really good one! It was totally exciting to come up with something new for her."

The diet even reversed Brian's unwillingness to initiate. "I'm so glad to see that Brian is doing more of the seducing now

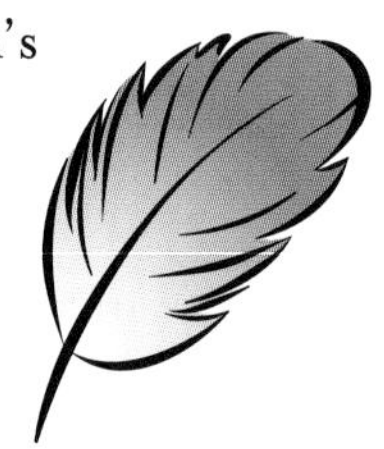

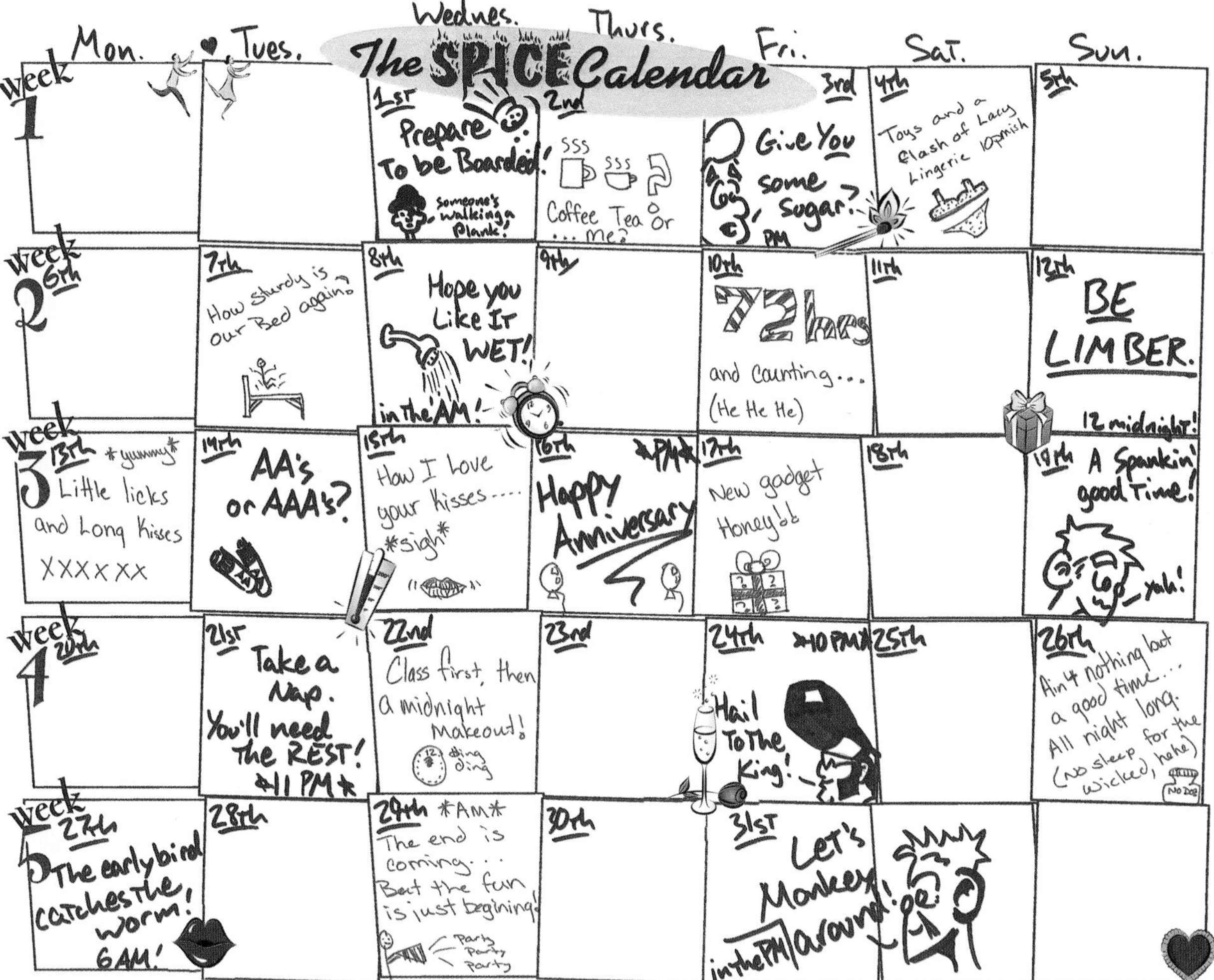

"During the diet, there was a subtle buildup of anticipation on a daily basis, and it had been a long time since I felt like that. In fact, the anticipation was so great that it made the actual event that much more exciting!"—Brian

because usually I'm in the lead," Amy says. "It's great that he feels comfortable doing it. It was kind of nice that he had these spices he can try. He knows I'm up for anything."

And they used a lot of different spices. Brian says, "We used a lot of combinations. Sometimes midstride, we would switch around and do other spices. Like I'd be doing a spice on her, and she'd say, 'I've got one!' So it kind of evolved from that point. There was one night we probably did three spices apiece."

Amy and Brian had amazing success on the diet. Just goes to show you that sex is a powerful tool. As Amy says, "I was thinking, 'Hmm . . . how can I do this just to blow his socks off?'" And Brian says simply, "I can't get enough of her!"

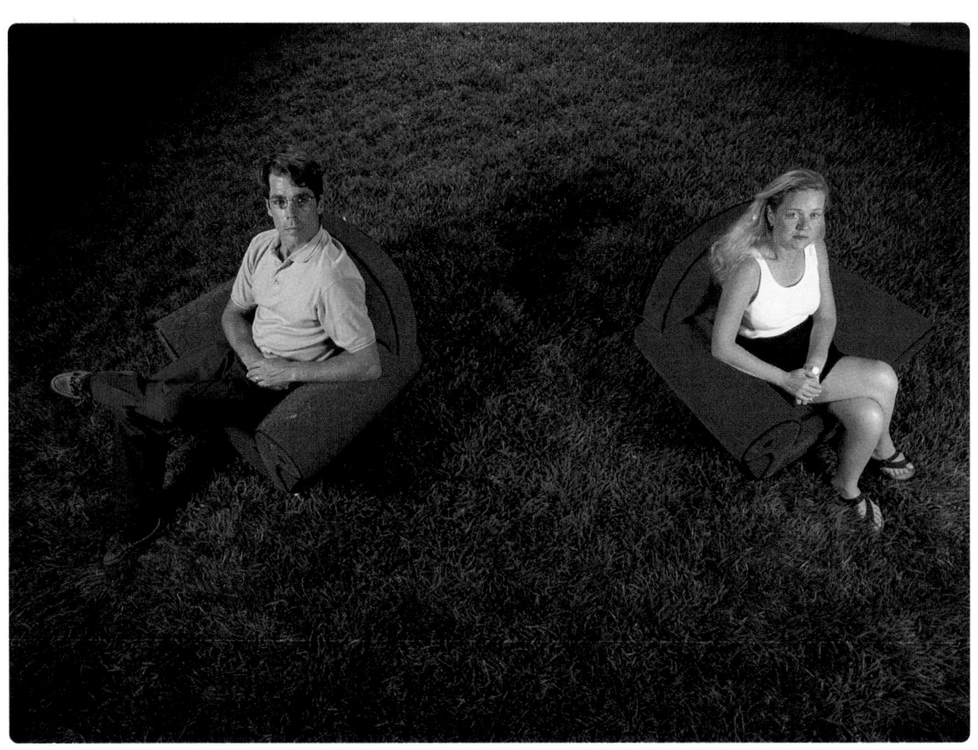

BEFORE THE DIET

"Andrew works so much, it feels like we are totally disconnected. We're like two separate islands."—STEPHANIE

Against All Odds

STEPHANIE & ANDREW

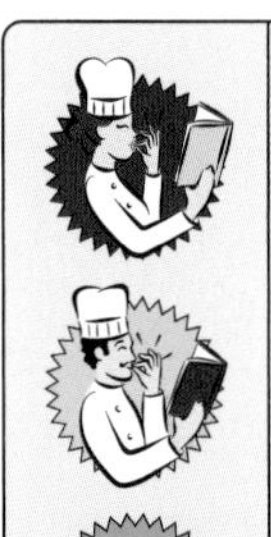

SHE: 30s, stay-at-home mom with a degree in law

HE: 30s, business owner

STATUS: together 19 years, married 16 years; 3 kids

Stephanie's after quote is quite an endorsement, isn't it? But even more than that, Stephanie's words hint at the enormity of the transformation she and Andrew experienced on the diet.

When I met them, Andrew and Stephanie had reached a crossroads. "Andrew works so much, it feels like we are totally disconnected,"

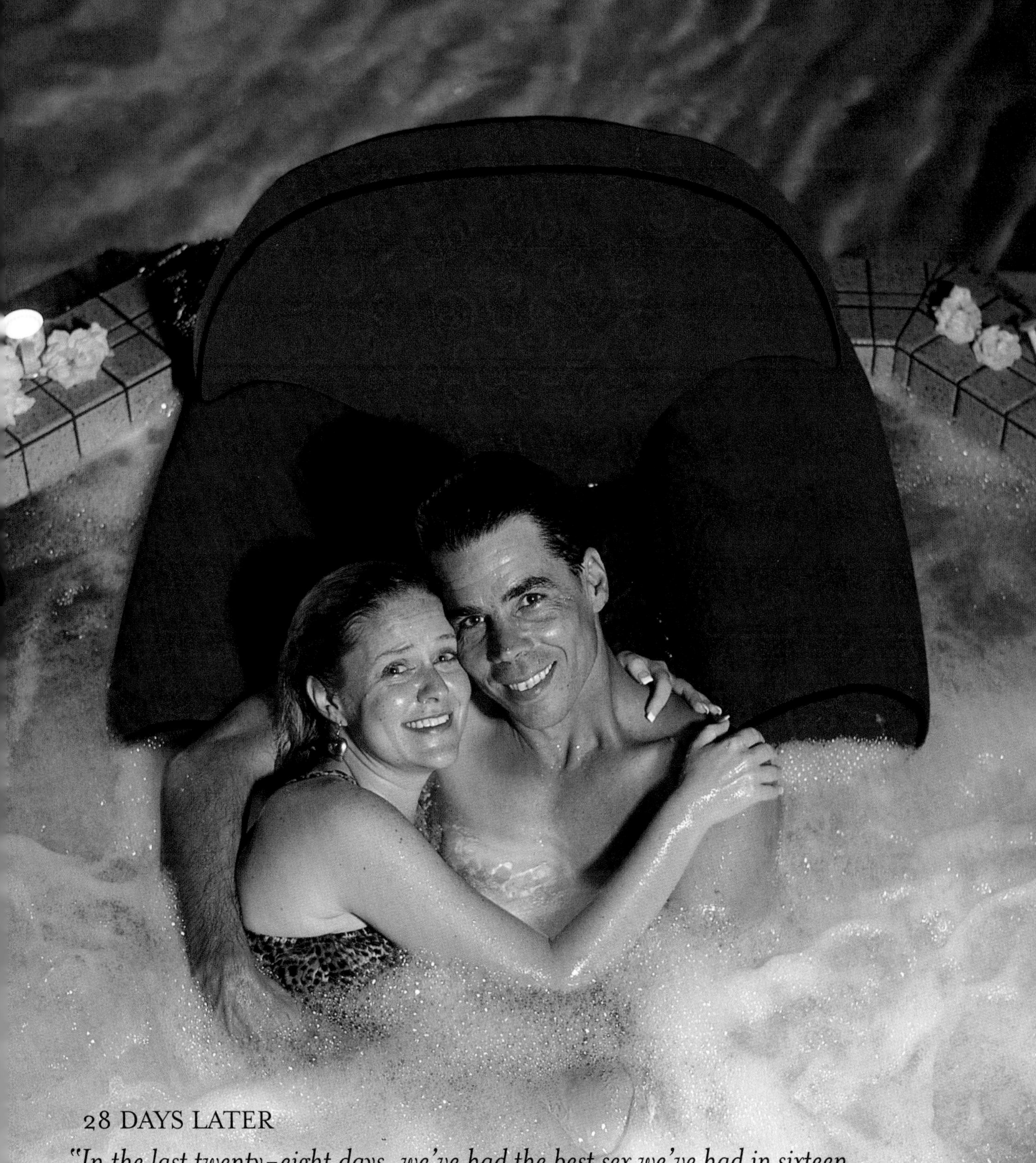

28 DAYS LATER

"In the last twenty-eight days, we've had the best sex we've had in sixteen years—quality, frequency, everything is there. It's like we went back in time ten years."—STEPHANIE

Stephanie explains. "We're like two separate islands." Even the photographer, Rick Dahms, commented on this distance between Andrew and Stephanie. He told me that the tension in their house was so thick, you could cut it with a knife.

Have you ever felt like you and your partner were on two separate islands? When the communication and intimacy have broken down to such a degree that you are completely without hope that things could possibly ever change? Jeff and I have certainly felt this way, and I'm sure we're not alone.

Both Stephanie and Andrew explain their having drifted apart in terms of Andrew's work being so consuming. As owner and operator of his own construction company with sixty employees, he has become successful and, by all standards, very wealthy. But in order to keep these balls of success in the air, he has to work—constantly.

Andrew describes his feelings this way: "You know why I come home so tired and don't even want sex? Because I work really hard. And you know why I work really hard? To provide for my kids." But behind his explanation I can hear his desire to change—change *something*—so that he has more energy to devote to his relationship.

"When you're having frequent sex you just can't help but feel more desirable in every way. And I'll tell you this: He's coming home from work a little earlier than he used to."

—STEPHANIE

Stephanie feels she is the one with the greater sex drive and waits for Andrew to initiate, but he's often too exhausted to do so. And yet Stephanie's indomitable spirit never waivers. In fact, Stephanie has multiple sclerosis, a condition that in her case does not impede her from leading an active, normal life. As she says, "You have a choice when you're diagnosed. You lay down or you stand up. I chose to stand up." She is not going to let anything stand in the way of fully accessing all the pleasure and enjoyment possible out of sex and life in general.

Going into the diet she and Andrew were optimistic but realistic. "When you've had sex with the same man for a number of years, you can always try something different. There's got to be one thing on the list that a person hasn't done yet," says Stephanie.

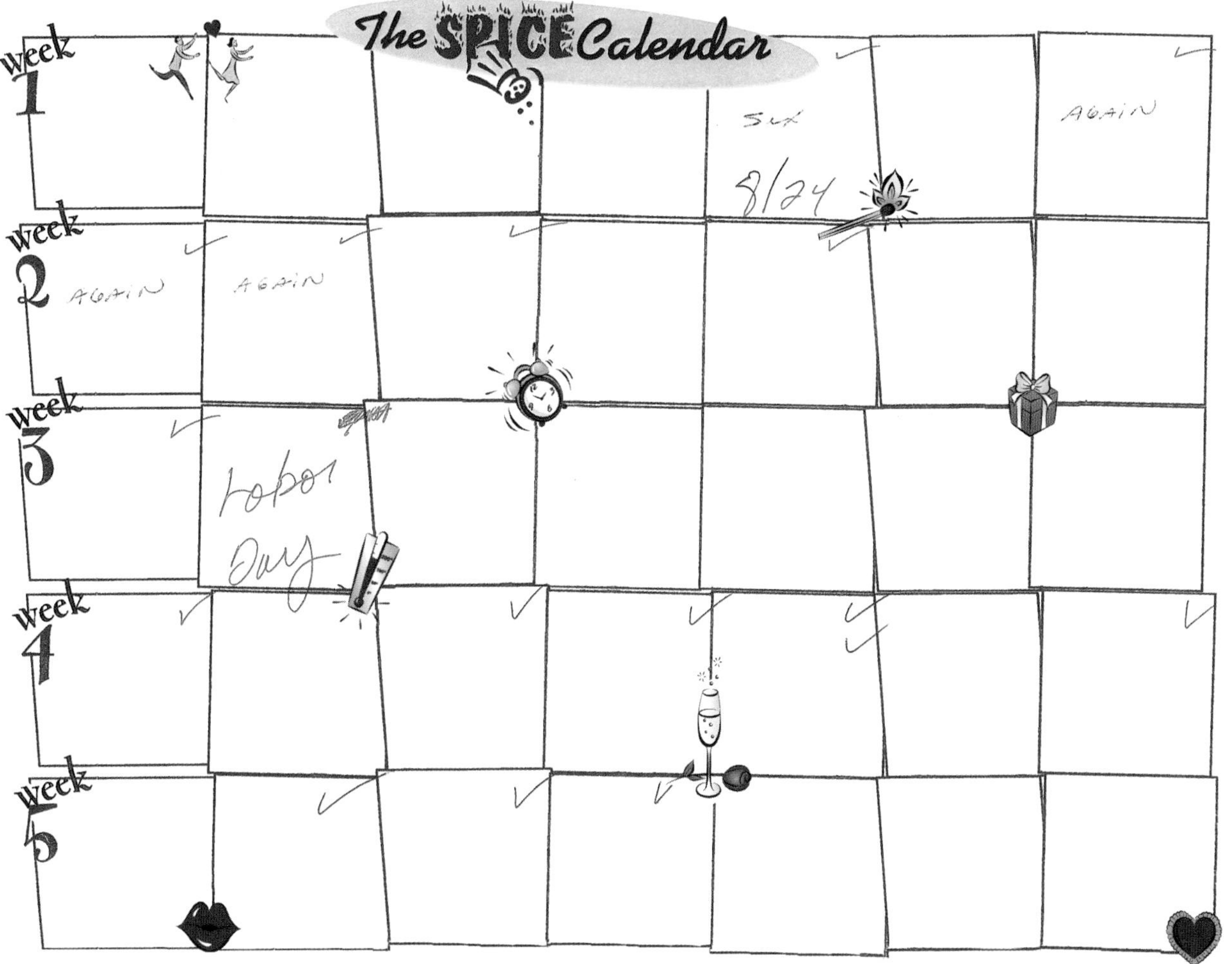

"The calendar is a great way to kind of break that 'I have trouble initiating' cycle. It opens up an avenue to be the seducer."—Andrew

On the diet, things began to change in a major way.

For one, Andrew gave Stephanie the biggest, longest, most intense orgasm of her life. As Stephanie says, "It was very powerful. It kept going on and on. I asked Andrew, 'Have you ever had an orgasm so hard and so long that you thought it was your last one ever?' I call it the 'screaming, last-forever orgasm.'"

But Stephanie certainly returned the favor by giving Andrew the best oral sex of *his* life. "One night," Stephanie explains, "he said to me 'That's the best blow job I've ever had in my life.' Want to know what started it? The scarf spice . . ."

Although Andrew was able to make time for more romance and intimacy, his heavy workload didn't disappear. But instead of falling asleep

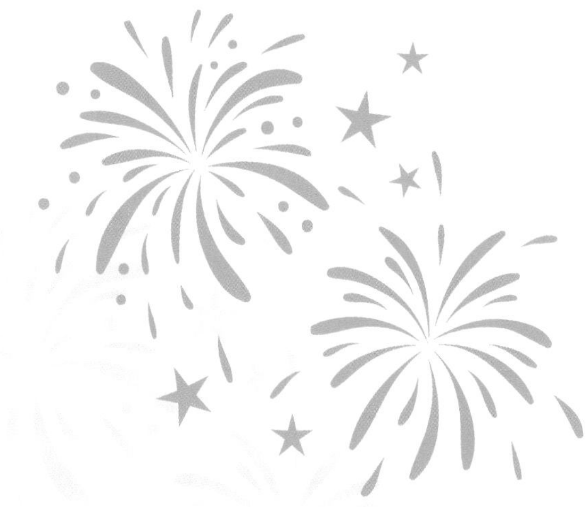

when he got home, he prepared by drinking coffee in the afternoon. "I grab a cup of coffee in the afternoon and that gives me motivation and helps me drum up some reserve energy so that I'm not so tired when I get home in the evening."

The overall change in Andrew was palpable—even his secretary noticed. Stephanie recalls, "One day I was talking to Andy's secretary and she asked me what I did to Andy last night. She said, 'He came to work in such a good mood!' I said, 'Oh, nothing.' What was I going to say? 'Let's see, I blew his brains out and then we had regular sex and then we did the oil spice'?" (They also got their sense of humor back!)

Andrew felt the frequency turned everything around. "When you have sex five or six days a week, your mind is racing about how you're going to make it different," he explains. "I think that some people need a little bit of a push to do what they enjoy and this diet gives you that." Stephanie agrees, "I never knew he liked sex so much. Now instead of going to sleep as soon as his head hits the pillow, he pulls me over to his side of the bed and says, *'What do you want me to do with this hard-on?'*"

As Andrew himself says, "A satisfied woman is a happy woman." Trying to make Stephanie happy seems to be Andrew's greatest goal.

I think most couples have probably felt the kind of emotional and sexual distance that Stephanie and Andrew describe. In fact, their before photo could be Jeff and me two years ago. Just take a look at the difference between their before and after pictures. That's the power of frequent sex!

"A satisfied woman is a happy woman. My wife said to me, 'Have you ever had an orgasm so hard and so long that you thought it was your last one ever?' She's been going crazy on this diet."

—ANDREW

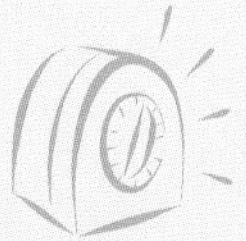

YOUR SOCKS BETTER BE IN THE HAMPER IF YOU'RE "THE FIVE-MINUTE GUY"

"If you're having sex once a week, you're a five-minute guy. You're just like, 'Oh my God, this is great.' Boom—you're done. There's not a whole lot of satisfaction going on. But halfway through this diet, you're the forty-five-minute guy. I mean, sex should take longer than forty-five minutes—playing around, doing other things. But physically it's hard. If you're only having sex once a week, I don't think you really build up any stamina. Your need for a release is so bad, it's over pretty quick. But when you've just had sex the night before, it just logically makes sense that it's going to last longer.

"And then you can get into the experimentation. Now you have time to play and you can do two or three positions. The original five-minute guy doesn't have a whole lot of time to be experimenting or playing around. The simple definition of the term *premature ejaculation* is an ejaculation that occurs earlier than desired. I mean, say you are having sex for ten or fifteen minutes and you have your orgasm. But you didn't want to. Prior to the sex diet, if you're the five-minute guy or ten-minute guy, whatever it is, you're not building up a sweat during sex. You're not even getting into each other. And it's over. And then you're waiting for another week. But halfway through the diet, you're getting sweat going. And you look at your clock and you're like, *'Oh my God, it's been an hour?!'* You feel like, 'Ho-ho!'

"I'm happy to say my wife is a satisfied woman, thanks to the diet. When a woman is not satisfied, she's going to have issues. Nothing her guy does is going to be right. His socks weren't in the hamper, and she's furious. But if you're having sex four times a week for a half-hour each time and she's having a couple of orgasms, she's not going to give a damn if your socks are on the floor or on the ceiling!" —ANDREW

BEFORE THE DIET

"With two kids and so many work responsibilities, we're sometimes just too busy and tired for sex. It's hard to remember that we're still the most important thing."

—CHRISTIE

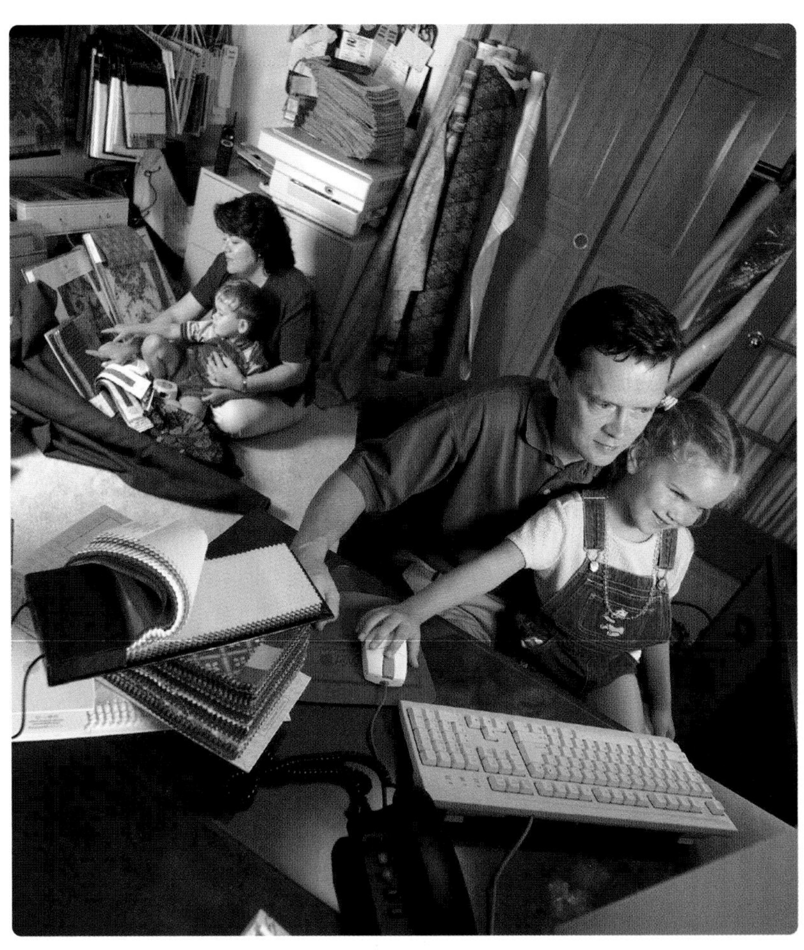

Isn't It Romantic

CHRISTIE & GLENN

SHE: 30s, owner of a design business

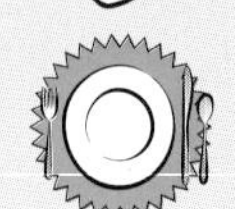

HE: 30s, engineer

STATUS: been together 8 years, married 7 years; 2 kids

For me, witnessing Glenn and Christie go through the diet and watching them reinfuse that wonderful romantic tension into their relationship was really touching.

Glenn and Christie have two young children who, like most kids, are demanding and require a lot of time. Of course, they love their children dearly, but before the diet,

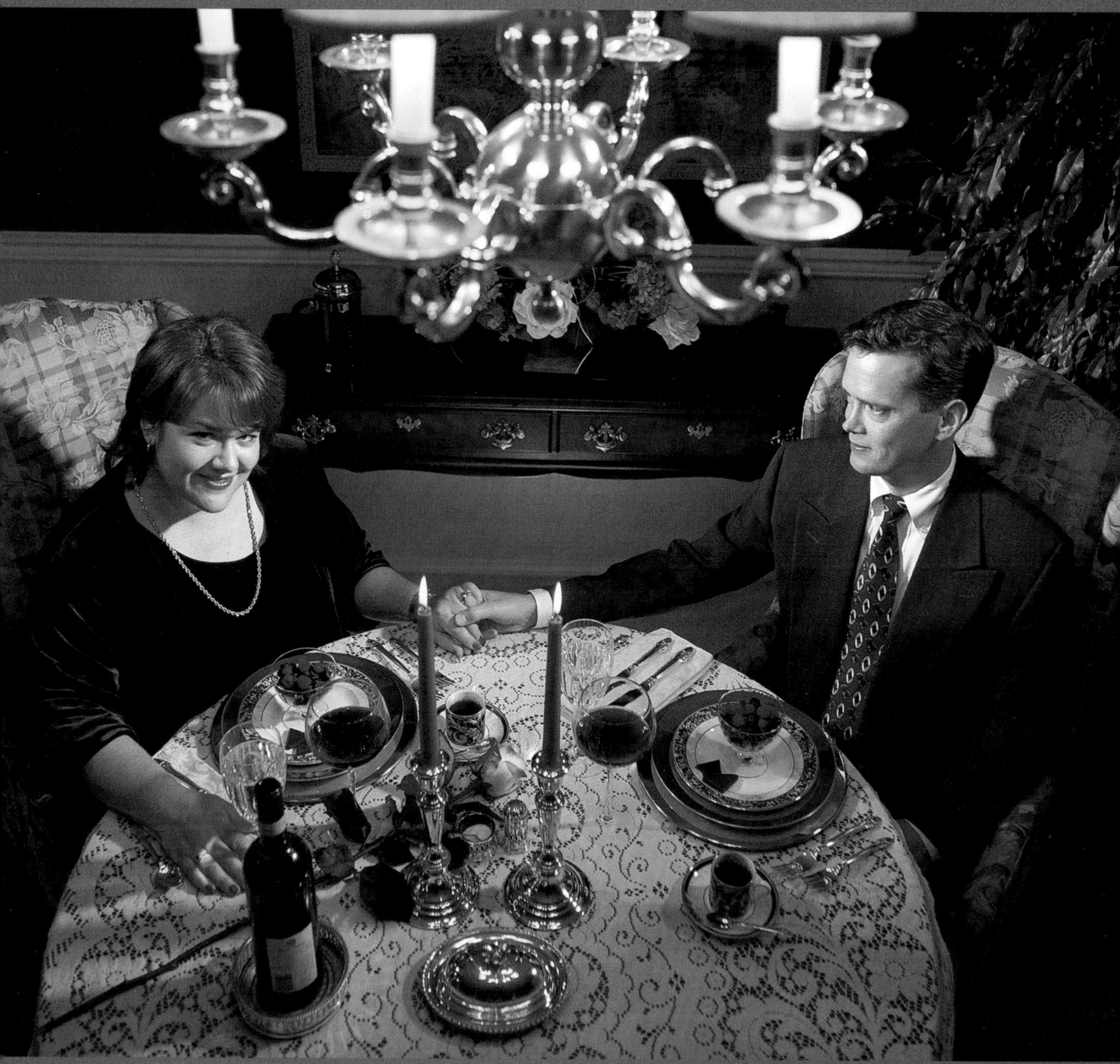

28 DAYS LATER

"Being on the diet energized us and made us feel like we were dating again. We're getting dressed up and having romantic dinners together just like we used to do. It was so fun. We loved it!"—Christie

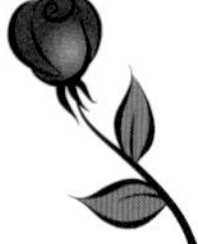

both Glenn and Christie were trying desperately to carve out time for each other. Sound familiar?

The first step they took was scheduling sex. As Glenn says, "If it weren't for scheduling, it wouldn't have happened because we would have been too tired. But with me, a schedule's important—I'm an engineer. The calendar helped us stick to four times per week and also helped us to plan. The last week we set aside *all* our free time just for us!"

"We look at this whole diet as an adventure. We just had fun with everything we did."
—Christie

They scheduled not only sex nights, but long, romantic evenings as well. As Christie says, "It had been so long since we dressed up and went out for the evening." They needed to treat each other and their relationship as special. Take a look at their after photo: Can't you see the romantic rapture in the air?

Going on the diet "was like going on an adventure together," says Christie. The diet was also successful for them because "both of us were making an effort. You don't feel like it's *one*-sided."

And one-sided it surely was not. They both went wild trying different spices—by the end of the four-week diet, Glenn had done fifteen spices for Christie and Christie had done nineteen for Glenn! As Glenn says of one combo spice he tried on Christie, "It drove her crazy because she felt that it was a little bit too rushed, but at the same time, it was the most incredible orgasm she ever had!" When he adapted another spice, Glenn says, "I did that in the bathtub instead of on the floor, and she liked that one a lot—anything that involved massage was very exciting."

Out of the nineteen spices that Christie did for Glenn, his absolute favorite was I'm Famous for This. "I had written on the calendar, 'Meet me in the bedroom at 10:00 P.M. for a hot surprise.' Then I lit some candles and blindfolded him." The more she dazzled him, the hotter Glenn got. "He was having a lot of fun with it. He kept getting more and more excited!" says Christie.

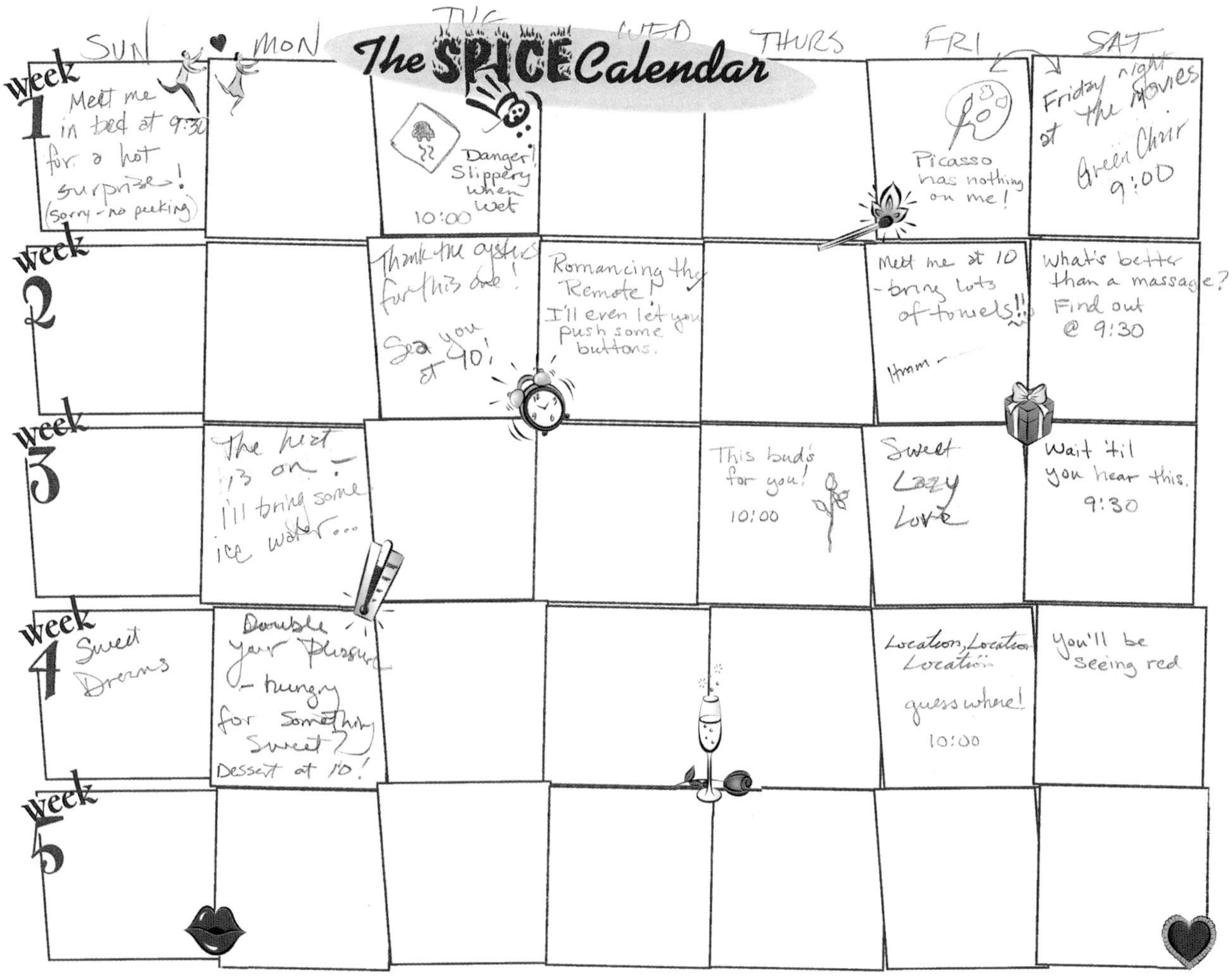

The SPICE Calendar

	SUN	MON	TUE	WED	THURS	FRI	SAT
week 1	Meet me in bed at 9:30 for a hot surprise! (Sorry – no peeking)		Danger! Slippery when wet 10:00			Picasso has nothing on me!	Friday night at the Movies Green Chair 9:00
week 2			Thank the oysters for this one! See you at 10!	Romancing the Remote! I'll even let you push some buttons.		Meet me at 10 – bring lots of towels!! Hmm –	What's better than a massage? Find out @ 9:30
week 3		The heat is on – I'll bring some ice water...			This bud's for you! 10:00	Sweet Lazy Love	Wait 'til you hear this. 9:30
week 4	Sweet Dreams	Double your Pleasure – hungry for Something Sweet? Dessert at 10!				Location, Location, Location guess where! 10:00	You'll be seeing red
week 5							

"We tried to write things on the Spice Calendar that really built the suspense up. You read it and wonder, 'What does *that* mean?' That part was really fun."—Glenn

Like so many couples, the diet brought Glenn and Christie closer. They added the romance, bedazzled each other with spices, and let the diet work its magic. "We realized that even though we do have so many responsibilities and so many things to do," Christie concludes, "*we're* still the most important thing."

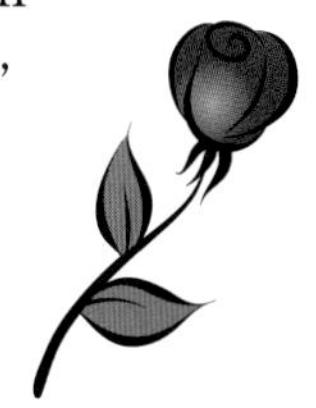

"Even our three-year-old son noticed the change. One day he said to Glenn, 'There you go, falling in love with Mommy again!'"

—CHRISTIE

BEFORE THE DIET

"We have a great relationship, but I would like to improve my performance and add a little more variety. My wife is heavy into variety, so I really need to provide her with more of it."

—DAVID

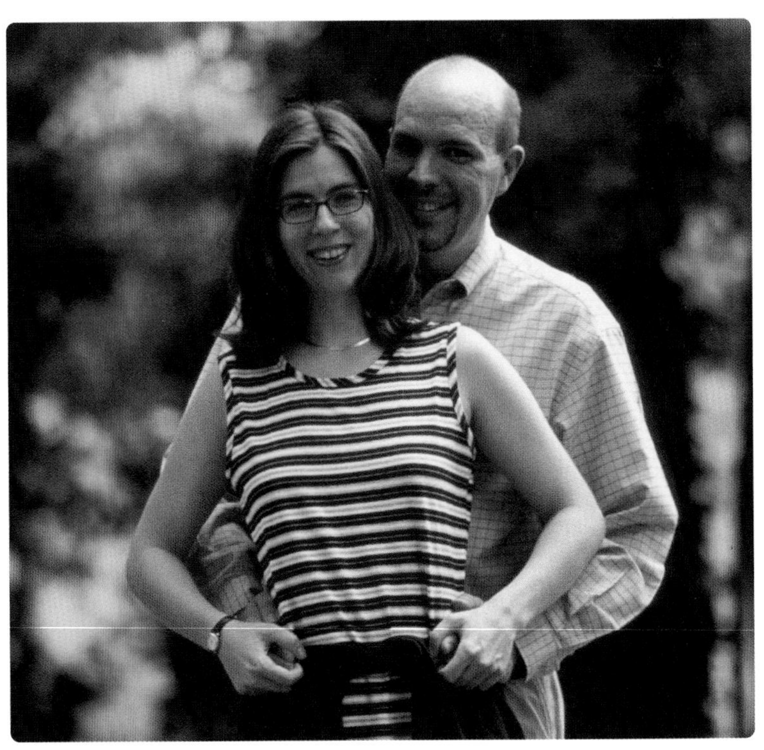

One Good Romp Deserves Another

DAVID & LUCIA

SHE: 20s, co-owner and operator with David of a design firm

HE: 30s

STATUS: together for 10 years, married for 6 years; 1 daughter

Most couples would drive each other crazy if they both worked and lived together—talk about 24/7! But not David and Lucia—they are a marvelous exception to this rule. They run their own design firm, and both say it's a labor of love. "Before our daughter was born, out of every seven days, we spent only three or four hours apart," David explains.

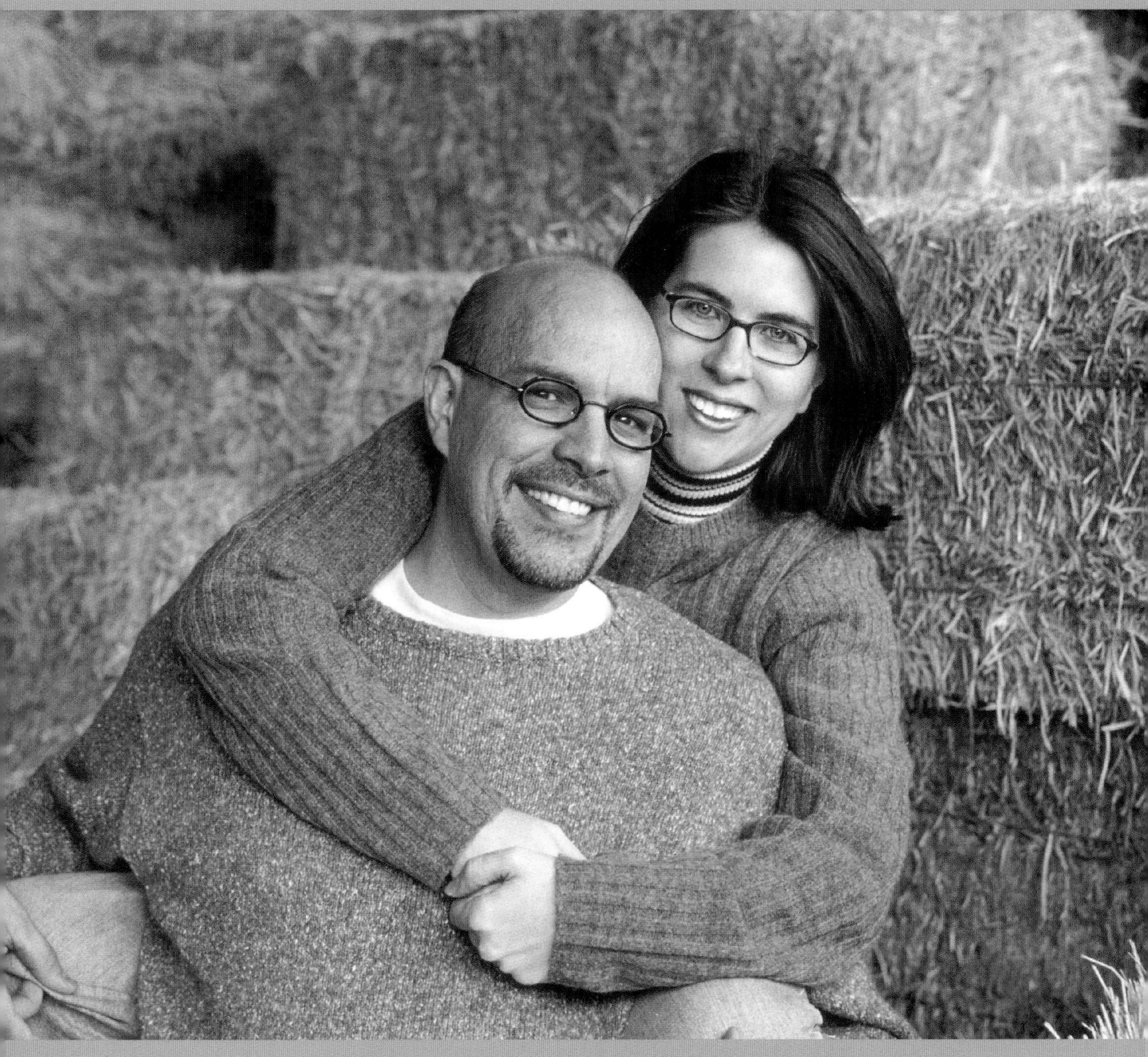

28 DAYS LATER

"The emotional intimacy that we both feel is the best thing that's come out of the diet. We've really enjoyed that. I mean, we've been connected for a long time. But now we're definitely more reminded of that deep connection." —David

"We worked together full-time, we played together full-time, and spent our nights together. And so many people have said to me over the years, 'How can you stand to work with your wife? I couldn't possibly stand to work with my wife the whole day!' And I think they're nuts. If I had to sell apples, I'd want to be standing out on a street corner *with my wife* selling apples. We have a great, great time together—all the time."

When you work together and live together, there is an immediate and undeniable challenge to keep the boundaries clear: Where does work end and the fun of the relationship begin?

When their daughter was born a year ago, life became infinitely fuller for both of them. "When we would make love, we'd sometimes look over at our daughter and it's just such a sweet feeling," Lucia says. "It's very wonderful to be making love and see the product of your love there before you."

"I have to tell you, we absolutely become more tense with each other when we don't have sex. I'll say to my wife, you need a good romp. And she'll look at me and agree. Having a romp solves all sorts of problems."

—David

But as it often does, their sex life dwindled dramatically after the baby was born. "Things slowed down for sure," David says. "I think one of the primary things that could make our relationship better would be to get back up to our college romp level. Yeah, we need to work the romp meter up." And that's where the Great American Sex Diet came in.

David is very aware of the difference in their relationship when they aren't having sex as frequently. "I have to tell you," he says, "we absolutely become more tense with each other when we don't have sex. I'll say to my wife, you need a good romp. And she'll look at me and agree. Having a romp solves all sorts of problems. And a romp for us includes what we call an ASM, aka after-sex massage. It's a natural part of it. We have romps and ASMs and it just really improves our outlook. It gives us a feeling of calm and satisfaction. For us, it's a way to relieve tension and bring us close together again."

One of the aspects of the diet that appeals to them is the wide range of seduction spices in the menu. As David remarks, "My wife's favorite ice cream at Baskin-Robbins is vanilla fudge, but she only orders it one out of seven times she goes. She is heavy into variety, so I really need to provide her with more of it." And, boy, did the diet ever give them that. They experimented with lots of new techniques and really enjoyed the toy spices. Lucia tells me that she really "zinged" David with the Finger Zinger spice!

From the start, it was clear that David and Lucia share a great sense of fun and carry it into their sex life. As David says rather proudly, "The diet helped me make time for the hunt. I make time to eat three meals a day, and I found I could just as easily find time to have sex four times a week. Or sometimes even five or seven!"

"I like the fear of getting caught. And different locations. Yeah, I like the hillside thing. I like the dressing room thing. I like the airplane thing. That's fun. When we were dating and we were staying in her parents' house, I'd always sneak into her bedroom. That was a joy."

—David

Being on the diet made them realize how important it was to carve out time for just the two of them. "We decided to have two date nights each week where we will definitely, positively get naked and experience joy," David says. A delighted Lucia adds, "We've always known that it was a good idea, but we hadn't implemented an actual date night before. But now every Thursday we're going to get child care and go out, no matter what."

I was moved by how David and Lucia were able to define themselves more clearly as lovers than business partners. Once again, I was taken aback by the power of the diet to create change. Not only were they successful on the diet, they also managed to conceive another child—Lucia is pregnant again!

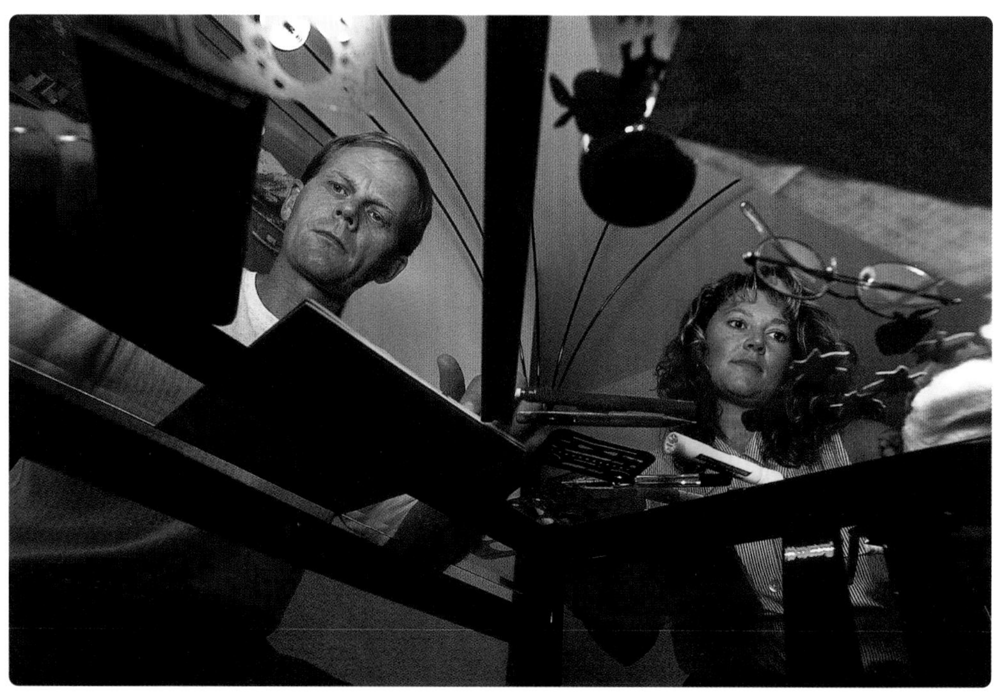

BEFORE THE DIET

"We bring our work home every night, and we're often too tired for intimacy by the time we're done. Sex just gets pushed to the back burner."—HEATHER

Just Like Clockwork

HEATHER & LARS

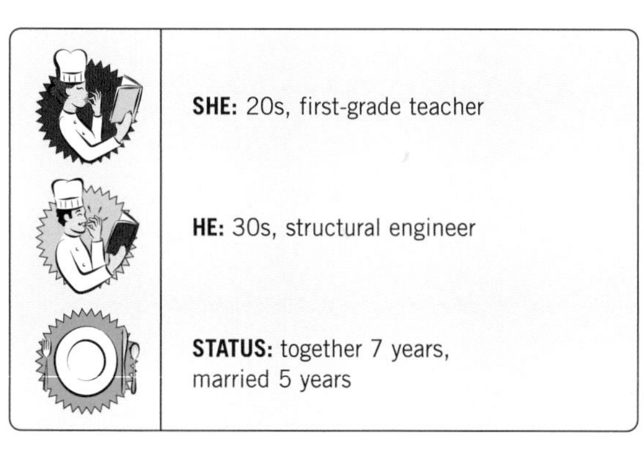

SHE: 20s, first-grade teacher

HE: 30s, structural engineer

STATUS: together 7 years, married 5 years

Lars and Heather consider themselves workaholics, but after the diet, you could call them sex-aholics! Before the diet, I could tell just by listening to them that they structure their lives around work and that success is important to them. As an engineer, Lars has a personality that is driven and systematic. And while Heather is softer and more feminine,

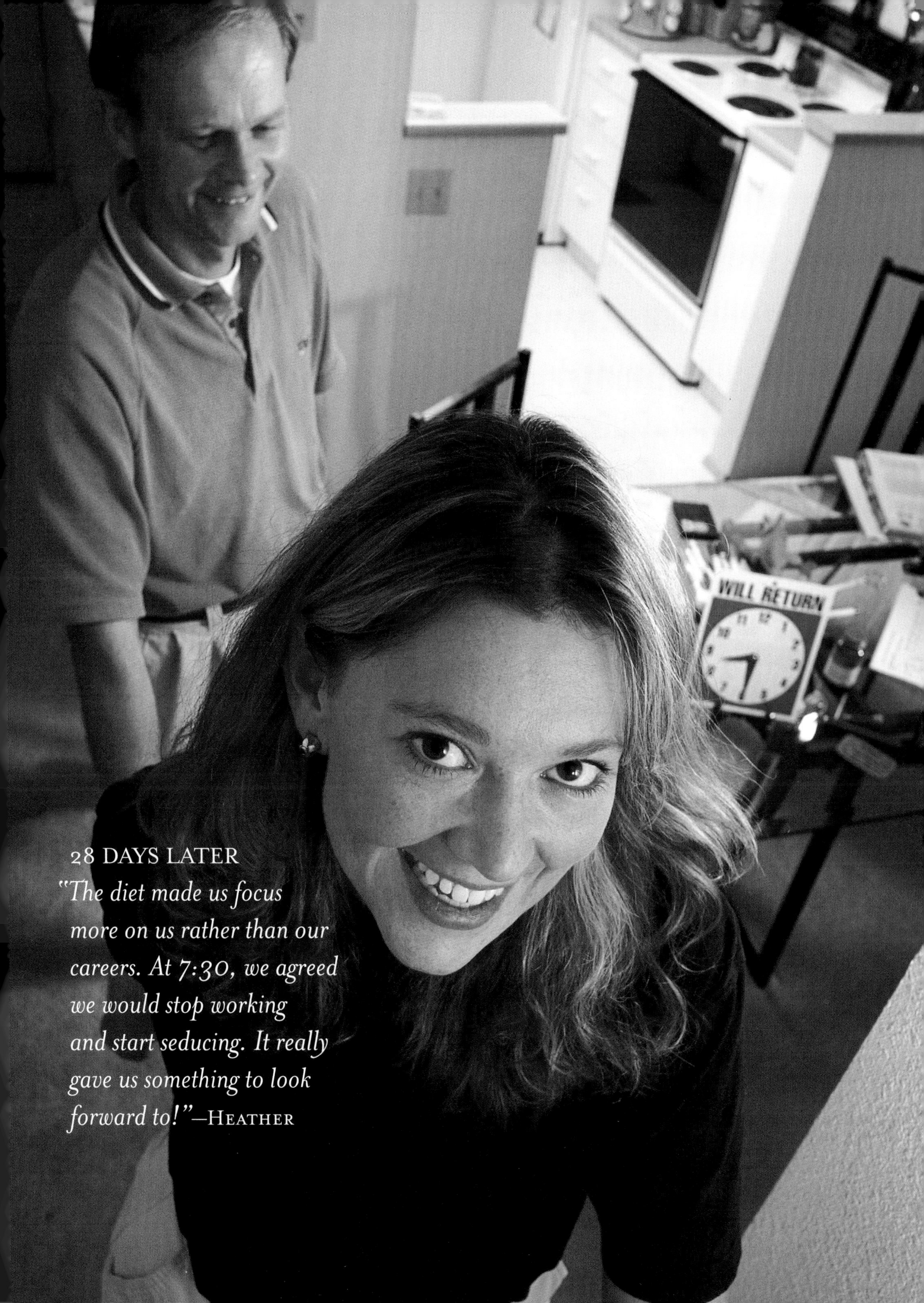

28 DAYS LATER
"The diet made us focus more on us rather than our careers. At 7:30, we agreed we would stop working and start seducing. It really gave us something to look forward to!"—Heather

she, too, likes to structure her days and considers herself a "type A"—probably one of the reasons they get along so well!

They began the diet hoping to add some variety to their sex life. Heather was also concerned that sex was taking a back seat in their relationship because they so often brought work home. As Heather says, "Normally we would work until eleven and then go to bed. And Lars is so practical, he'd never stop in the middle of what he was doing to make love so intimacy always got pushed and pushed and pushed to the back burner."

Well, that certainly changed on the diet! They got so into the anticipation and the spices, they couldn't wait for the day to end so that they could make time for romance. But one night that wait was practically endless! As Heather recalls, "One whole day, I kept waiting for him to do a spice because I thought he was scheduled to do it. Finally, we'd crawled into bed and I'm lying there, still waiting and waiting. And I finally asked, 'Aren't you going to do a spice?' And Lars said, 'Heather, it was supposed to be your turn.' And we went back and forth and then I got up and looked at the calendar on the refrigerator and it *was* my turn! We'd both been waiting and anticipating all day long for the other person to do something."

Even though they experienced that one minor scheduling mishap, they both loved the idea of scheduling sex. It fit in with their planning personalities. As Lars says, "When you schedule sex you know whatever else you're doing, you're going to drop it." And Heather responded to the scheduling as well. "We were really watching the clock. We would both be doing our work, and we'd constantly check to see if 7:30 had arrived. When it did, it was like, 'Let's go!' We couldn't wait to try our spices."

In fact, Heather was so inspired by the Spice Menu that she even devised a rating system.

HEATHER'S GUARANTEED RECIPE TO KNOCK HIS SOCKS OFF

Instructions:
Combine all these spices, then heat until he reaches full boil.

What's the Number for 911?
+
Lingerie Parfait
+
The Heat Is On!
+
The Chef's Favorite
+
Toasted!
+
Lip Service
=
One Happy, Satisfied Man!

The SPICE Calendar

	Sunday	Monday			Thursday	Friday	Saturday
week 1			Wear your favorit pair of shear panties, be ready @7:30	Every man would like to be you tonight You lucky dog!	My vibes will knock your socks off.		I need my vitamin C. And vitamin U!
week 2	Wet t-shirt contest today at 3:00.		VISA This one is going to cost you. Bring your credit card			"Tool Time" Staring Lars the tool-man Holte	Seduction @ seven, encore @ nine.
week 3			You're In the HOT seat buster! Don't be late!	2 for 1 tonight @ 7:30 pm	You won't find this at SEARS...	I'm going to do it til you beg me to stop	
week 4		Who Says There's Nothing Good On...	You will ache with pleasure.		Tonight you Panties should be satin		This will burn a hole on your memory! Designed by Laura herself!
week 5							

"Using the Spice Calendar was exciting, because you were planning ahead and being kind of secretive. You wanted to write the perfect little teaser on the calendar just to make it even more enjoyable and fun!"—Heather

"I'd give the spices one, two, three, or four stars," Heather explains. "The combo Lars did for me the first night of the diet got four stars!" Because he had such success with them, Lars was a big fan of combos. "Using a combination of the spices worked well for me," Lars said. "It was like going to a restaurant. You start with an appetizer, then you have a main course, then you have dessert."

One night, Lars was treated to a *six-course* meal by Heather: "I really wanted to knock his socks off," she says, "so I did *six* spices for him on the same night!"

As you can imagine, Heather's surprise treat for Lars was a four-star success! He was blown away by her creativity and so was I. A six-spice combo . . . *now there's a girl after my own heart!*

BEFORE THE DIET

"Our life is basically centered around our daughter. We get caught up in the family—gotta do this, gotta do that—and we forget about each other."

—KaeCee

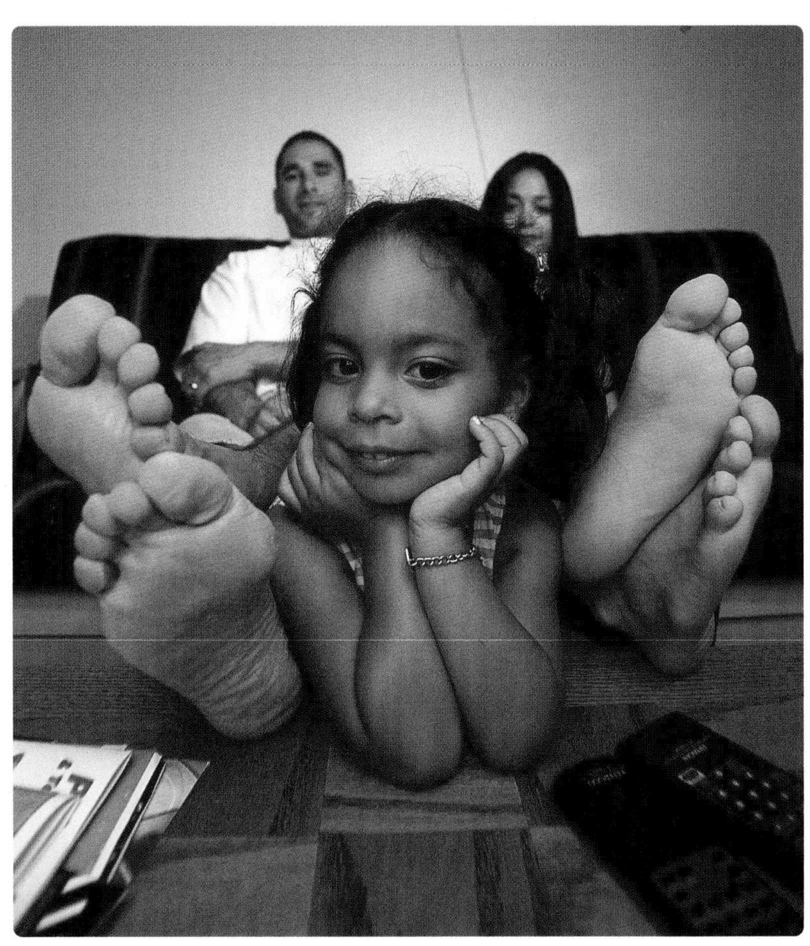

Web of Desire

KaeCee & Paul

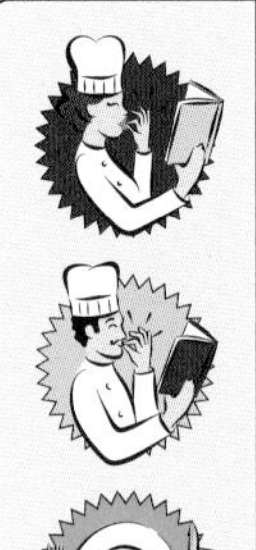

SHE: 20s, configuration manager

HE: 20s, waste management worker

STATUS: together 3 years, married 1 year; 1 daughter from her previous relationship

Still newlyweds, KaeCee and Paul were already feeling like the honeymoon had ended. "Our honeymoon was awesome," Paul notes. "There was definitely a lot of sex, but as soon as we got home, we didn't have sex for a week. I was like, 'What's going on? Is this what happens when you get married?'"

Although they go to bed by nine every night

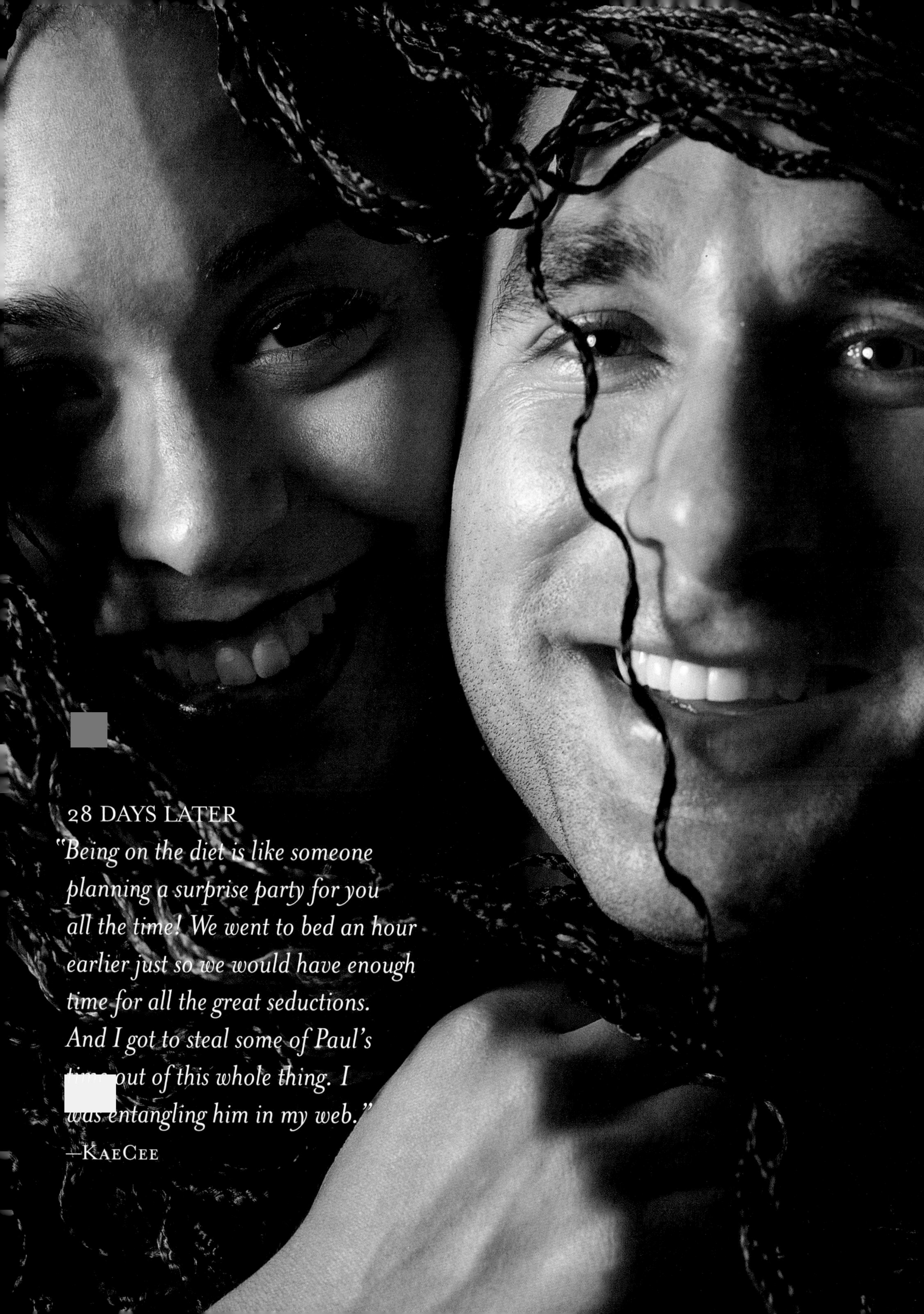

28 DAYS LATER

"Being on the diet is like someone planning a surprise party for you all the time! We went to bed an hour earlier just so we would have enough time for all the great seductions. And I got to steal some of Paul's time out of this whole thing. I was entangling him in my web."

—KaeCee

(since Paul has to get up at 3:30 A.M. to get to work), KaeCee and Paul were determined to stir up their sex life. "I like to do it in the evening," admits KaeCee. "But he's pooped at night." Another obstacle in their path to great sex is having to wait until their daughter goes to sleep. KaeCee agrees, "We kind of get caught up in the family thing. We forget about each other. Paul watches TV and I worry about getting my daughter a bath and reading her a story."

Paul's evening ritual complicated matters further: He comes home, takes a nap, then watches TV and goes to bed. When they were on the diet, that all changed. First to go was Paul's television watching. "I said to him, come on, turn off the TV," says KaeCee. Next, they went to bed an hour earlier, which helped a lot in the fatigue department. As Paul says, "We didn't just go to bed at the usual time; we went to bed earlier because we had planned on it."

And once they were in bed, it didn't take much to keep them awake! They had a lot of fun with the Spice Menu. One night Paul drew KaeCee a hot bubble bath, but found they had run out of bath foam. He improvised instead and used Dawn, the dishwashing liquid. "It made great bubbles," Paul says jokingly, and it also made the whole mood more playful and fun. As KaeCee says, "Being on the diet is like someone planning a surprise party for you all the time!"

Paul didn't stop at giving KaeCee baths. As he became more aware of KaeCee's need to be romanced, he planned more surprises for her. "I learned that she likes to have special things done for her. Before I would just be lazy—you know,

"I learned that she likes to have special things done for her. Before I would just be lazy—you know, wanting to do the wham-bam-thank-you-ma'am. But now I know that she likes to have extra attention."

—PAUL

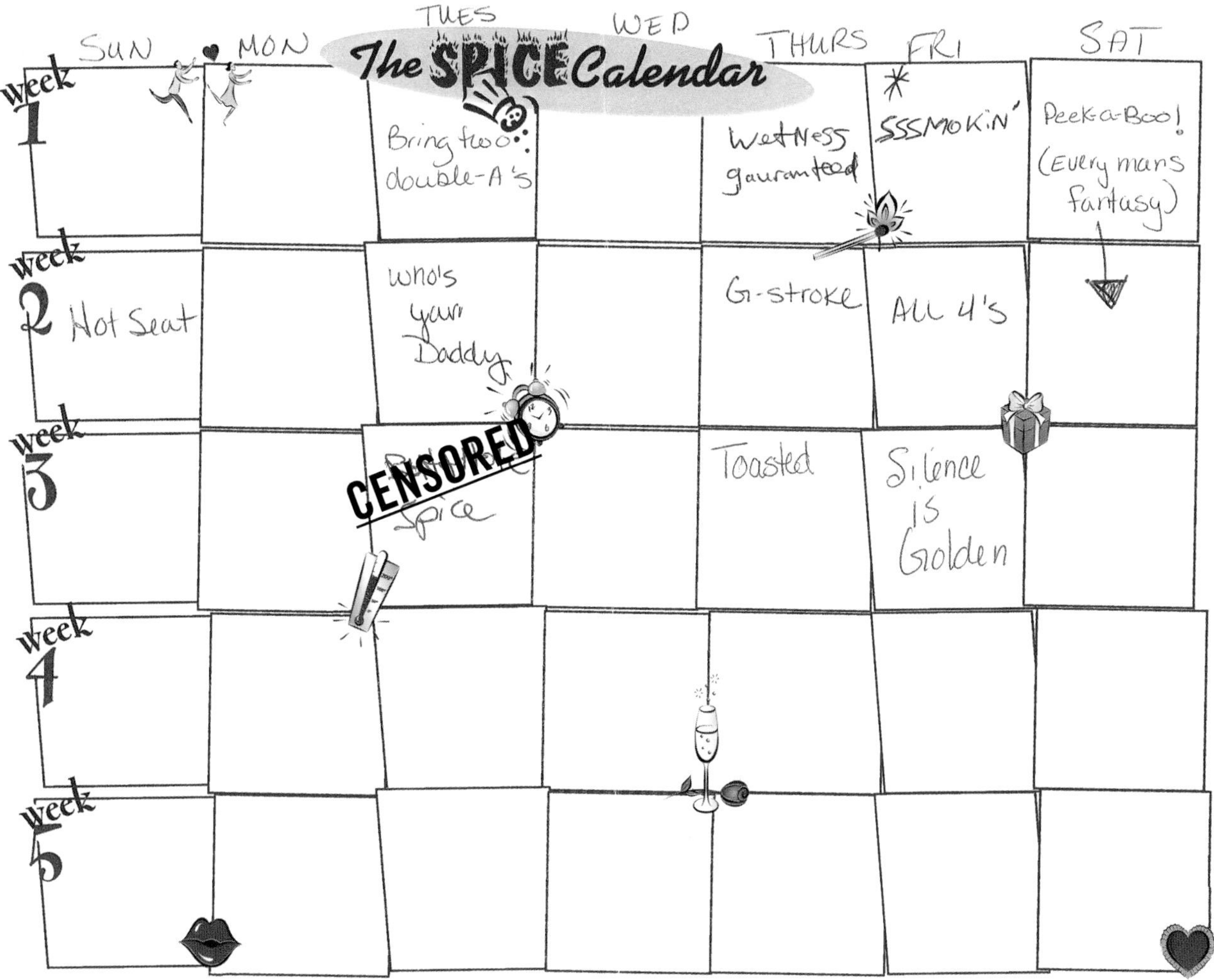

wanting to do the wham-bam-thank-you-ma'am. But now I know that she likes to have a massage and extra attention." Once he figured this out, Paul and KaeCee were back to their honeymoon schedule of sex four times a week!

I can relate to Paul. I never miss my favorite show, *Sex and the City* (what else?), but when I find myself night after night in front of the TV flipping channels, I remind myself that most of these shows are hardly on my must-see list.

TV is zone-out time. Although a lot of people watch it to relax, I think it's very important to keep a balance. So the next time you're thinking of turning on the tube, turn *on* your partner instead!

BEFORE THE DIET

"Food is part of the way I express love. After all these years, I still love making a great meal for Don and watching him enjoy it."

—Donna

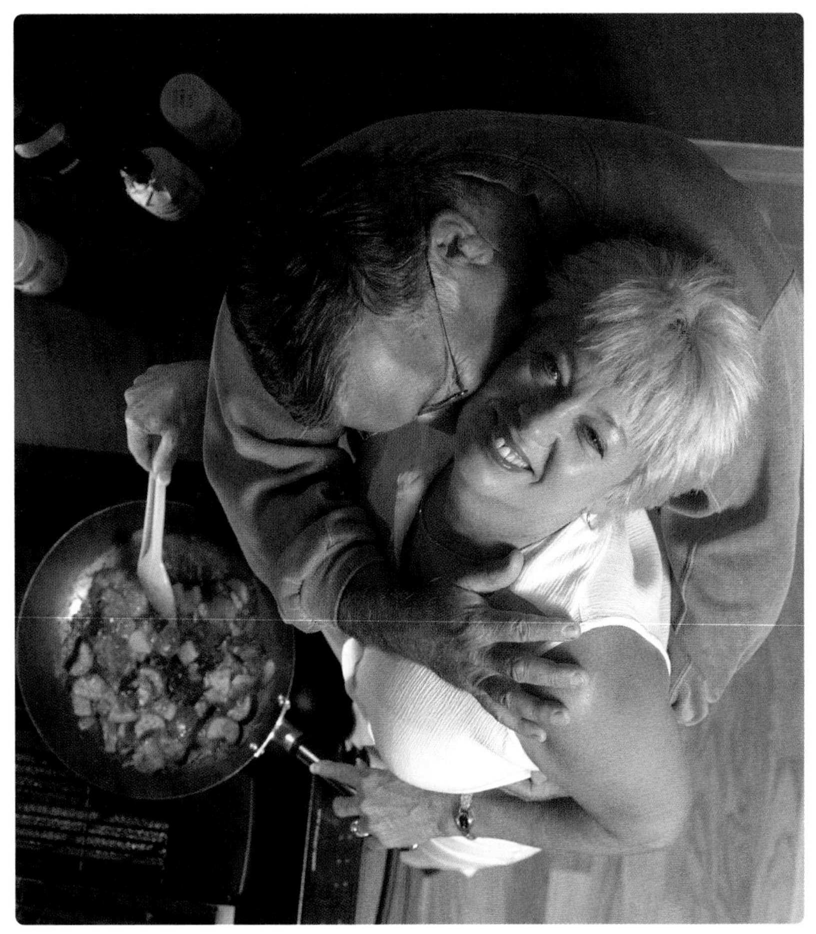

Love Feast

Don & Donna

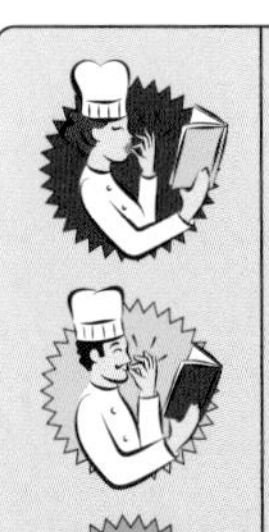

SHE: 50s, owns insurance agency

HE: 60s, retired teacher

STATUS: together 30 years, married 28 years; 5 kids—1 daughter together, 4 sons from his previous marriage

Sexual confidence is one of those much-sought-after characteristics that can make the best of us green with envy. When I met Donna, I was simply in awe of her sexual confidence. In our discussions about sex, she stated quite frankly that she doesn't see a reason to have sex unless she's going to have at least two orgasms. In fact, a couple of years

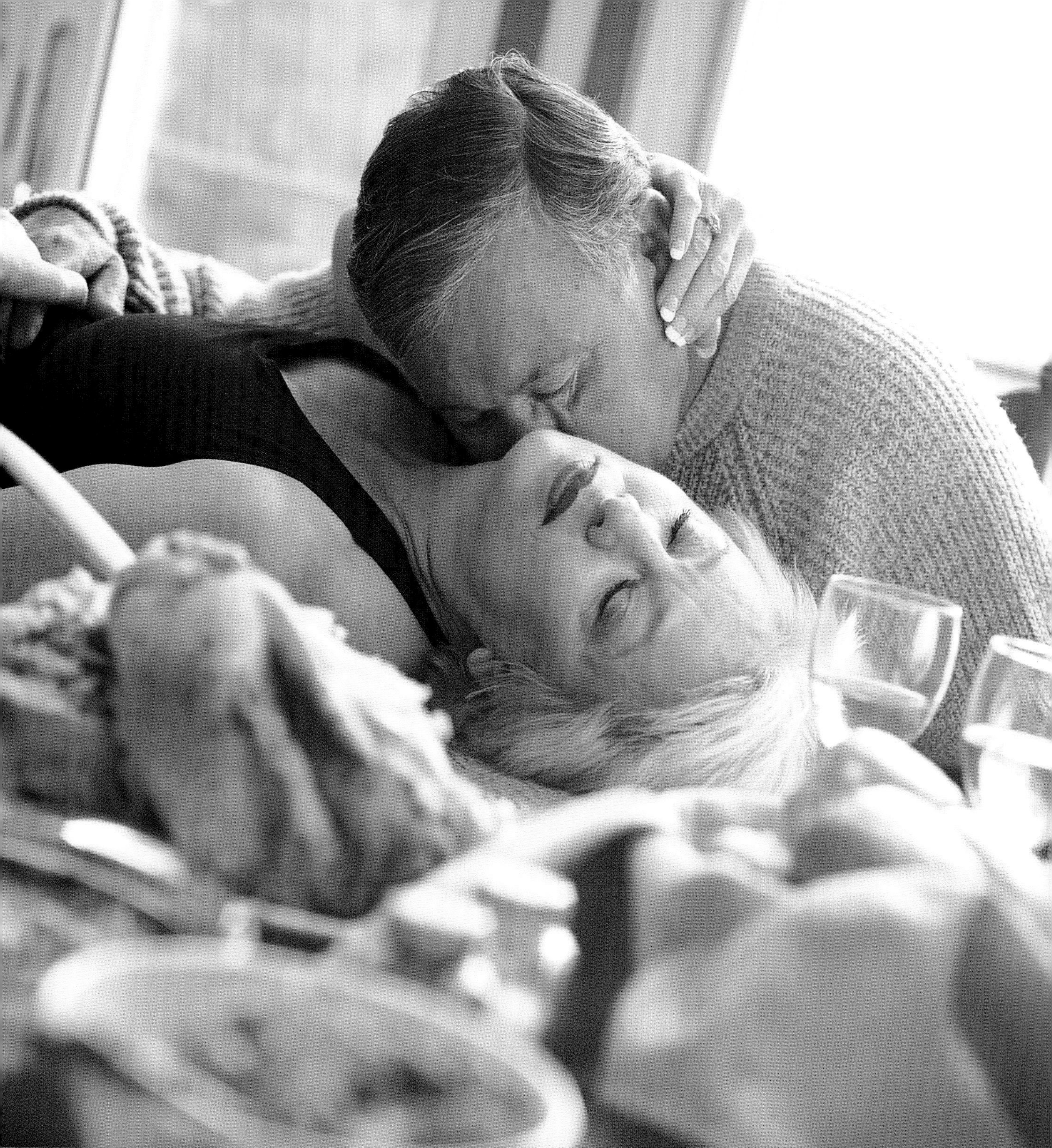

28 DAYS LATER

"This made us realize how much we enjoy sex and how important it is. The diet just kept getting juicier and juicier!"—Don

ago, when she noticed that it was suddenly harder to have her usual multiple orgasms, she immediately consulted her doctor and discovered that it was menopause-related. She quickly had the problem taken care of with hormonal cream. There was no way Donna was going to be cheated out of her orgasms. What a woman!

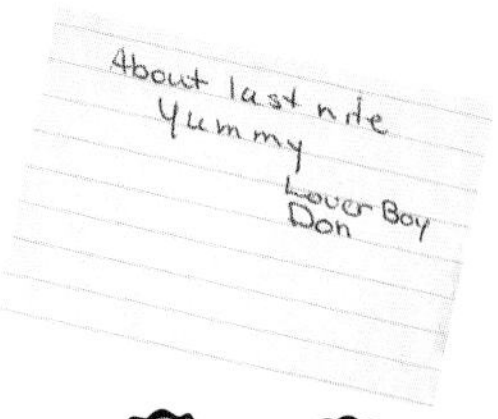

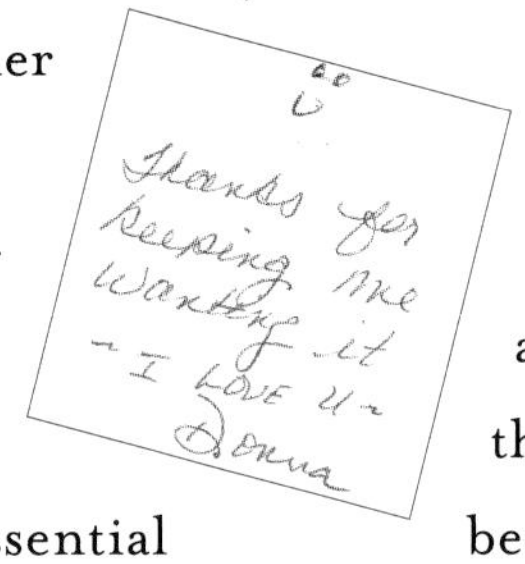

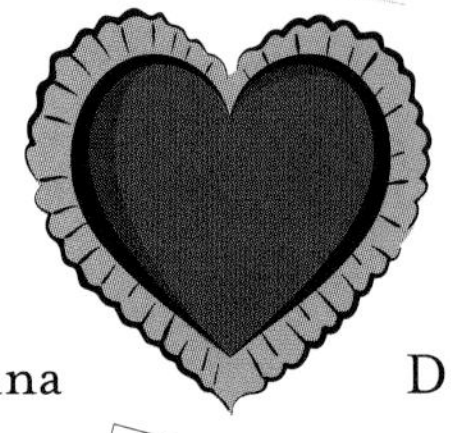

And Don is just as exciting a personality as his wife. Though he was a teacher for over twenty years, I like to think of Don as the quintessential Renaissance Man. He's taught kids, owned and operated a fruit stand, and worked as a photographer, creating multimedia pieces in which he synched his photos with sound.

Don and Donna were one of those couples who went from great to greater—emotionally, spiritually, and sexually. They met over thirty years ago, when Don was Donna's high school biology teacher (okay kids, you can stop that giggling now!), and, yes, they waited until two years *after* she had graduated to go on their first date. "When he kissed me," Donna says, recalling the dramatic moment, "I was very shocked because he used to be my biology teacher. But we were always mesmerized by each other and so as time went on, we started dating and that was the end of it." Or the beginning.

They have always found time for sex. Donna's philosophy is very clear: "It's always healthy to have sex because then you relax more and get satisfied. You also get closer to each other and don't get uptight and fight. I think a lot of people are fighting because they may need a good screw."

Like I said, Donna is a self-confident straight-shooter. When I ask her why she wants to try the Great American Sex Diet, she says, "I hope that it will rejuvenate us sexually. Because even though we have sex twice a week, we want to be more creative—it gets old hat after a while." They also want to "build each other up." As Don says, "Sex just helps the juices flow. It's a good tonic."

After they began the diet, Don immediately noted a shift in Donna. "I could tell she was enjoying the romance of it in a different way." When they tried a couple of spices, Donna

"We're aging together. And we dim our lights. We don't have them all the way off, but we dim them and that's arousing in itself. And we have music on. We like to create a mood."—Donna

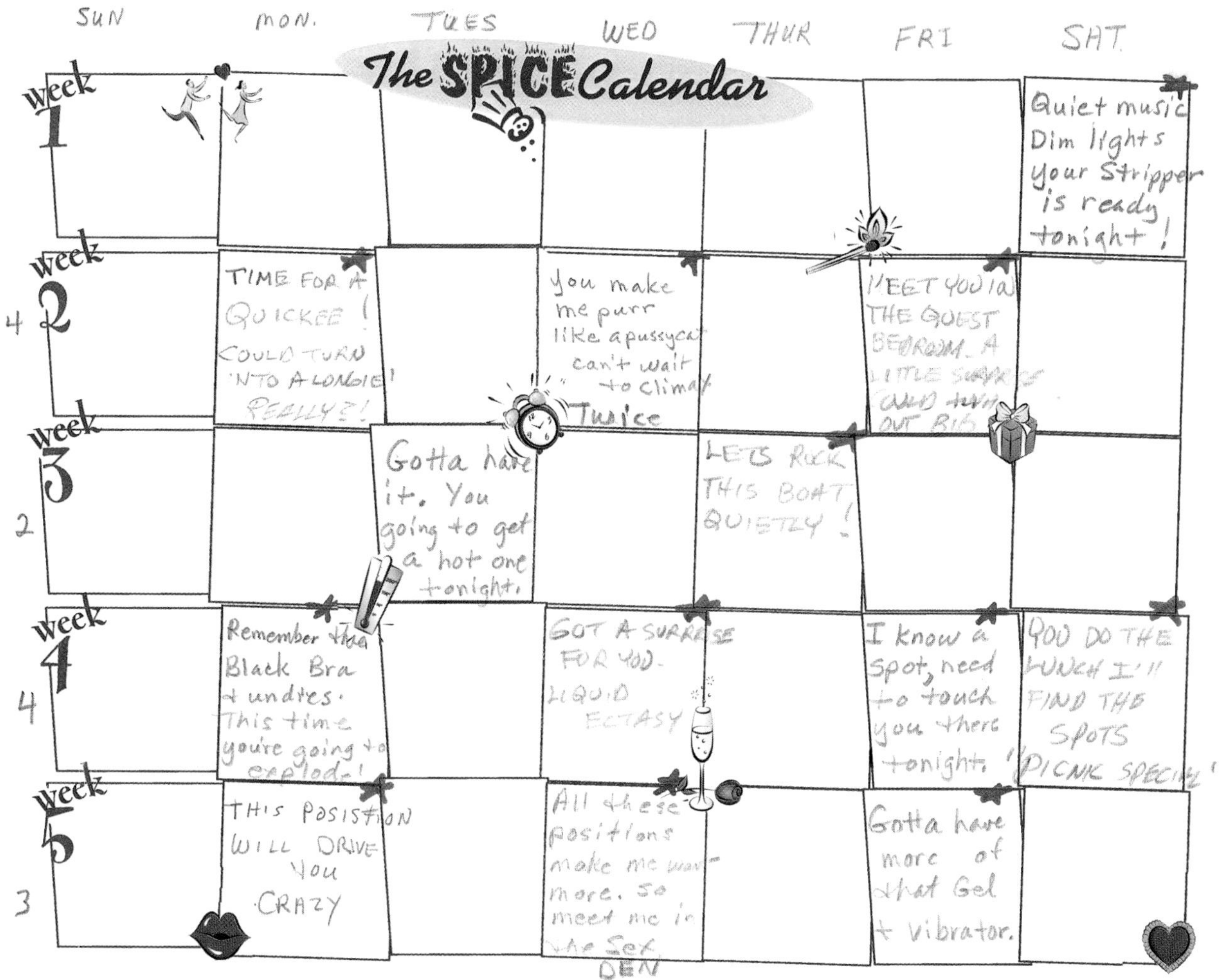

"When she wrote 'You make me purr like a pussycat . . . can't wait to climax twice' on the calendar, that really got me going!"—Don

says Don made her "purr like a pussycat."

They both played with the toy spices and Don in particular enjoyed experimenting with vibrators on Donna. "At this point, when we get going, it gets pretty intense, so we just kind of let the hormones take us where we want to go," Don explains, trying to put into words how sexually charged he and Donna became doing the spices. Donna found that she did a few sexual positions she hadn't done in a *long* time. "Don said that was a 'whoa'—you know, one of those things that you don't do anymore. We went forty-five minutes on one of them!"

Needless to say, Don and Donna found their route back to nirvana. As Don says, "We can still look at each other and know that there are no distractions. I just get to look at her real close, and *oh boy.* Those are the love moments that lead us into the sex moments."

BEFORE THE DIET

"We've had a very strong relationship for twenty-eight years. As you mature and grow together, you realize it's not the material things that really count—it's the spiritual things. It's the real love that bonds you."

—KIRK

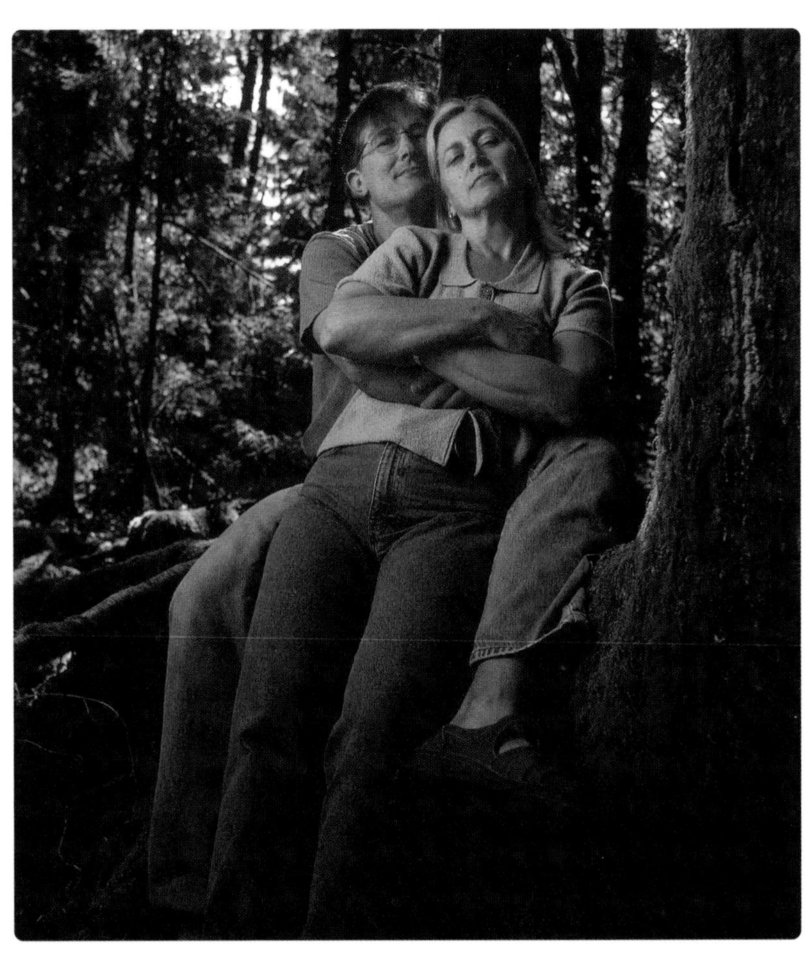

Jungle Boy

SHERRY & KIRK

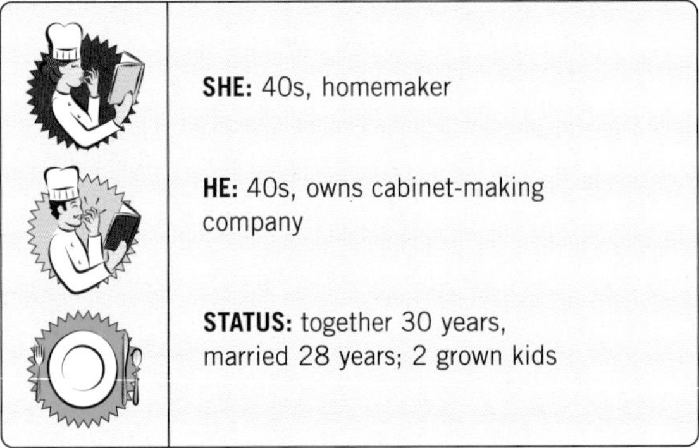

SHE: 40s, homemaker

HE: 40s, owns cabinet-making company

STATUS: together 30 years, married 28 years; 2 grown kids

I really envy Kirk and Sherry as a couple. What they've done with their lives is amazing. This is a couple who makes you say, "I wish I could be more like them. How do they do it?" And they make it look so easy! There is just something between them that's hard to define but impossible to miss: When you're in their presence, you can feel the love between them,

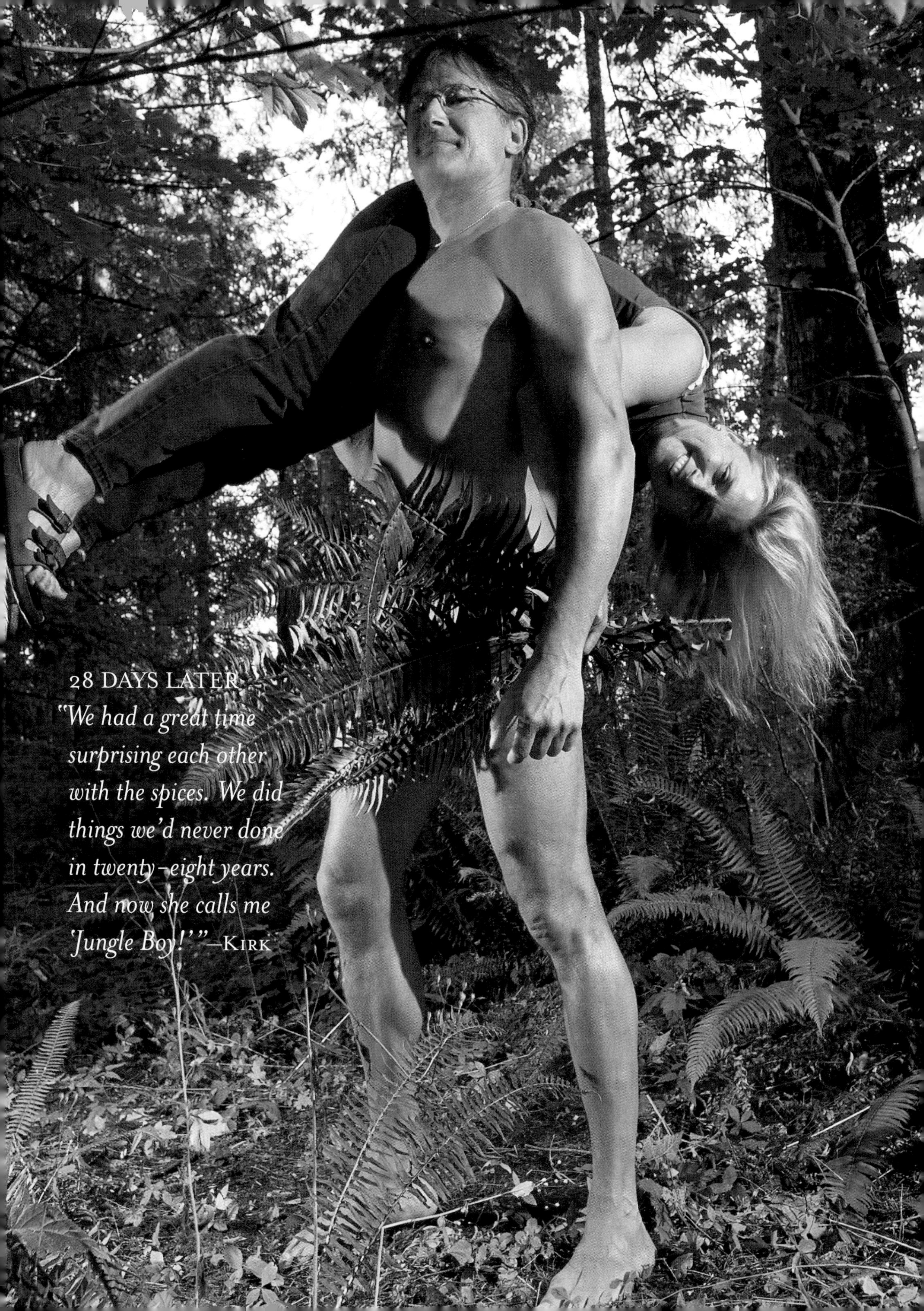

28 DAYS LATER

"We had a great time surprising each other with the spices. We did things we'd never done in twenty-eight years. And now she calls me 'Jungle Boy!'"—Kirk

which I know is rooted in a solid-as-a-rock foundation. The strength that pours out of them as a couple also reaches across any room and embraces anyone in their path!

Only in their forties, Kirk and Sherry have been together most of their adult lives. They had children young and are still young enough themselves to enjoy a very active life together—no empty nest syndrome for these two! Through their years together, they've built a very strong relationship that has weathered many storms. As a professional builder, Kirk is especially attuned to making a foundation strong and vital. He and Sherry even built the homes of their two adult children. "We feel a responsibility toward our kids," Kirk explains. "We brought them into the world, so we kind of felt like we needed to do more than just kick them out of the nest. I'm glad we were able to give them the start we gave them."

Kirk and Sherry have always had a great sex life, but like many couples who have been together a long time, their biggest challenge is trying to experience change as a positive rather than as a negative. You reach a point where, as Sherry explains, "it's easy to take each other for granted." Kirk says, "Over a period of time, it's the same old routine—over and over. Not just sex, but life in general."

So how do they keep the spirit of fun alive? They keep their doors wide open. I feel total admiration for not only Sherry's character and values but her ever-changing, continually blossoming sexuality. At a time when many women fall into a rut or get set in their ways, Sherry continues to stretch her sexual boundaries. And the diet helped her to stretch them even further. It brought out a sense of experimentation and playfulness in both of them.

Sherry set the tempo early in the diet by placing a leopard G-string in Kirk's gym bag. "I'm looking for my underwear after my workout, but can't find them anywhere," he

"Sherry thought she was very conservative. But now she's running around the house naked!"—KIRK

(S) = Sherry
(K) = Kirk

The SPICE Calendar

Week	Sun	Mon	Tues	Wed	Thurs	Fri	Sat
week 1	13th of Aug (S) Hidden Treasure in Hot Pursuit (combo) / (K) Late nite Thursday	(thighs whispers)			It's a (S) Jungle IV Here— (Fun with Fruit)	Late nite (K) Raiding the Refrigerator (Have it your way)	
week 2	(S) Finger Zinger / I'm going to touch you in places you didn't know you had!!	(K) Reclining "on" the Big Boy! (Erotic Rush)	(K) Thats the spot / Bring a pillow			Frid (K) Aft-Cabin Quickie (Round + Round) more to Cum (see Note)	(S) Designated Driver (Erotic Rush)
week 3	(S) Now this is a message / Body to Body message / (K) Dangerous when wet	(K) Surprise at top of Stairs (Location Spice)	(K) Lick'ity Split (From the Kama-Sutra) Candles + wine + music		(S) Double Your Pleasure / Sweet-Torture		
week 4				(K) Getting the Feel of Putting / Watching Golf Channel	(K) Total Control (Blindfold)	~~Pearl Lingus~~ who says there's Nothing Good ON (Video) Candida Royalle	Pearl Lingus / Blind Fold / Sept 10
week 5							

"One night, she wrote 'Pearl-Lingus' on the calendar. I knew she was going to surprise me with something different. She blindfolded me, then started doing something really unusual. I didn't know what she was doing, but pretty soon it started feeling really good!"—Kirk

recalls. "When I pull my shirt out, I see this leopard silk thing pinned to it, and I didn't even know what it was. I didn't know if it was a woman's panties or bra or what! And then I see a note attached that says, 'Go ahead and put them on.' I'm thinking, 'Yeah, right, I'm putting these on in front of all the guys? I don't even know if I'd put those on at home!'"

Sherry was very disappointed when Kirk came home without his G-string on. "He took me out to dinner and we talked about it when we got to the restaurant," she explains. "I said, 'Well, gee, if you had read the *inside* of the note, you would have put them on!' So he

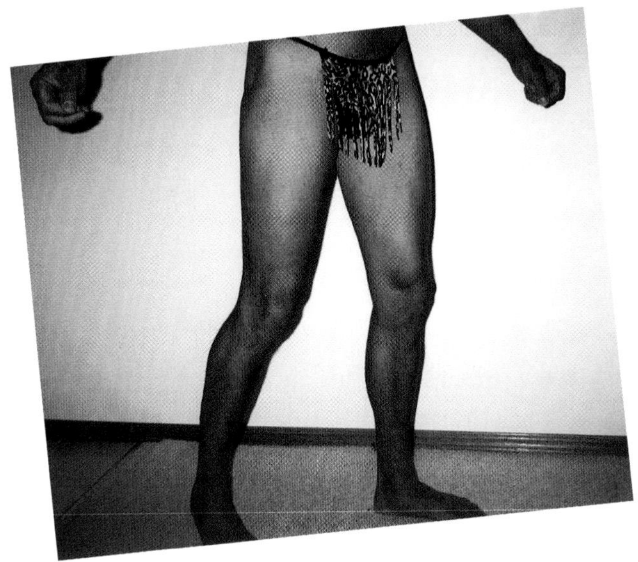

"I'm going to quit my job and just become a sex symbol." —Kirk/Jungle Boy

runs out to the car and finds the note, which says, 'Don't be worried about the other Jungle Boys, they're just jealous!'"

"Once I read the note and figured out they were men's underwear, I went straight into the men's room to change," Kirk says. And when he walked out, Sherry says he had a big smile on his face! As you can see from the after photo, this playfulness and experimentation awakened the "Jungle Boy" in Kirk. (Check out the photo above, too!)

Things reached another boiling point when Sherry rented an erotic video for the first time in her life. Kirk had been wanting to do this for all of their twenty-eight years but never wanted to push Sherry. On the diet, Sherry was suddenly game. When they were in the video store picking out the video, Kirk said to the salesgirl, "Isn't this sex diet great? My wife's renting me videos!"

As soon as they started pulling out of the store parking lot, Sherry said, "Now, honey, don't speed because you're so excited about getting home to watch these!"

"I was so excited, because this was something I never in my wildest dreams thought she'd do for me," Kirk says. "And when we got home, we popped in one of the videos and watched it about halfway through. But what happened after that was even better than the video!"

Kirk and Sherry's adventurous spirit continues to inspire and amaze me. After twenty-eight years, *they've still got it.*

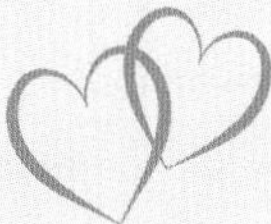

WITNESS TESTIMONY

Kirk and Sherry and the previous couple, Don and Donna, decided to do something different and go on the diet at the same time. Each couple was amazed at the other's transformation. Here are Don's observations on the experience.

"Sharing the diet with another couple was fun. It brought out the romance in all of us, and broke down our inhibitions. It made our friendships a little deeper, too. I really noticed a difference in Kirk and Sherry when they were on the diet. They just wanted to touch more. They had a spark in their eyes when they looked at each other and would smile with their own private communication. I think it really rejuvenated them. They had a lot of surprises along the way. A lot of the stuff they did was pretty amazing, because, in nearly thirty years, they had never been so experimental. I think they've found out that they were in love with each other even more than they thought. And that's what a good sex life does." —DON

"The menu opened up my mind to do other things that I wouldn't normally do, that maybe I thought would be kinky. But then you learn to open up and experiment with new things and it's really fun. We had a great time surprising each other."—KIRK

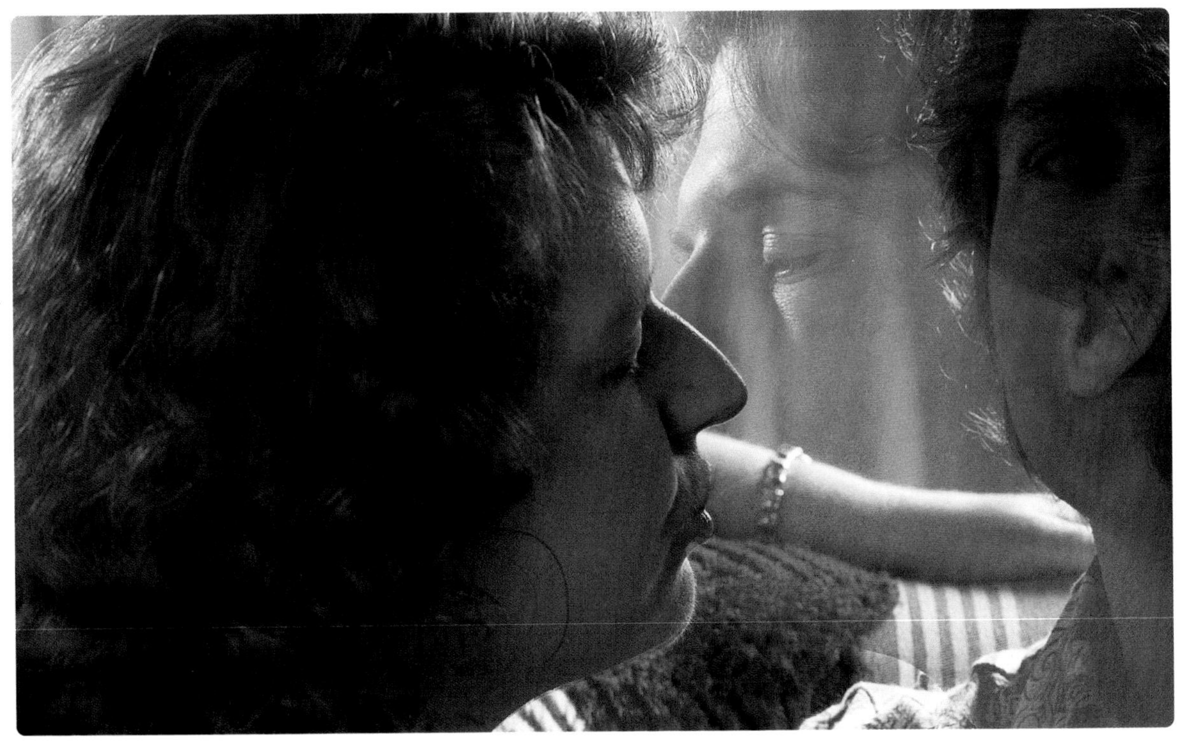

BEFORE THE DIET

"We have very conflicting schedules. And by the time we do everything we need to do, there's no time left for us."—Paul

Diet Detour

Erika & Paul

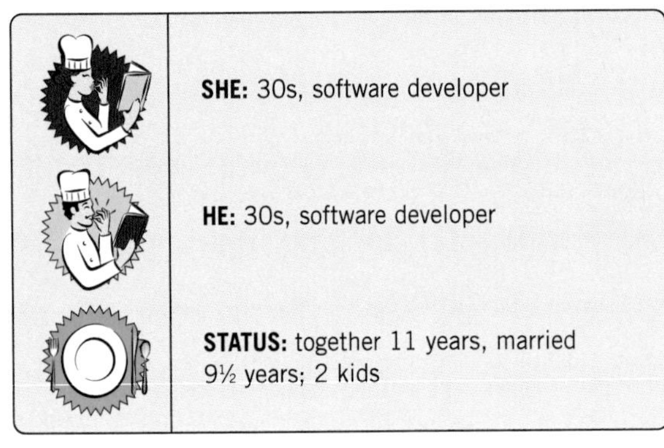

Paul and Erika, unfortunately, were unable to complete the diet due to health reasons. However, they did begin the diet with vigor and enthusiasm and seemed bound and determined to get out of their rut and learn to feel more connected, especially sexually. Like so many couples, Paul and Erika say that part of the problem is that they fall into communication ruts. "We try to work them out instead of just shoving them under the rug and letting them build up. But sometimes it just cascades into other problems," explains Erika.

Take a look at their before photo: They're together but apart. They had such busy lives (especially Paul) that everything came between them. Serious about their relationship, they sought out counseling, yet they still weren't able to get their relationship on track. Then they turned to the Great American Sex Diet, figuring it was the perfect way to surprise each other more and find more creativity. They were also interested in seeing how the increased frequency would affect them. "Going from two times to four times a week seems like a stretch, but we wanted to try," says Erika.

Paul says that Erika's energy, or a lack thereof, has always been a problem. He says that Erika often doesn't have the energy "to want to participate" in sex. In fact, about four and a half years ago, Paul had become so frustrated with Erika's low desire that he thought of actually leaving, but he ultimately decided against it. As he says, "I was raised in a family where you never said good-bye. That's just unheard of. I would rather sever one of my limbs." Yet he does admit having felt enormous frustration with Erika's lack of interest in sex.

On the diet, Erika had began to turn around her low desire and initiate more frequently, including trying new spices on Paul. But two weeks into the diet, Paul became ill—just as they were beginning to see wonderful results! One night as Paul was walking by their bathroom, Erika called to him: "She turned to me while she was getting ready for bed and said, 'You've got to get better. We've got to get back on the diet!'"

Unfortunately, this illness was no temporary interruption; it developed into pneumonia, and Paul needed all his energy to recuperate. To complicate their ability to complete the diet even more, as soon as Paul was up and walking around, he had to travel to Russia on a goodwill mission to deliver food and clothing to children in remote villages. No easy trip, this was a major undertaking, showing not only Paul's enormous commitment to his work but also his compassion and dedication to helping people.

Even though Erika and Paul weren't able to complete the diet this time, they told me they really want to give it another try in the future, and I have no doubt they will be in the next edition of this book!

BEFORE THE DIET

"It's hard finding time for just the two of us without any other people around—children, pets, or anyone. It's kind of difficult when they're pounding on the door, saying, 'What are you guys doing in there?'"

—DYAN

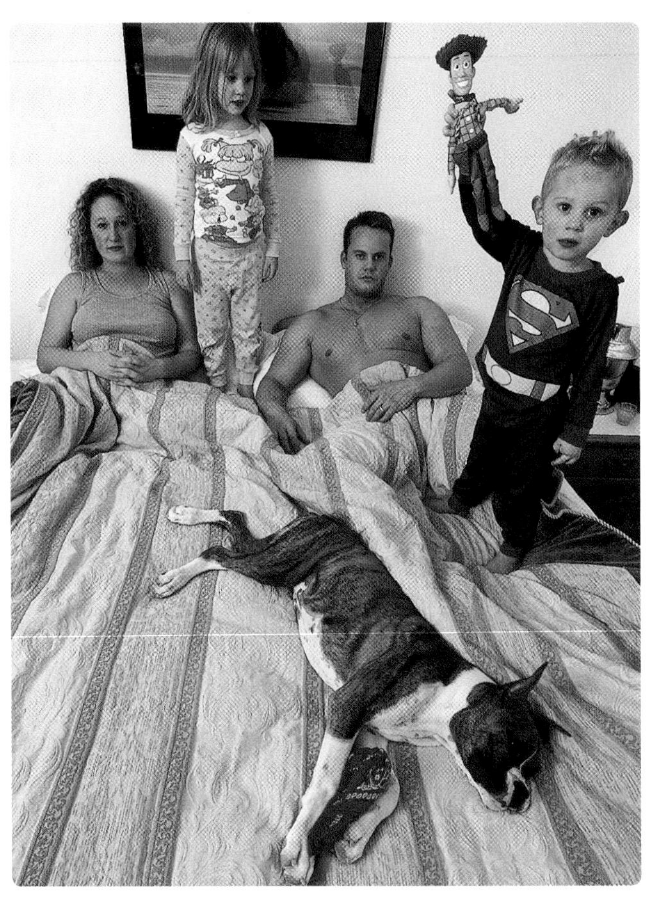

A Kiss Is Not Just a Kiss

DYAN & SHANE

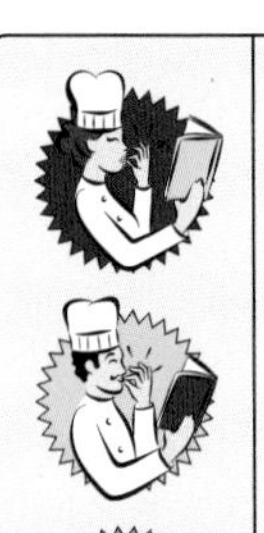

SHE: late 20s, day care owner

HE: late 20s, hydraulic sales, professional body builder

STATUS: together 13 years, married 6 years; 2 kids

In today's world, it is rare and charming to meet couples who not only were high school sweethearts but also virgins when they married. The love between Dyan and Shane is so obvious and tangible that I noticed it as soon as I spoke with them. Since that day, I've continued to be impressed by the specialness of their bond.

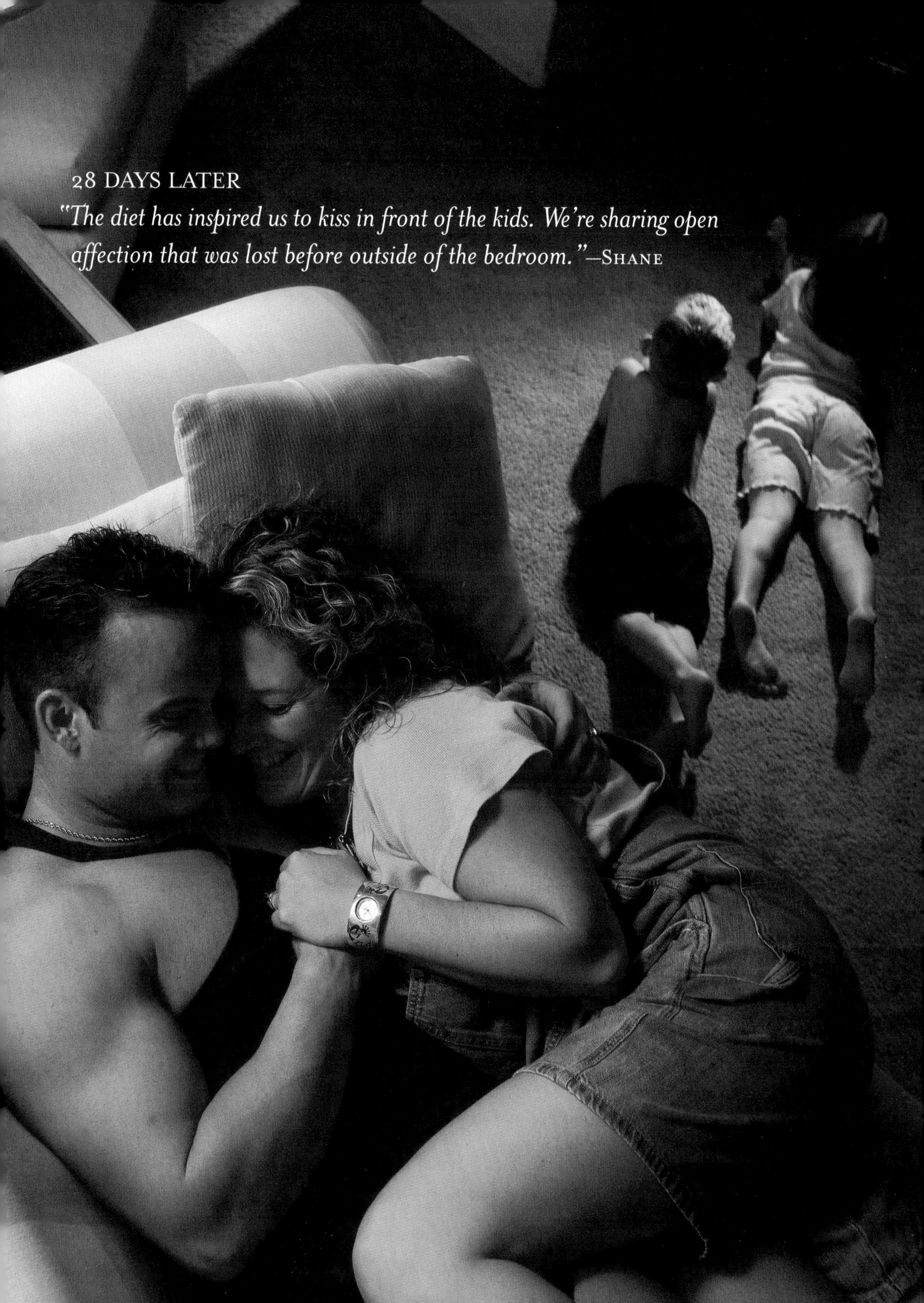

28 DAYS LATER

"The diet has inspired us to kiss in front of the kids. We're sharing open affection that was lost before outside of the bedroom."—SHANE

The biggest obstacle to making love as much as they would like is their two children. If they could, they'd make love every day, but before the diet all they could manage were sporadic moments of pleasure.

Most of the time Dyan waits for Shane to make the first move. Dyan explains that when they are not being physically intimate (like when Shane is training for a body-building championship), "I feel a loss of connection with him. I feel there's a big void and it becomes very tense between us. And then I start thinking that I must not be attractive to him anymore. You know, you think the worst."

For his part, Shane gets frustrated and would like Dyan to initiate more. So when they began the diet they were looking for a way to jump-start their relationship.

Interestingly enough, their major breakthrough revolved around something quite simple: kissing in front of the kids. As owner of a day care center, Dyan is surrounded by at least sixty-five kids a day, in addition to her own children. Before the diet, she was anxious and reluctant to show any affection toward Shane in front of the kids. But what she discovered on the diet was that her children responded really positively to seeing their parents kiss and hug. "The kids were playing in their bedroom and we were on the couch kissing," Dyan recalls. "They came out to check on us three different times. It was so cute!"

Dyan is excited and much more at ease with this open attitude toward affection, and I've got to say I am thrilled. To me, when parents are open about their love and affection, it's a positive: Kids grow up with a warm, healthy attitude toward sex and love between adults. Now, in their house, whenever they say good-bye to one another, there is always a group hug and kiss!

Shane also believes in the power of kissing, not simply as great foreplay but also as a path to creating that special intimacy that leads to deeper, more heartfelt sex. He says, "Being on the diet brought us back to the dating stage. It gave us something to look forward to and was like having a Friday night date *four nights a week.*"

And they absolutely *loved* their secret menus. On their anniversary, they stayed overnight in a hotel and pretty much shocked each other by doing five spices (that means having sex five times!) in twenty-four hours! Talk about taking advantage of being away from the kids!

"When we got to our suite, there was supposed to be a bottle of champagne on ice waiting for us, but it wasn't there yet," Dyan recalls. "So we went into the bedroom and ripped each other's clothes off. Shane did the Total Control spice on me and I

The SPICE Calendar

	Sunday	Monday	Tuesday	Wednesday	Thursday	Friday	Saturday
week 1			22	23 Lunch is on me! "literally"	24 Nooner "Ready or not here I…"	25	26 Sex Marathon!! Room Service Tonight!
week 2	27 *6 yr Anniversary I'm not sore yet!	28	29 Are you up for a little squeeze play action?	30	31 Here kitty kitty kitty	1 I want to hear you beg!	2 Shave for me!
week 3	3	4 Caution: Things may get sticky		6 It's hump day! Wear your favorite undies	7	8 Meet me in the pool at 10. Suits	9 Home Alone!! ? Hmmm?
week 4	10 Slippery When Wet		12 Wear High Heels!	13	14 You won't want me to stop!	15 Bring Handcuffs	16 Are you feeling nasty?
week 5	17	18 Multiple treats ahead!	19 Honey I'm a sure thing!				

"When someone seduces you, it's instant proof that somebody wants you and you're desired just the way you are. You may not be happy with the way you look, but there's your proof right there."—Dyan

just about flew off the bed. Things got pretty wild . . . and *loud*, too. When we came out of the bedroom an hour or so later, the bottle of champagne was there. The room service guy had dropped it off in the middle of our marathon session, and we didn't even hear him! But I have no doubt he heard *us*. I'm still blushing about that one!"

Funny moments such as this one helped Shane and Dyan keep the spark alive. But the key to the diet's success for them was their decision to kiss in front of the kids. "We're sharing open affection that was lost before outside of the bedroom," Shane says. This will no doubt impact their children's future relationships forever, giving them strength, security, and confidence. Everybody in their household wins.

BEFORE THE DIET

"We're so far apart right now with the kids and all the things we have to do, sex is probably the furthest thing from our minds. Hopefully the diet will give us the time to be closer together."

—MIKE

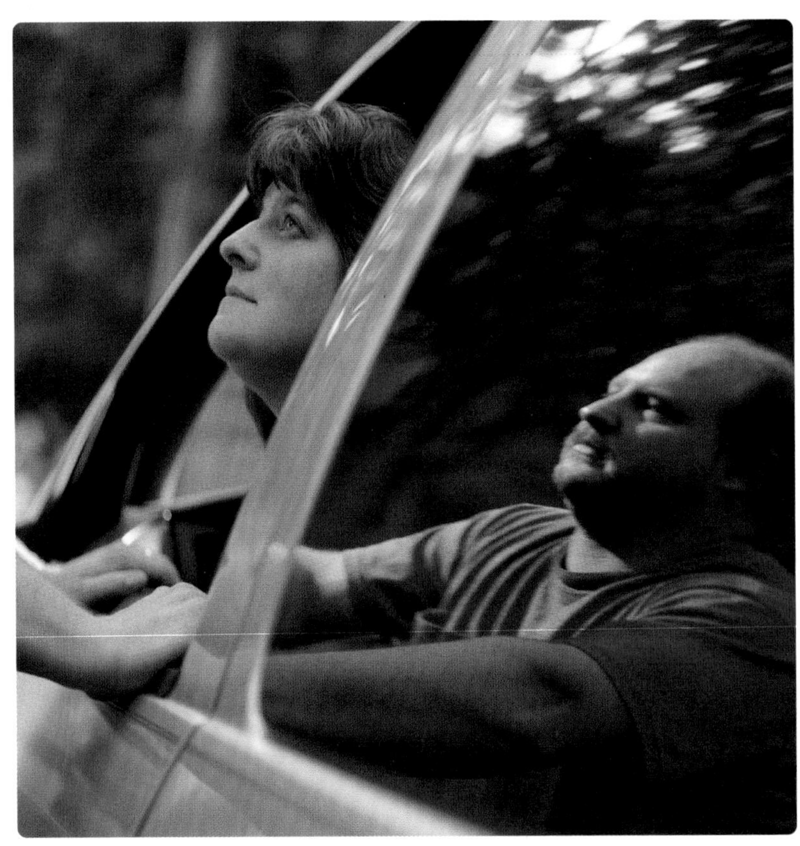

Foxy Roxy Is Back

ROXANNE & MICHAEL

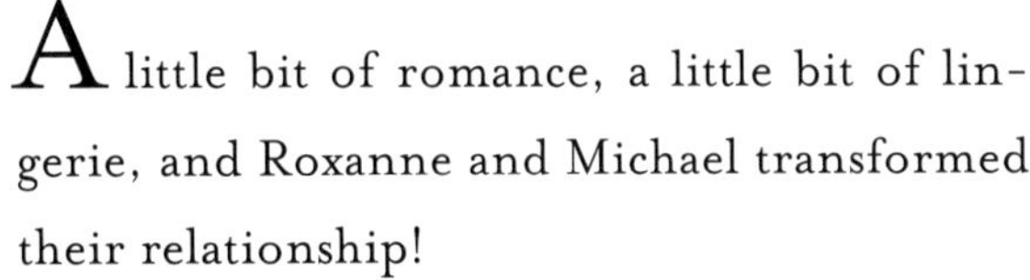

A little bit of romance, a little bit of lingerie, and Roxanne and Michael transformed their relationship!

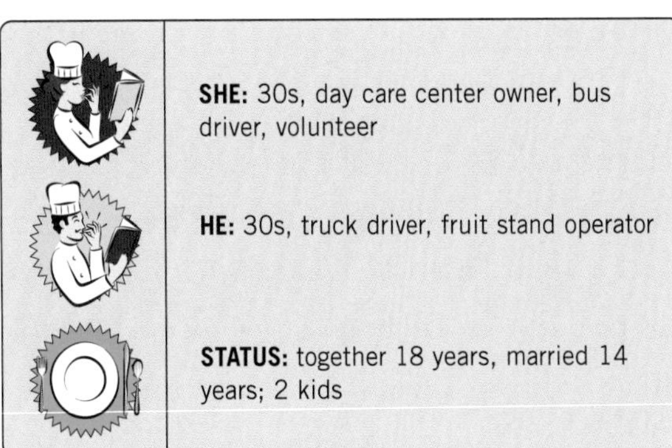

One of the most striking things about Michael and Roxanne is the fact that they both work at least eighty hours a week on average. Now, these two are busy! As Michael says in frustration, "We're so far apart right now with the kids and all the things we have to do . . . Hopefully the diet will give us the time to be

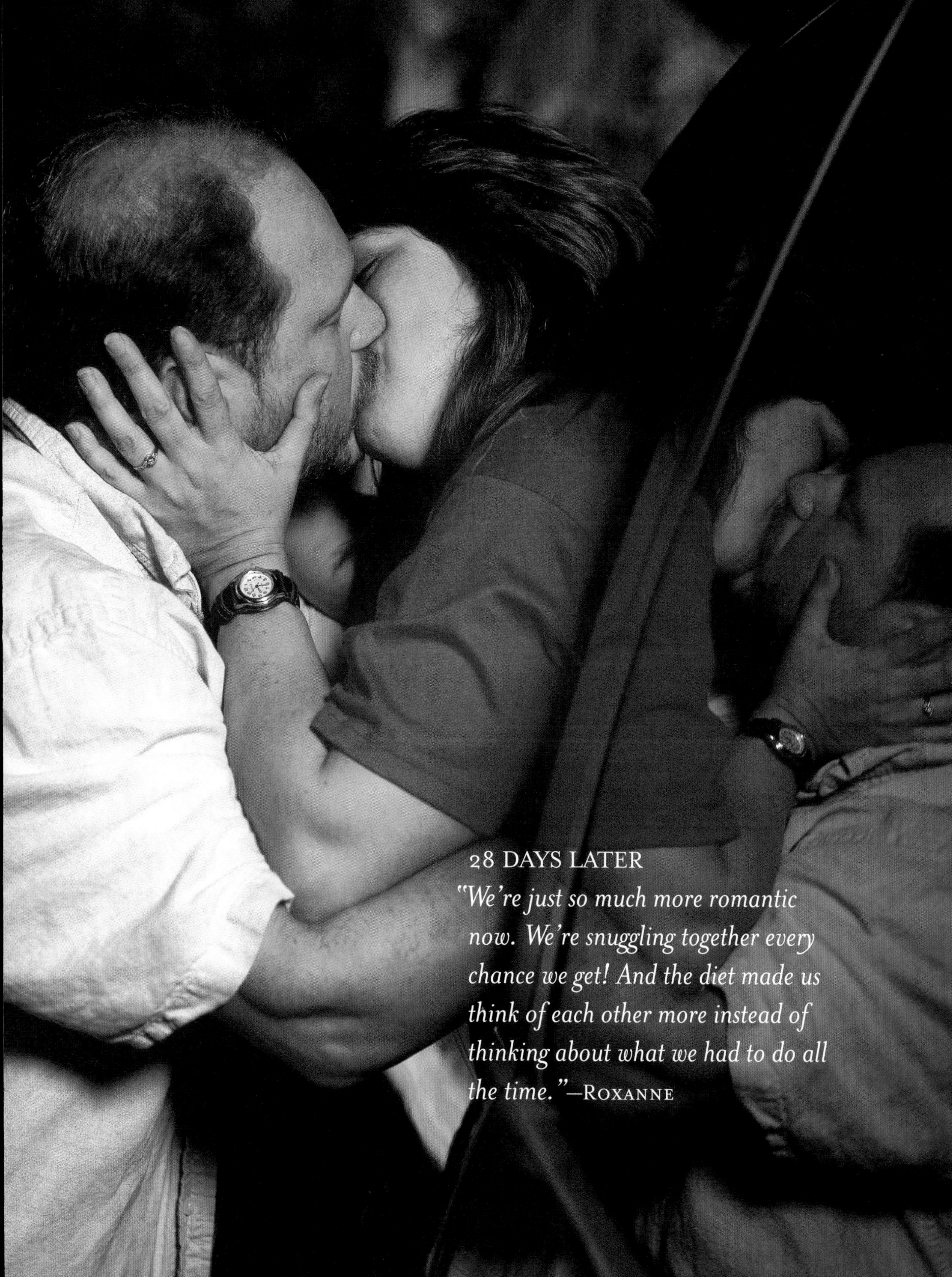

28 DAYS LATER

"We're just so much more romantic now. We're snuggling together every chance we get! And the diet made us think of each other more instead of thinking about what we had to do all the time."—Roxanne

closer together." But he remains hesitant about scheduling sex. He says it feels like "something else to do—more work." Like so many of us, he still harbors that wish that sex would just happen spontaneously. I explain that if you wait for that spontaneous sex to happen, you may find yourself waiting for a long time!

Roxanne, on the other hand, is very optimistic about scheduling. For her, the hardest part of keeping a relationship alive is "making time for sex." Because she's so tired and stressed by the end of the day, she finds herself "hiding, hoping that he's not going to want it."

Another factor that made her want to avoid sex was her weight. In the past year she had given up smoking and stopped working out as frequently as she used to and consequently, she'd gained weight. "I began to think he can't possibly think I'm sexy if I'm shaking all over," Roxanne explains. "I didn't want him to look at me because I don't want anything shaking that isn't supposed to be shaking."

I've met and talked to countless women whose self-esteem is directly tied to their weight. When they gain weight, their self-esteem plummets. And with that, so does their comfort with themselves sexually. But being on the diet helped Roxanne turn around her attitude. When I asked her about the last twenty-eight days, she said, "It was sexy. As Michael said, 'Everything's all good!'"

Both she and Michael got totally into the spices and became particularly drawn to any spice that contained water or oil. Their absolute favorite was Dangerous When Wet—they really made a splash with that one!

Michael and Roxanne do have a serious side and were quite sentimental about how the diet brought them closer together. As Michael says, "We're thinking of each other more instead of ourselves." I think this is no small feat in a day and age when we are so bombarded with information that tells us to "take care of yourself first!" I mean, how is a relationship going to work if you don't put your partner before yourself? Isn't that what we all want from our lover?

Michael and Roxanne also became

"When you have a secret Spice Menu, you both know where you're getting your ideas from. That way, your spouse doesn't think, 'What kind of loony pervert are you?' when you try something different. It's okay and legit to do wacky things because it's on the menu."

—Roxanne

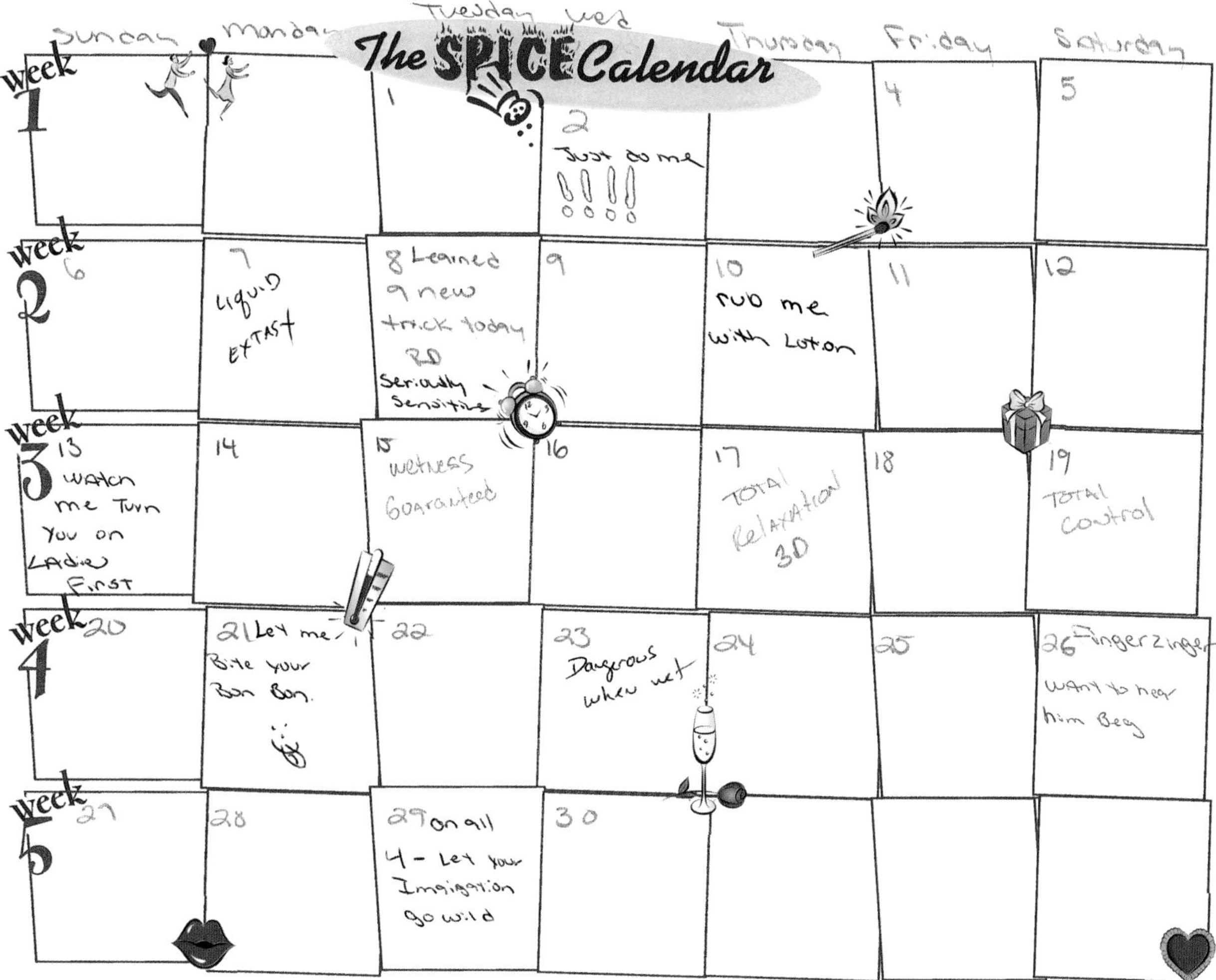

"Every morning I write myself a honey-do list and, believe you me, I get my list done. If I don't put lovemaking on there, it ain't going to get done!"—Roxanne

more romantic with each other. Roxanne found herself writing love notes and taping them to the refrigerator, or putting them on the wipe-off board. She also bought him special little gifts. One gift she bought she actually wore: new sexy lingerie. "Because I had gained weight, I hadn't been wearing any. And I thought, you know what, I'm just going to buy a bigger size because I know I'm going to look good," she says. "And now I just feel sexier!"

Michael and Roxanne opened up their relationship and took it to another level. Michael says about relationships in general, "My whole theory is that the more physical contact you have, the more closeness you have to each other." And Roxanne's parting words? "Have fun and *bon appétit!*"

BEFORE THE DIET

"We work between twelve to fourteen hours a day, so it's hard finding intimate time for each other."

—WALT

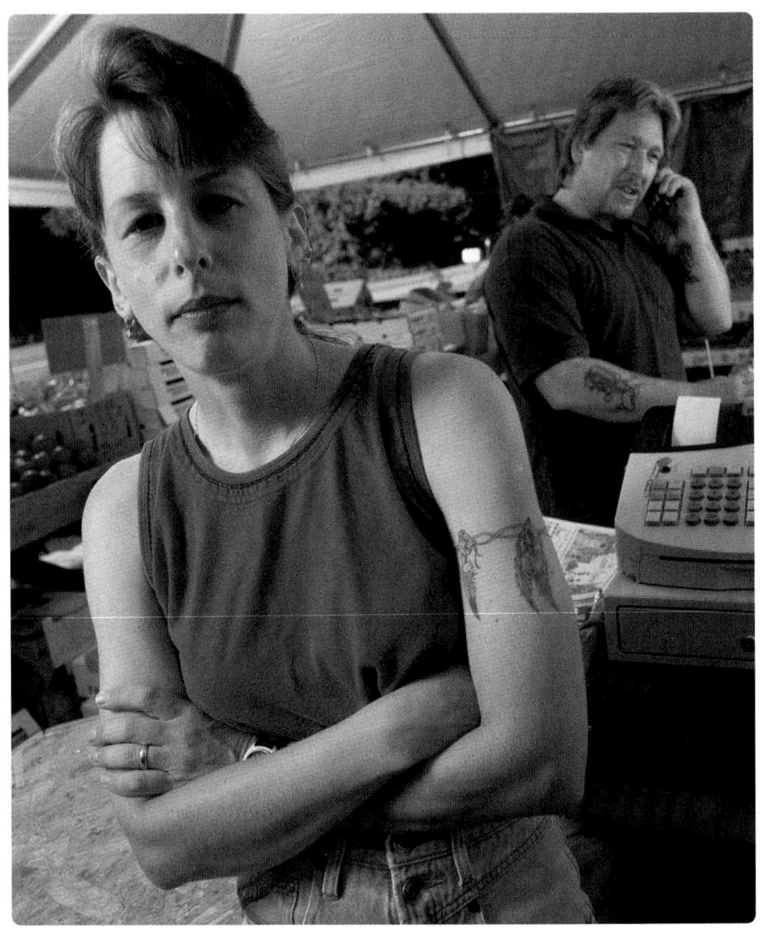

Peaches and Cream

RANA & WALTER

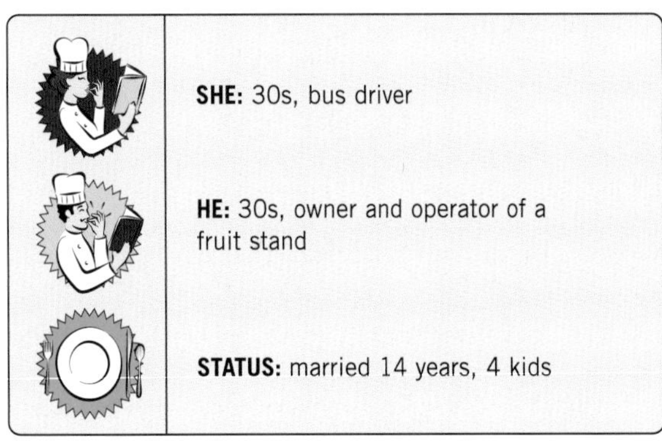

SHE: 30s, bus driver

HE: 30s, owner and operator of a fruit stand

STATUS: married 14 years, 4 kids

Rana and Walt are one of those couples who just bubble with energy—that is, if you ignore their sex life. But, boy, did that turn around on the diet!

On the diet, Rana and Walt went from having sex once a month to twelve times a month. Why? With four kids and hectic schedules, they used to have difficulty finding

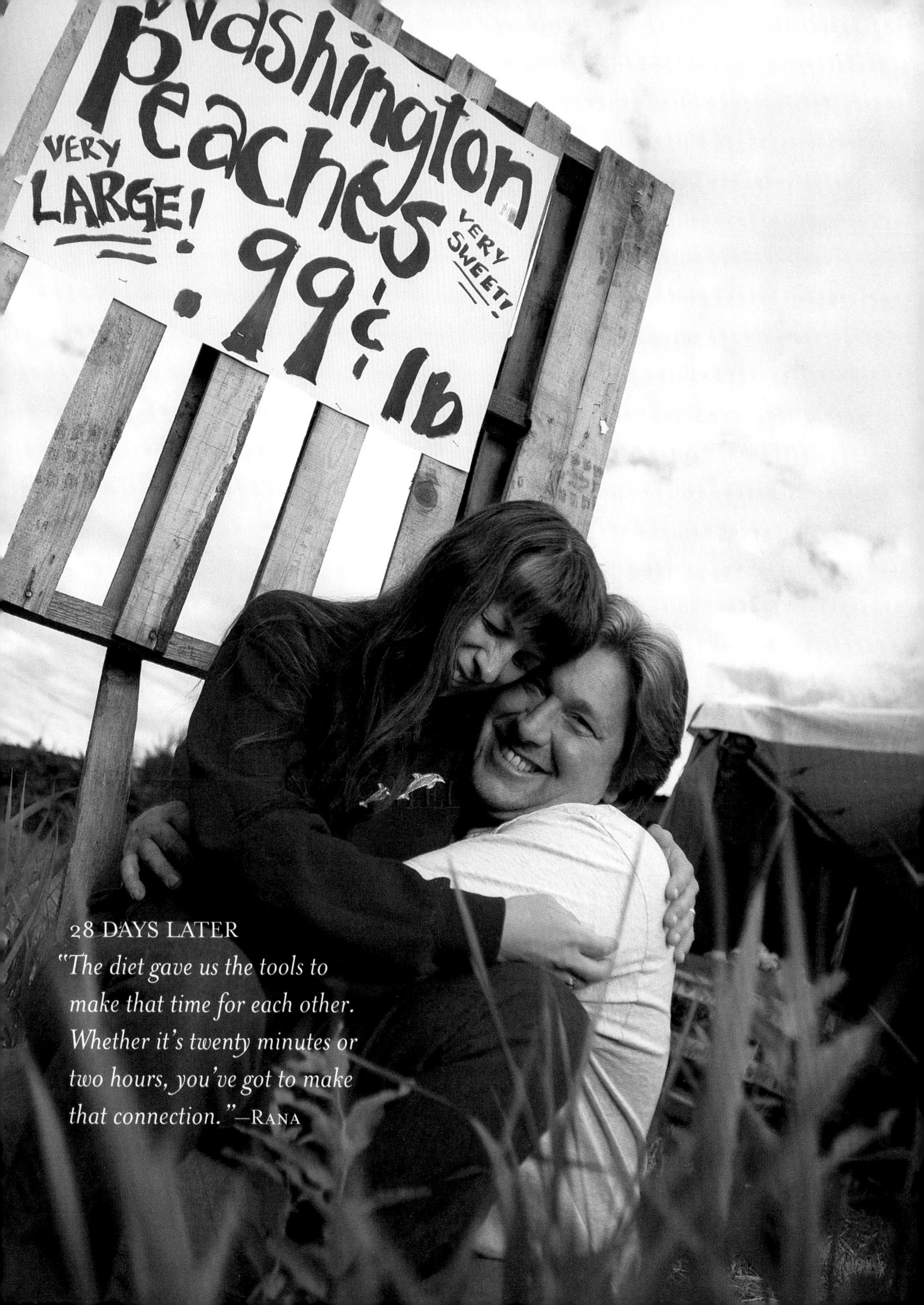

28 DAYS LATER

"The diet gave us the tools to make that time for each other. Whether it's twenty minutes or two hours, you've got to make that connection."—Rana

time to breathe—much less breathe life back into their relationship. And when they did manage to squeeze in a few minutes for a romp, Rana says there was an aspect of boredom that had crept in for both of them. Walt agrees: "It seems like you get to a point where everything is ho-hum. And sex is just another night of sex." But the Spice Menu forced them to think outside the box and be creative. "The menu gave me new ideas and new things to do," Walt says. "And I appreciated that because it took the pressure off. I loved trying spices like Hocus Poke Us and the Clock Technique. I had an ear-to-ear grin when I'd get done—and so would she!"

Hocus Poke Us not only made Rana sing with pleasure, it also made Walt realize they needed a new bed. "Our bed was too short. So we ended up grappling for each other all over the place. It was a gas trying to get everything coordinated. You know, you've got to have a sense of humor about these things!" I could hear the hilarity in Walt's voice—you just know they were having a blast with that spice!

"There are so many things on the menu that turn me on. When I'm feeling tired, I can actually look at the menu and it brings me back up. And the next thing you know, my imagination is running wild."

—Walt

Being on the diet helped Rana feel more sensual, too. "To be in the mood, I've got to Crock-Pot all day," she explains. "I have to simmer. And just knowing we were going to do it later that night helped me to do that." Like so many women I've spoken with, Rana relied on the anticipation of having sex to get her in the mood. Knowing they were going to make love heightened their anticipation and made them breathless, waiting for their intimate time together. Unlike some couples who really got into scheduling sex, Rana and Walt used the calendar differently. "Scheduling sex made me feel like I was at work and writing out an order," Walt explains. "Like I just wrote a fruit order and now I've got to fulfill it. For me, I like more spontaneity. Put some peaches on the rack and let's make some cream!"

Though Walt and Rana chose to use the calendars in an unconventional way, filling them out *after* they had sex, they still had

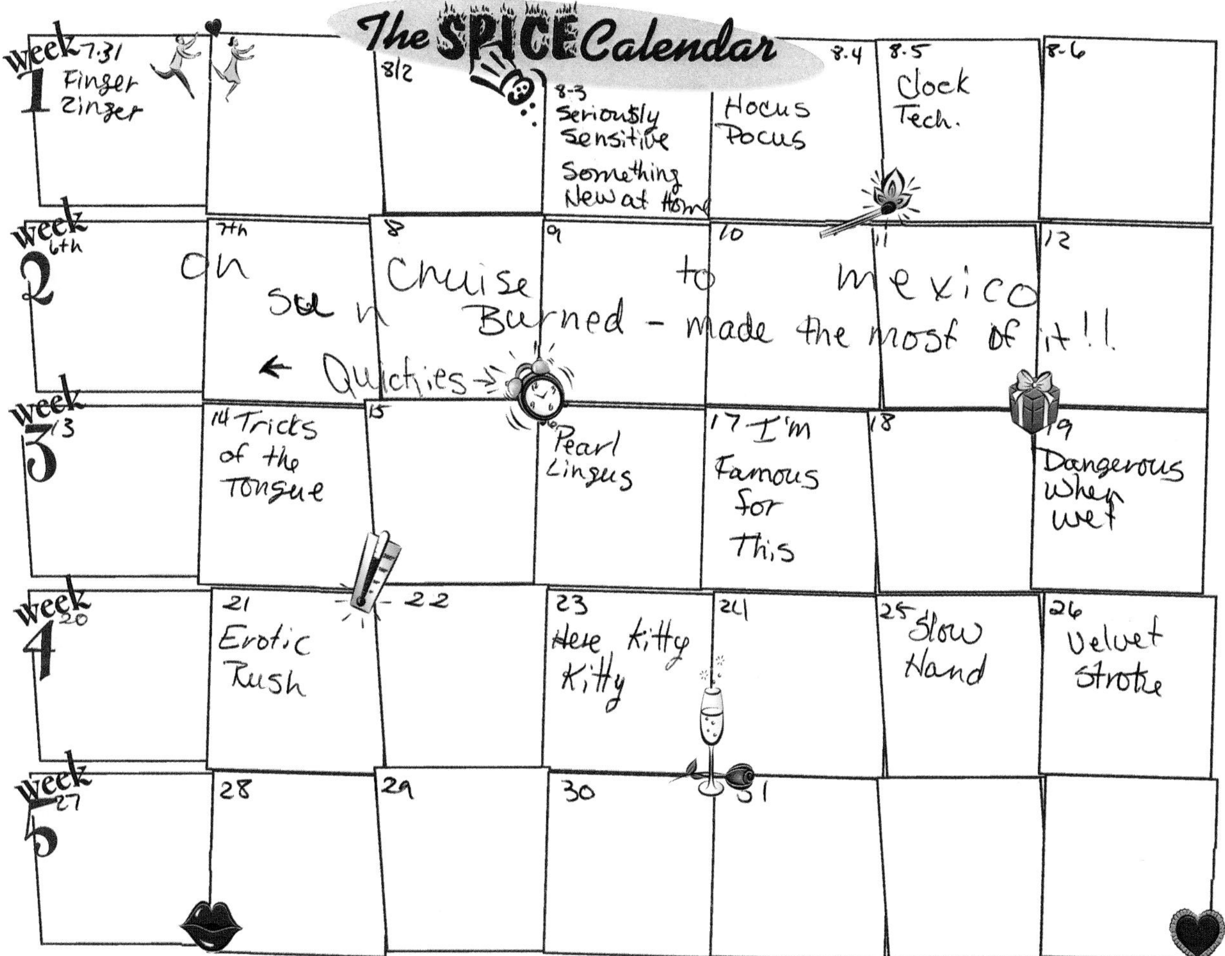

"We used the calendar to keep track of what spices we surprised each other with instead of to actually schedule them. Afterward I'd say, 'What was that spice called, honey?' Then I'd write it in for that day."—Rana

frequent sex! They made love *twelve times* more than they normally do and consider themselves to be highly successful on the diet. "I've learned that intimate moments are very important, and you need to have them more than once or twice a month," Rana says. "When the work and the school and the parenting responsibilities are all over and done with and everybody goes home, it's just the two of you and you've got to have something. And now I realize I want to take that time for just us."

Walt also had a revelation of his own. "After having so much sex for four weeks, I don't think we'll ever go back to having sex once a month," Walt declares. "Never again."

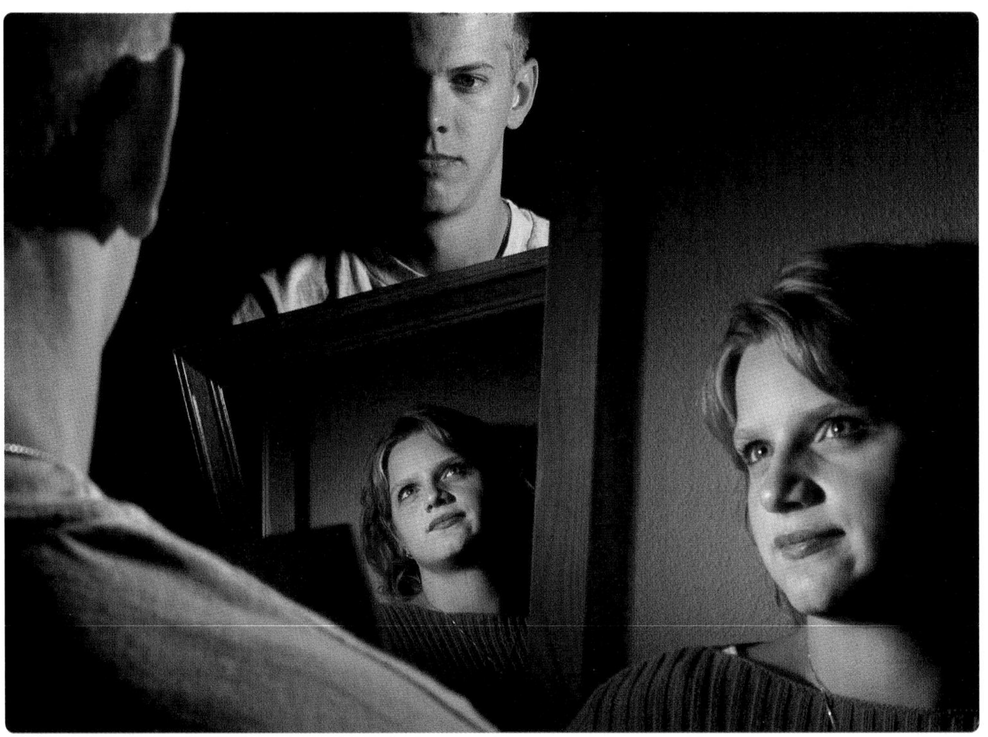

BEFORE THE DIET

"When we met on the Internet, there were all these other people there and for whatever reason, we picked each other. It was like being on one side of a mirror and not knowing what was on the other side."—SARA

Next Click, Wonderland

SARA & SCOTT

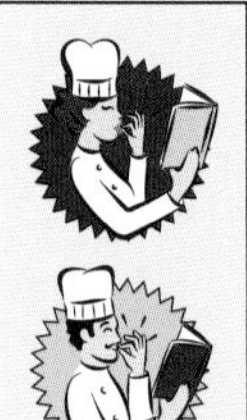

SHE: early 20s, preschool teacher

HE: early 20s, network engineer, volunteer fireman

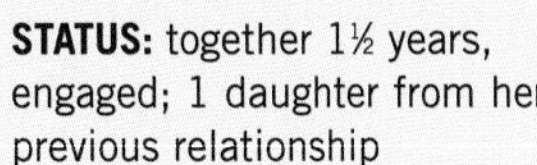

STATUS: together 1½ years, engaged; 1 daughter from her previous relationship

When most of us think of young couples, we think their hormones are raging and they're having tons of wild, crazy sex. But the truth is, like couples of all ages, young couples can also run into barriers that block their ability to fully get into and enjoy sex. This was the case with Sara and Scott.

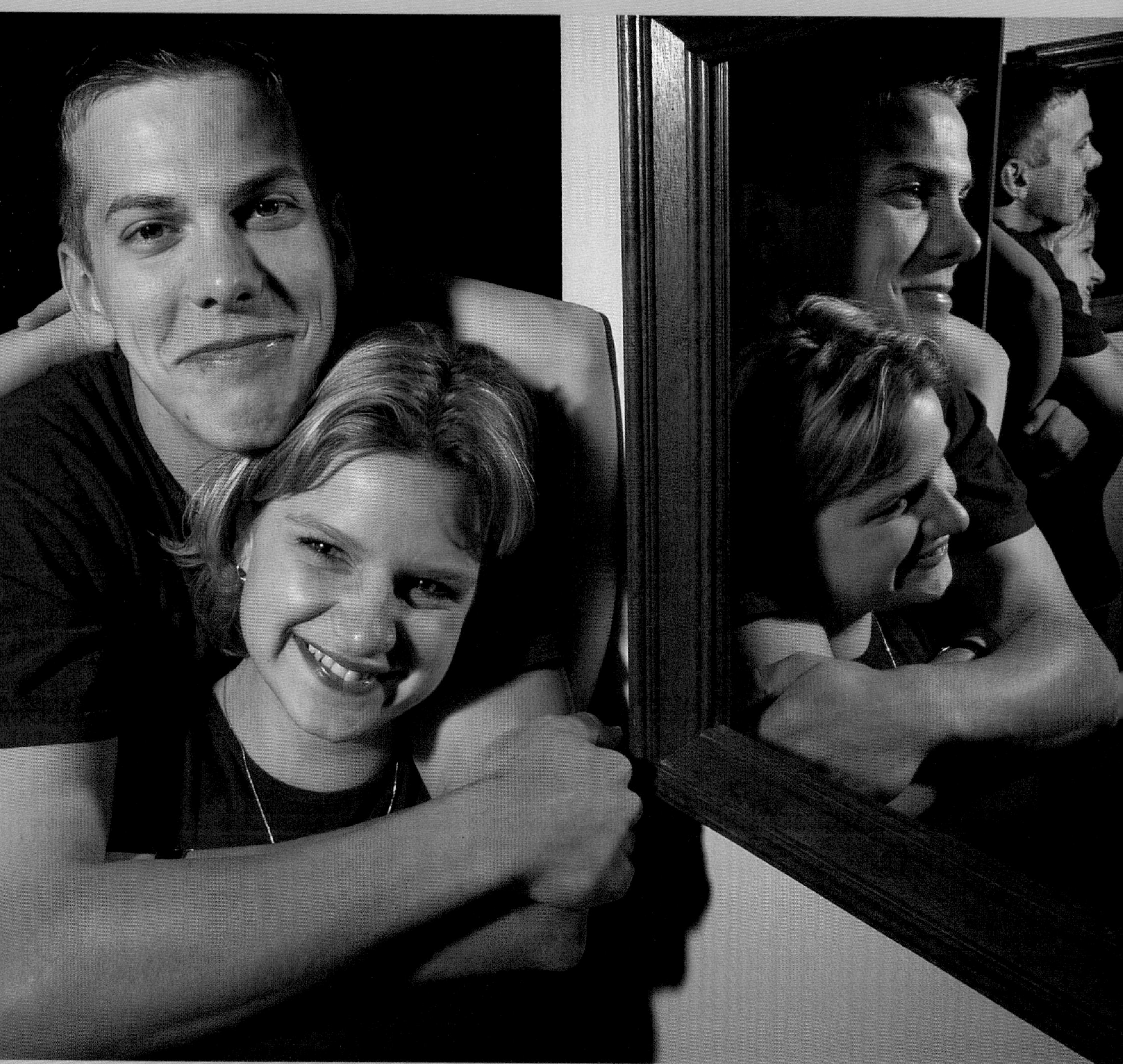

28 DAYS LATER

"To us, the diet was all about changing and spicing up our sex life to build a better relationship. And you can definitely see a difference in ours. It's like night and day. We've grown closer than we've ever been before."—SARA

Sara and Scott met more than a year and a half ago in a very contemporary setting: in a chat room on the Internet.

For Sara and Scott, meeting this way felt like "Alice in Wonderland . . . meeting people through a looking glass." "For whatever reason," Sara explains, "we picked each other even though we didn't have a clue what each other looked like. It was like being on the other side of a mirror and not really knowing."

Now, you may think that two people could never actually meet and fall in love if they met in cyberspace. But I've been hearing about more and more examples of that. The only problem, as far as I can tell, is that here is a couple who after an initial burst of wild sex had settled into a pattern of predictable sex. Can you imagine being twenty-three and running out of ideas for the bedroom?

Part of their pattern emerged when Scott, who had always initiated sex, got tired of waiting for Sara to initiate. But rather than talk it through with her, he began withholding sex "to teach her a lesson." At this point Sara's self-esteem had already become an issue for her. As Sara says, "I'm carrying twenty extra pounds that I've been unable to lose since having my daughter, and I'm a total eat-for-comfort person," she says. The less sex they have, the more likely she is to look to food as a way to fill the gap left from less intimacy with Scott. To further complicate their struggle for intimacy, Sara and Scott share their apartment with a roommate and Sara's three-year-old daughter, so privacy and time alone is not always easy.

They decided to start the diet because they wanted to get their relationship back on track. And they both wanted to add variety and creativity to their standard routine. But there were some speed bumps along their road to success. Sara recalls, "When we first started the diet, Scott was on the computer all day and all night. I finally just went crazy, and we had a huge fight about it."

This fight actually became a communication breakthrough and the key to Sara and Scott's triumph on the diet. "When we both calmed down, I told him I understand he has busy weeks and has

"When we're sexually active, I feel much better about myself. I'm just happier, and I carry myself differently. I don't feel like I have to crawl into my fat clothes every day!"

—Sara

to work at home, but that doesn't mean I have to take the back burner and wait for him to come around," she says. "He understood, and we really talked it out. Every week and every day after that has been absolutely wonderful."

Though they didn't use the Spice Menu often, the frequency really motivated them and they say the sex was "totally awesome" on the diet. They used different places around their home—the kitchen counter, the computer desk, the dining room table—to spice up their usual routine—and it worked! "The diet got us back to how creative we used to be at the beginning," Scott says. "Not that we're old fogies, but we had started doing it the same way in the same place every time. This really got the creative juices flowing!"

On the diet, Sara discovered a "secret weapon" of her own. "When Scott doesn't want to have sex, I know how to unlock the door now," she says. "If I'm willing to do a certain kind of spice, then he's willing to stop whatever he's doing and enjoy it, period. I'm not kidding. He might continue to work, but then ten minutes later, he's chasing me around the house. It's absolutely hilarious. I haven't told him this yet because I don't want him to think that I've found out his secret."

No time is a bad time for Sara and Scott—they fit it in! "Now we notice we've got twenty minutes before our roommate's going to be home," Sara says. "Or we've got half an hour before Brittany's going to wake up from a nap. There have been quite a few times where it's just so spontaneous and so just *wow*. We're like, 'That was very cool—we need to do this again tomorrow!'"

For Scott and Sara, the fight they had the first week of the diet was the key to twenty-eight days of great sex. As for Scott, he said, "I learned that I had to have some understanding and listen to Sara when there are issues and problems. It helped us both realize that we need to make sure that we set time aside."

"One of the spices is called Side Saddle, and it really surprised Scott when I did it. After we were done, he was like, 'Nobody's ever done that for me before.' And I'm like, 'Shut up! You're kidding me.' He said, 'No, I'm totally serious.' And I was just completely shocked. That was very cool."

—Sara

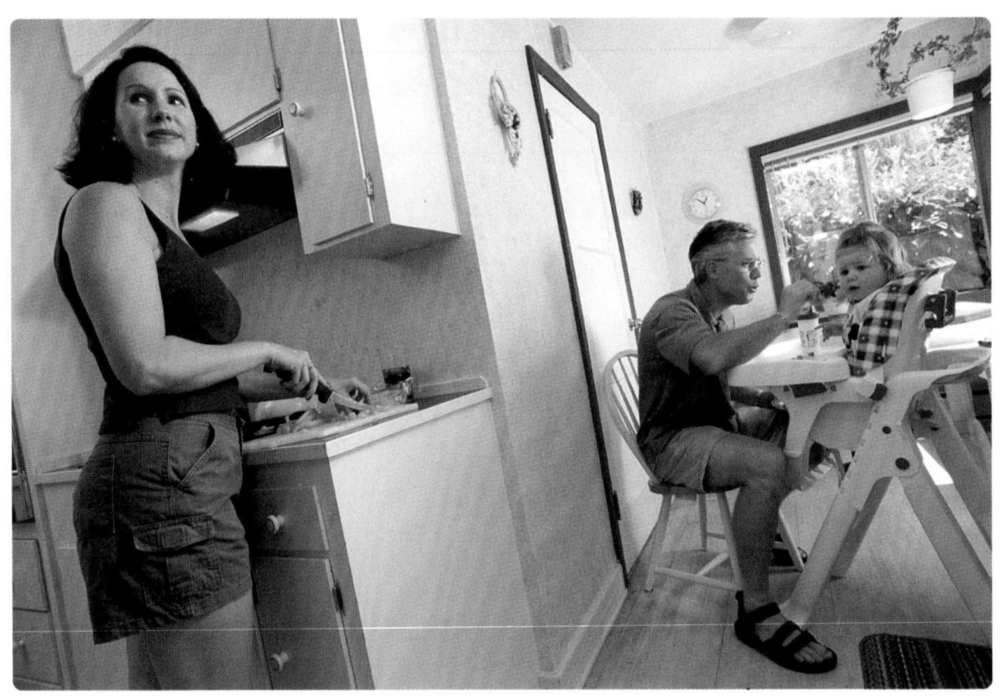

BEFORE THE DIET

"Our baby has definitely affected our love life. You give it all to your kids . . . everything you have. And then you have nothing left to give to your relationship."—CAMERAN

Master of the Universe

CAMERAN & BRIAN

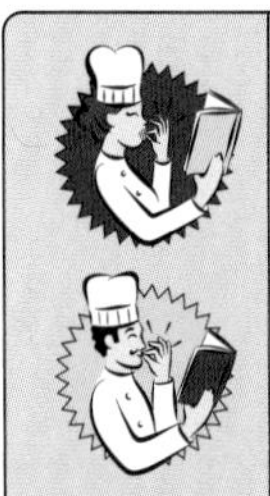

SHE: 30s, assistant supervisor at a credit union

HE: 40s, sales rep for beverage company

STATUS: together 7 years, married 4 years; 1 child together and 1 on the way; he has 2 kids from a former marriage

Take a quick look at the after photo of Brian and Cameran. What blows me away is the sense of easy, happy power Brian exudes. Why? Because after twenty-eight days of intimacy with Cameran, he feels totally empowered. He has become, as he says, Master of the Universe! I've seen this same

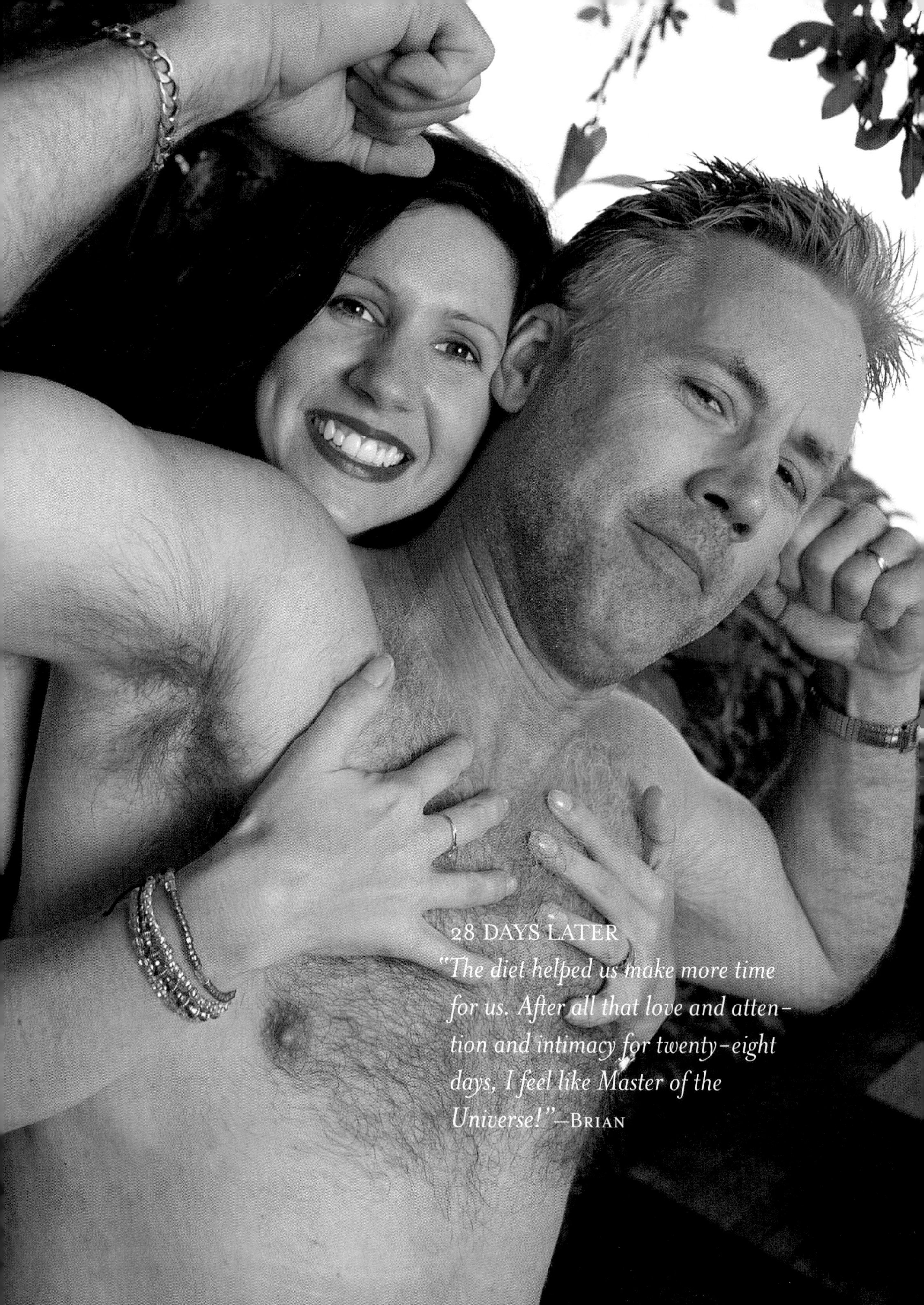

28 DAYS LATER

"The diet helped us make more time for us. After all that love and attention and intimacy for twenty-eight days, I feel like Master of the Universe!"—Brian

transformation in Jeff; I've seen something similar in myself. Seeing is believing.

With an eighteen-month-old baby, Cameran and Brian hadn't made sex the priority it once was in their lives. Add to the mix Brian's two teenage daughters who visit on weekends and there just didn't seem to be enough hours in the day to make time for intimacy . . . much less passion.

Cameran is quick to pick up the responsibility for her less-than-stellar sex life. She says, "We have sex about once a week, but I know it's not enough, especially for Brian. He'd like it seven days a week! But it's hard after having a baby and going through different things. It makes it harder to try to still feel sexy and keep it alive because you've got so many other things on your mind."

> *"I really like to schedule lovemaking, because if it's not on my to-do list, it might not get done. It was easier to make it a priority, because it was a commitment. And it was something to look forward to because I knew it was going to happen."*
>
> —Cameran

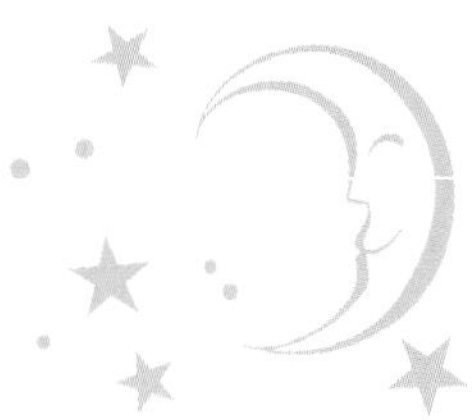

Brian says time—or lack thereof—is a major factor. "There are so many demands from work and the commute and the kids, we don't have much quality time for just ourselves," he says. "But we have to cut up the pie and leave a little bit bigger piece for us because intimacy helps make the pie complete."

This time pressure was exacerbated the first week of the diet when Cameran found out she was pregnant. Now, on top of their heavy schedules, she had to deal with morning sickness and fatigue. But she was a woman on a mission! "I raised up a level to meet his desire," Cameran explains. "Yes, the frequency of the diet was very hard for me, especially since I was pregnant and feeling exhausted. But I still did it. And it had an impact on the relationship. Brian was more affectionate, and it had a snowball effect where I was more affectionate."

Brian is quick to applaud his wife's efforts. "She's a real trooper," he raves. "Respicing our lives and making the time helped us get back to each other." And he surely felt the benefits! "Sometimes when I get up early in the morning, I like to have sex before I go to work," he says. "Then I go to work with a big old smile on my face, and the guys at the office will say, 'Okay, your wife gave it up today, right?' Then they'll give me a high five. I mean, *it's that obvious.*"

Even more obvious to Brian were the differences in his wife. "A few times in the morning, she surprised me and jumped my bones. It reminded me of a trip we took a few years ago in Hawaii, when Cameran was making the moves while I was still sleeping. I was like, 'Cameran, is that you? Are you the girl in my dream or my wife?' She did stuff like that again during this month. '*God, who is this?*' It was pretty cool."

Brian says the diet helped them get back to the way they used to be. "We always talked about the pre-married days. You know, we made love here and there, one or two times a day. And then the next day, it happened again. It's just like, wow, what happened to those days?" Now, happy days are here again, and Brian says he feels totally revitalized. "Something about lying next to my wife when she's not wearing anything just *charges* me," he says. "It's a really good feeling all over."

In my eyes, Cameran and Brian are both Masters of the Universe. It's no fun dealing with the early effects of pregnancy, and Cameran really pulled through and had the intense pleasure of reaping the rewards. As Brian says, "I think the most important thing is not the job, not the kids, not the family . . . all of those things come in a real close second. Couples have to solidify that they are the most important element of the relationship. And the diet helped us do that."

"When you have a baby, your body changes and you feel unsexy. But Brian's like, 'You're just the hottest thing. I see women every day and you are just perfect.' He really is wonderful to me."

—Cameran

BEFORE THE DIET

"Even though we own a chain of sex boutiques, we only have sex once or twice a month. Dan tries to seduce me every morning, but I always say, 'I'm sleeping—leave me alone.'"

—Shelli

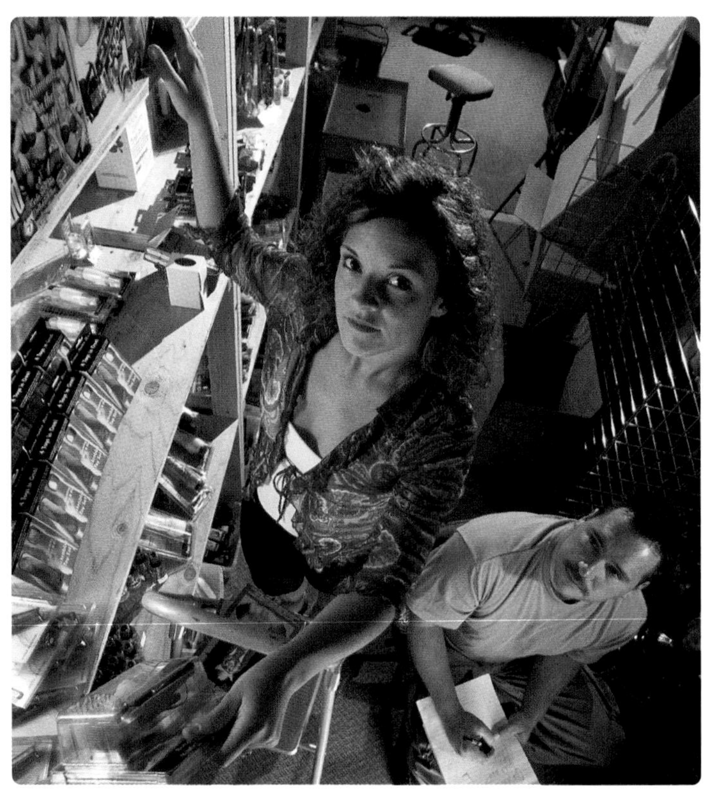

Deep in the Heart of Shelli

Shelli & Dan

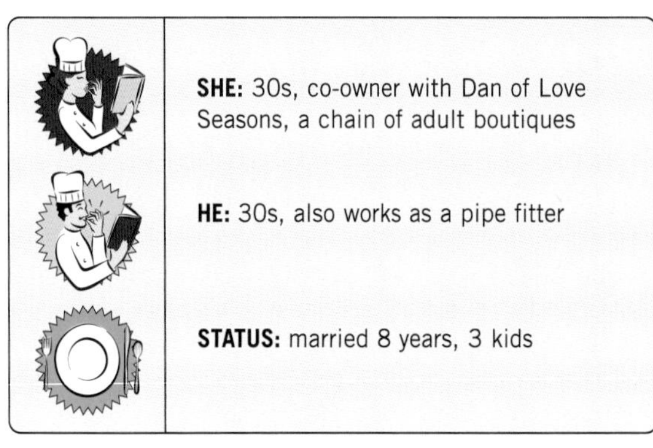

It's almost spooky how similar Shelli and I are. For starters, we both have made sex our business: I write sex books, and in her case, she sells sex toys, erotic videos, and various other items to stimulate and arouse the libido. And our similarities run deeper.

As she and I got to know each other and she began to talk more openly about her sex life

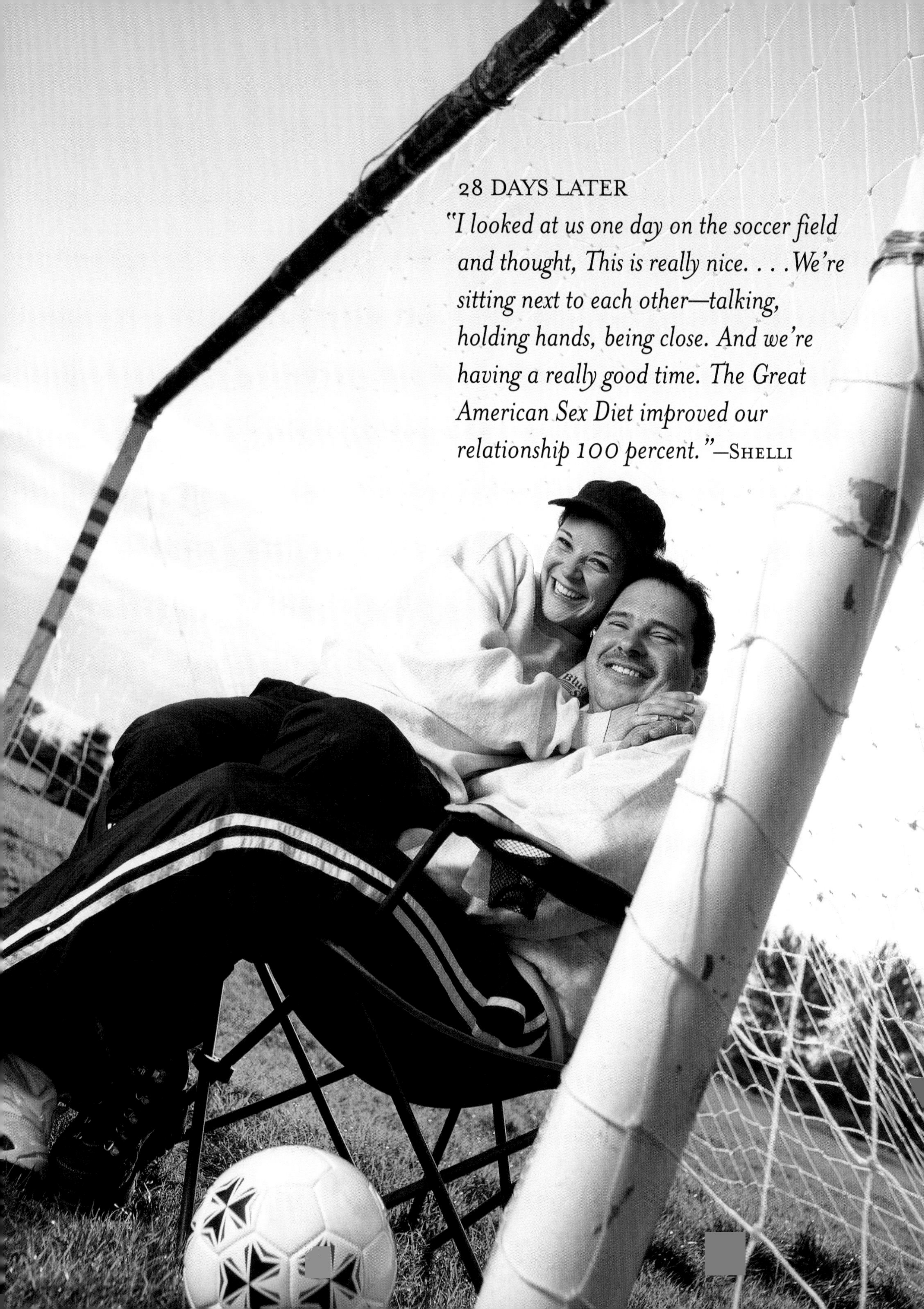

28 DAYS LATER

"I looked at us one day on the soccer field and thought, This is really nice. . . . We're sitting next to each other—talking, holding hands, being close. And we're having a really good time. The Great American Sex Diet improved our relationship 100 percent."—SHELLI

and her wish to make it better, she revealed to me that the main reason she was closed off from sex was because she had been sexually abused. "It kind of defines your sexuality and the challenge is trying to step outside of it," she says. "You have this belief that it's not okay to be sexy, to be sexual, and enjoy it."

I have an intimate understanding of Shelli's struggle because I too was sexually molested when I was young. For both of us, choosing a business that had to do with sex was a step to take this shame out in the open and resolve it. Ironically, its omnipresence in our lives built a kind of numbness to actually experiencing sex. As a result, Shelli, like me, has suffered from low desire. When Dan would make an overture, she would just say, "I'm sleeping—leave me alone." And she has to say that almost every morning.

However, once she and her husband began the Great American Sex Diet, Shelli realized how little effort it could take to change her attitude from not wanting sex to looking forward to it and needing it. As she says, "I know Dan wants to have more sex, but I didn't really realize that it wasn't that much effort. And the outcome just seemed to improve us 100 percent." She began to understand the connection between frequent sex and its rewards. "I had an eye-opening experience. Sex does need to happen more than once a month. Definitely. Because having it affected everything. When we had sex, we got along. We were happy. It made him happier. It made me happier. And I've got to tell you, last night Danny actually said out of nowhere, 'You know, you're really pretty.'"

> *"On the diet I learned that sex is not a duty. That's how I was looking at it before—like 'I got married, so this is what I have to do.' But I now realize it's something that I do need to do because it's right for us. It makes us feel connected, which has a domino effect on everything else in our lives."*
>
> —Shelli

For Shelli, this was a breakthrough moment. "That kind of said everything. The 'really pretty' thing hit me hard. This is a guy who doesn't throw compliments around.

He'll tell me I'm hot. He'll tell me I'm sexy—but not just say something as serious as, 'You're really a pretty person or a beautiful person.' That's just not him. And to hear him say 'you're pretty' and actually mean it, wow. Last night when I got that comment it was like, you know, this diet really did work."

On the diet both Shelli and Dan became more open and communicative, and this was a huge help to breaking her low desire and reconnecting them sexually and emotionally. As Shelli points out, "My marriage started getting better in the sense that I actually started talking to my husband. I looked forward to that half an hour a day on the soccer field. That's what it's all about for us. It doesn't have to be wine me, dine me all the time. It can be something as simple as finding the time to really talk. We're sitting next to each other—talking, holding hands, being close. And we're having a really good time. This is great."

Another thing Shelli considered "great" was Dan's new attitude around the house. "He steps up so much more and helps me do things," she says. "Before, he wouldn't take five minutes to start dinner. He'd just wait for me to come home so we could grab a pizza. But now he was putting the chicken in the oven without me asking. And he was helping out with the kids' homework and reading to them. This was pretty amazing because the man really is busy. He has a full-time day job and a full-time night job. So I've always been the one who kind of keeps the kids and the household going. And suddenly I noticed he was doing these little things that I think a lot of other people would take for granted but for me were huge stepping stones."

Clearly, Shelli and Dan committed to the diet and reaped enormous rewards from having frequent sex. But in the end, the diet for Shelli and Dan was about healing—healing a part of Shelli that had borne the burden of her pain for so long. On the diet, she was able to release this pain and discover the joy and pleasure that comes with fully embracing your sexuality.

"If I had continued to have sex with my husband only once a month for the next year, I don't know if I would have had a relationship."

—Shelli

BEFORE THE DIET

"We are very connected, so there isn't a lot of space between us. But we believe there's always room for improvement. We can always move in just a little bit closer."

—PATRICIA

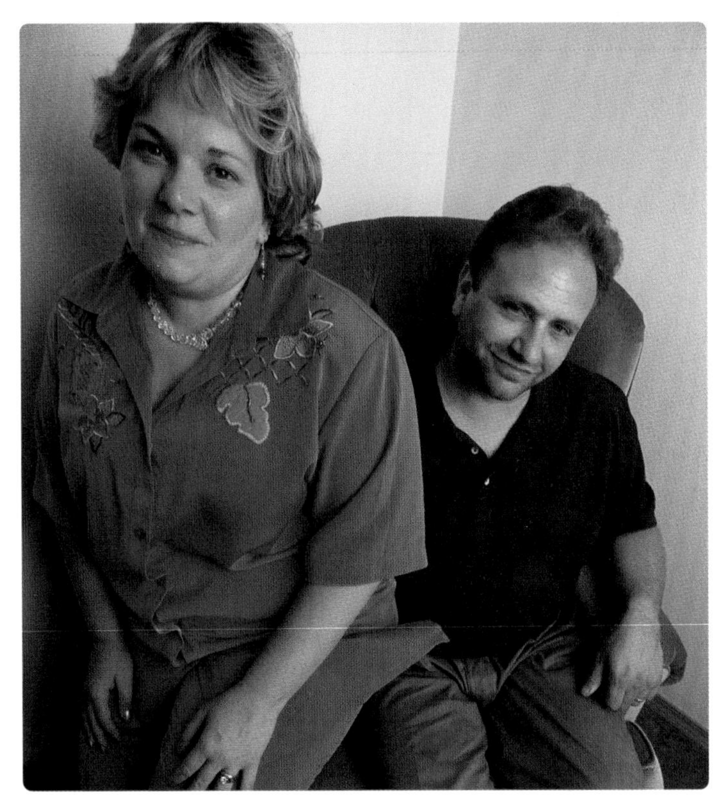

A Ghost Comes Out of the Closet

PATRICIA & TOM

SHE: 30s, registered nurse

HE: 30s, buyer

STATUS: together 15 years, married 14 years; 3 kids, 2 from his previous marriage and 1 together

Tom and Patricia have always had a good life with frequent sex. As Tom says, his wife of fourteen years is the "spice in my chile." So despite the stress of busy careers and raising three teenagers, they describe their relationship as very close. "There's no space between us," Patricia told me, yet they wanted to take their relationship to another level.

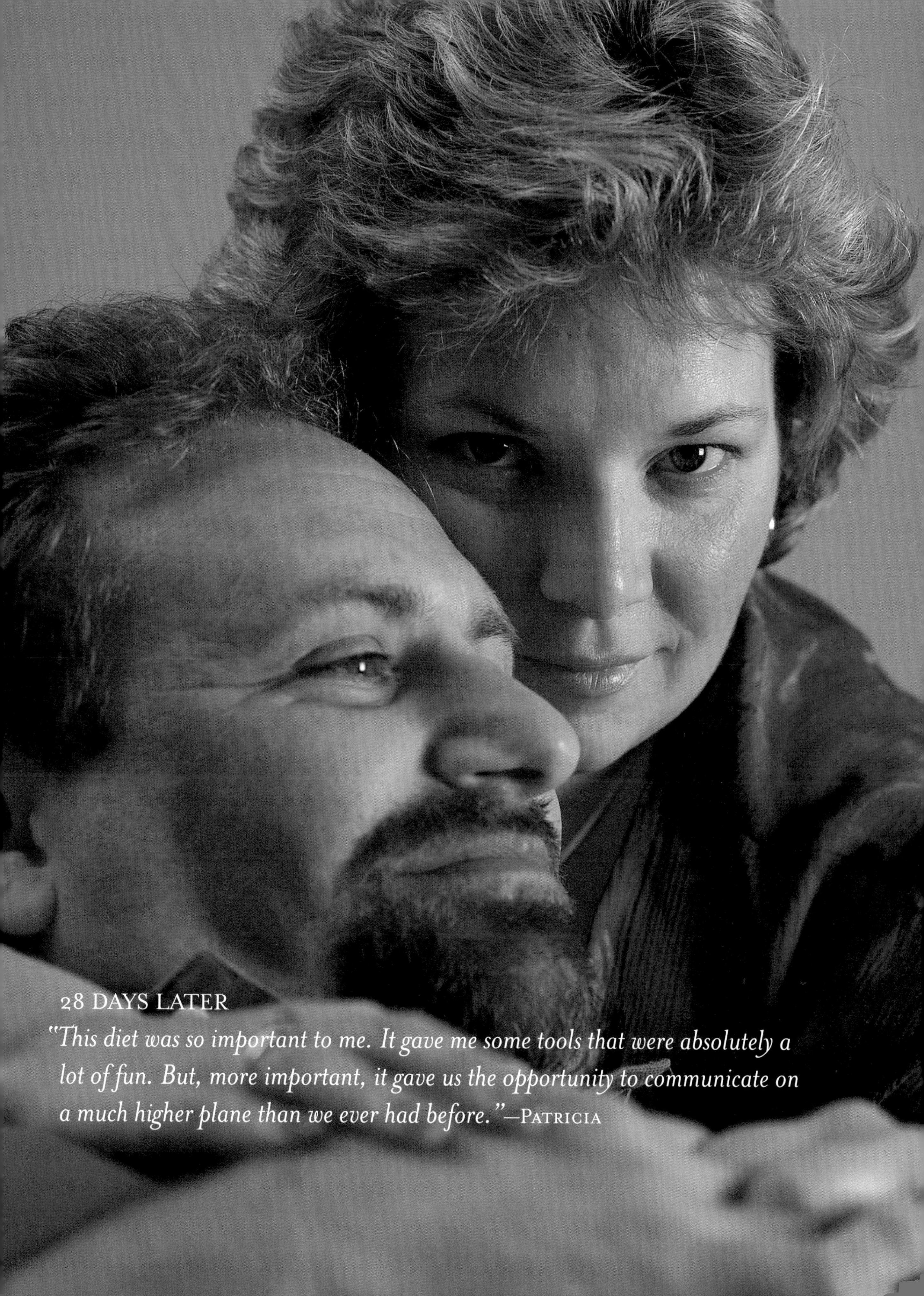

28 DAYS LATER

"This diet was so important to me. It gave me some tools that were absolutely a lot of fun. But, more important, it gave us the opportunity to communicate on a much higher plane than we ever had before."—Patricia

Their children have always been an enormous focus in their lives. "There were times," Patty admits, "when we even let the children sleep in our bedroom with us. And that was a mistake we made."

Until three months before the diet, Patty had a high-powered executive position and it was hard for her to feel both powerful and assertive at work and more relaxed and open once she got home. Yet in bed, she's never been the initiator. Before the diet she said, "There is no way. I can't do it," explains Patty. But once they began trying out the secret spices, all that changed. In fact, more than that changed: Tom and Patricia reached a magnificent breakthrough that transformed their already solid relationship.

Patty didn't see it coming and it virtually swept her off her feet. She says, "We've always had good communication but I was finally able to share something with Tom. It was ancient history, but it was something I had been carrying around with me for a long time in our relationship. Being able to verbalize that was worth all the past pain."

"Now I'm finally able to understand pleasing me is pleasurable for him. Just understanding that was a big eye-opener for me."

—PATRICIA

Although Patty chose not to share the exact details of the incident with me, she did tell me that it happened at a time when she had attempted something new in the relationship. "It happened when we were first married. I tried suggesting something new, and Tom's response was negative.

"A ghost came out of the closet and bit me," she continues. "I needed to be able to say how it felt for me at the time. At first, he was offended that I hadn't told him. He said, 'We've made a baby together. What's the matter with you?'" But in the end, this revelation brought them even closer.

For Patty, the biggest benefit of the diet came down to both her being able to share the old hurt with Tom and Tom being able to hear why it had been so hurtful for her. "Tom wanted to go back and do the moment over again so that I would never hurt or he would never cause me to feel less-than. And I guess I always knew that about him: his prime directive is to take care of me."

After the revelation, Tom says they had "a deeper understanding of each other. It was one more crisis that we lived through," and it made the relationship stronger.

Another—more physical—breakthrough came during the diet. Patty found her G-spot! When I heard that Tom and Patty had spent much of their time on the diet exploring her G-spot, I was a little surprised. In retrospect, I'm not sure why I was so surprised—when I found mine, I was so excited I didn't get out of bed for a week! For many years I didn't even believe that the G-spot existed. When the floodgates finally opened, my sexuality went to another level—and Patty said she felt the same way, too.

Yet for all the new enjoyment, Patricia still held back, troubled by her thoughts that she was being selfish by receiving all this pleasure. "When we were on our G-spot mission, Tom was really looking to put me at the center of this. And that was really hard for me. We had to have some pretty serious conversations about how selfish that felt to me. But now I'm finally able to understand pleasing *me* is pleasurable for *him*. Just understanding that was a big eye-opener for me."

> *"There is nothing more intimate than having intercourse with someone you love. But more than that you've got to be able to make love to their mind, too."*
>
> —Patricia

In the end, Patty and Tom agreed that the diet was "about being able to connect at a different level. When you're connected at a higher plane, a spiritual level, you can take chances, you can try all those things," says Patty. Of course they had a ton of fun, but their success all came down to that ghost coming out of the closet.

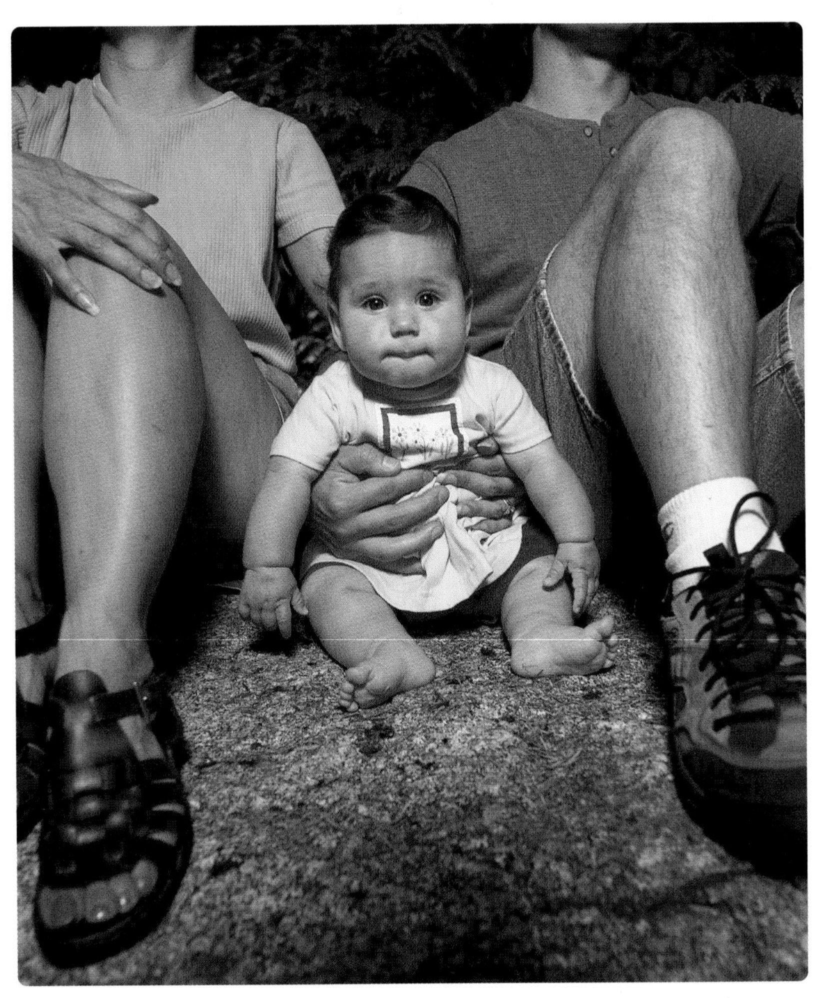

BEFORE THE DIET

"The baby has had a dramatic effect on our relationship. She's our entire focus."

—MARIE

Oh, Baby

MARIE & MICHAEL

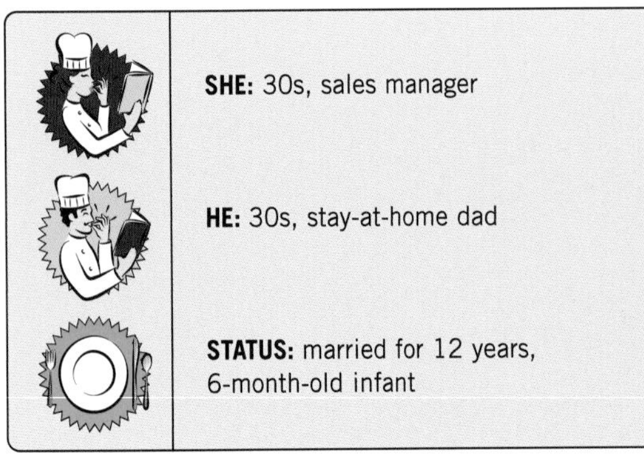

SHE: 30s, sales manager

HE: 30s, stay-at-home dad

STATUS: married for 12 years, 6-month-old infant

When Michael and Marie's bundle of joy, Gracie, came into the world six months ago, neither Michael nor Marie was prepared for the changes that their sex life would undergo. "For three or four months after I had her, I totally lost interest in sex," Marie recalls. "Adjusting to this whole new thing was

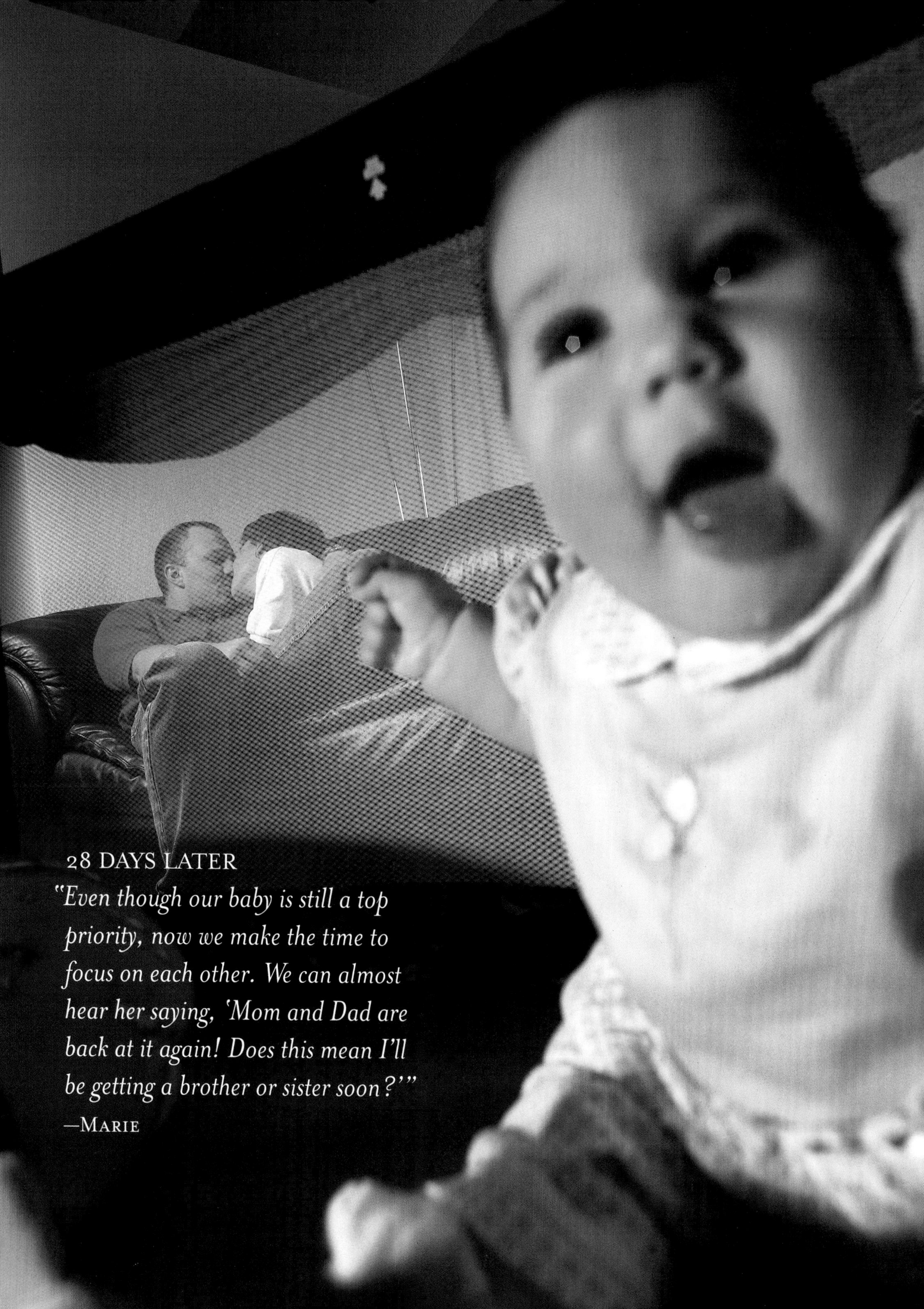

28 DAYS LATER

"Even though our baby is still a top priority, now we make the time to focus on each other. We can almost hear her saying, 'Mom and Dad are back at it again! Does this mean I'll be getting a brother or sister soon?'"

—Marie

exhausting. I was breast-feeding up until recently, and I had to sleep in a bra because I was leaking all over the place. It just felt very bizarre."

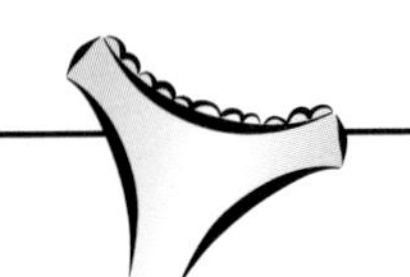

Michael, a stay-at-home dad, wanted to rekindle some of that old spark they once had. "We're extremely busy with the baby, so it seems like sex is very low on the priority list right now," he says. "By the time we get to it, all of our energy is depleted. I'd like to get to the point where we are planning lovemaking so that we can focus on *us* a little bit more."

And the Great American Sex Diet helped them do just that! In the four weeks they've been scheduling sex, Michael and Marie have faithfully made love four times a week. But they've had their share of obstacles. "My mom was staying with us for almost a week, so that made it a bit more challenging," Marie says. "But we were so committed, we were able to fit the four times a week in despite it all."

"A lot of times we were so tired, we would have normally put sex off until the next day. But since we had a schedule, we went ahead and made love. And it was worth it. It actually gave us more energy, not less."

—Michael

And their diligence has paid off, for they have already seen some amazing changes in their relationship. For instance, Michael lit candles for Marie all over the bathroom and bedroom—something he hadn't done in at least a year. And Marie says that she found the courage to put on some of the lingerie she'd banned since Gracie was born: "I hadn't felt sexy in a long time, and this helped me feel sensual again."

Michael also loved the fact that Marie was initiating sex, something she hadn't done in quite some time. "That was a nice change," he says. "It took a little bit of the load off me. It was great to be able to relax a little bit and let her take care of the planning."

Perhaps the most important lesson they've learned is that scheduling works. "We loved the scheduling, and we're going to continue to do it at least three

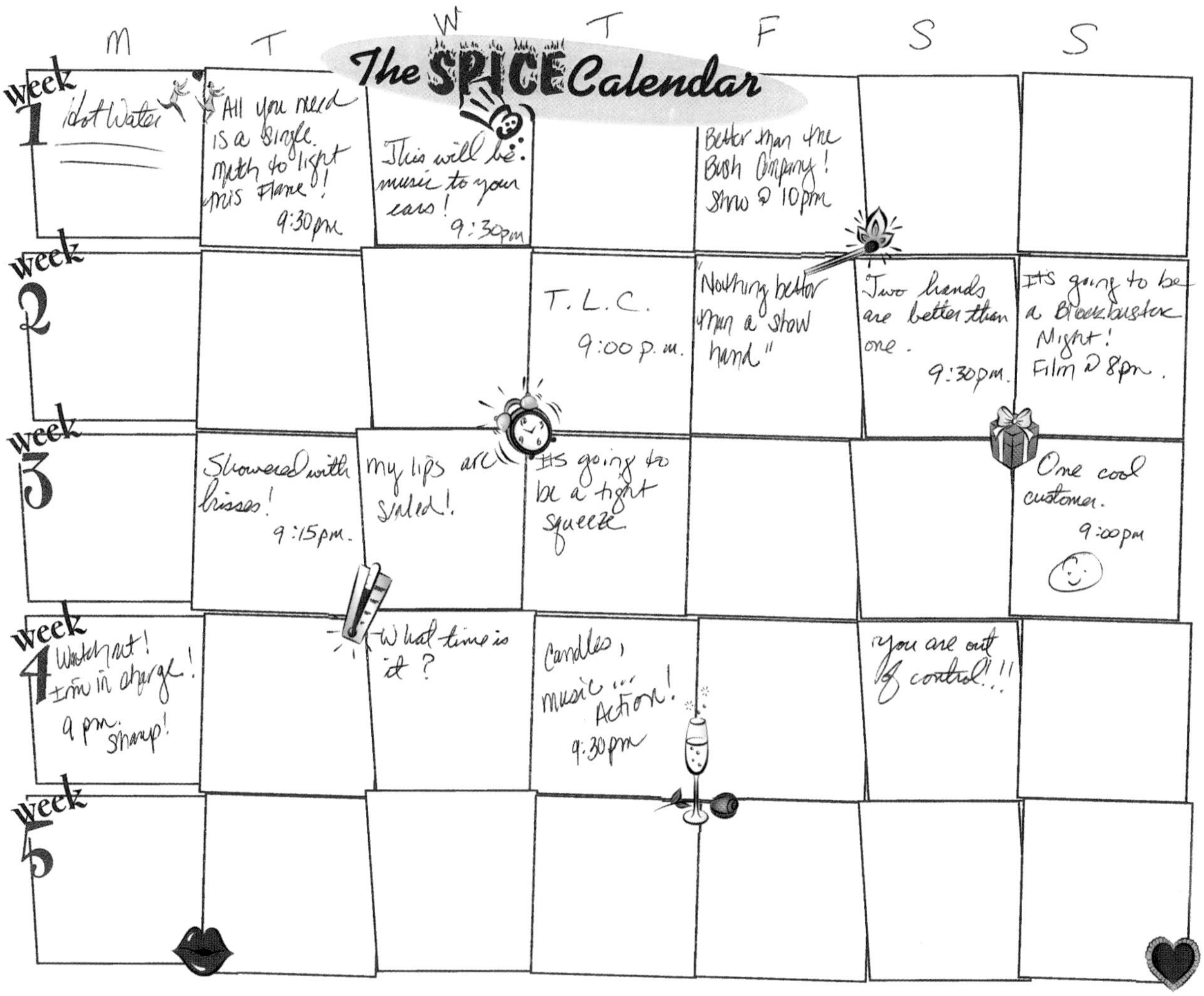

The SPICE Calendar

	M	T	W	T	F	S	S
week 1	Hot Water	All you need is a single match to light this flame! 9:30pm	This will be music to your ears! 9:30pm		Better than the Bush Company! Show @ 10pm		
week 2				T.L.C. 9:00 p.m.	"Nothing better than a show hand"	Two hands are better than one. 9:30pm.	It's going to be a Blockbuster Night! Film @ 8pm.
week 3		Showered with kisses! 9:15pm.	my lips are sealed!	It's going to be a tight squeeze			One cool customer. 9:00pm
week 4	Watch out! I'm in charge! 9 pm sharp!		What time is it?	Candles, music... Action! 9:30pm		you are out of control!!!	
week 5							

"We loved the scheduling, and we're going to continue to do it at least three days a week. The calendar made me see that if you make time for sex, there is *always* time for it."—Marie

days a week," Marie says. "The calendar made me see that if you make time for sex, there is *always* time for it."

Michael agrees. "A lot of times we were so tired, we would normally have put sex off until the next day," he says. "But since we had a schedule, we went ahead and made love. And it was worth it. It actually gave us *more* energy, not less."

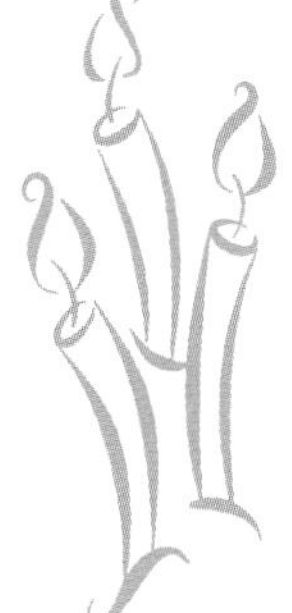

"Right after I had Gracie, I felt as big as a house. I hadn't felt sexy in a long time, and this helped me feel sensual again."—MARIE

BEFORE THE DIET

"Geoffrey is a computer guy. He's on the computer 24/7, no kidding. We get home, he's on the computer. I make dinner, he's on the computer. I go to bed, he's on the computer. What I'd really like is for him to spend more time on us."

—Tarah

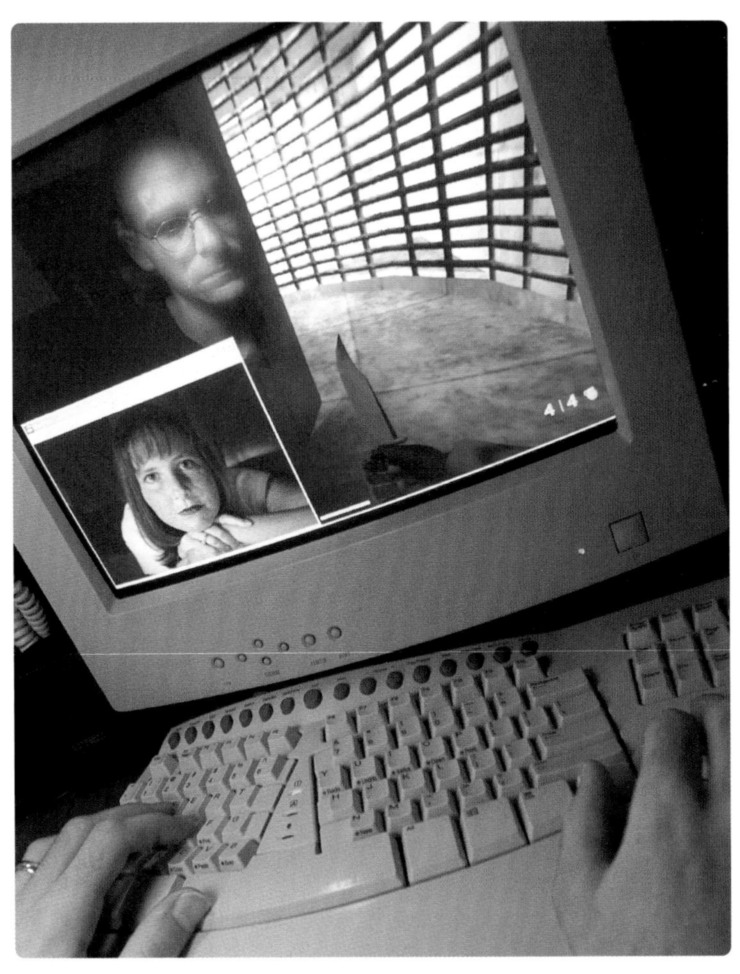

Short Circuit

Tarah & Geoffrey

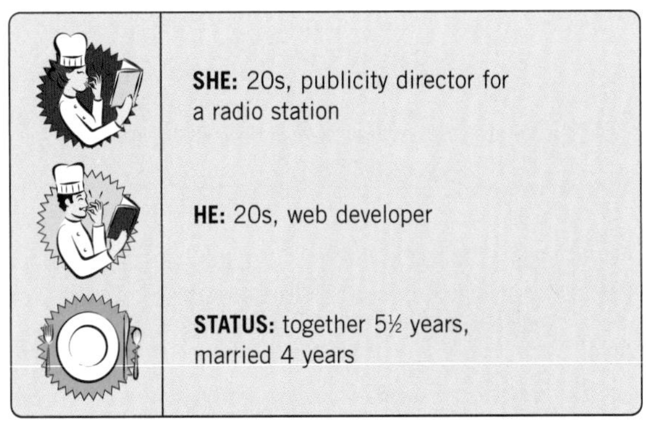

SHE: 20s, publicity director for a radio station

HE: 20s, web developer

STATUS: together 5½ years, married 4 years

When I first saw the before photo of Tarah and Geoffrey, I must admit I was a bit startled—I actually found it quite eerie. The computer seems to reflect not only their faces in a chilling way, but also a certain dimension of their dynamic. A young couple, Tarah and Geoffrey both seemed motivated to do the diet because sex had become predictable. As Tarah says, "After being married for four years, our sexual relationship had become routine." Tarah, who was a virgin when she got married, also felt a bit insecure. As she says, "I don't have a huge background. I'm not too creative and I don't know any neat tricks, and that has been an insecurity for me."

She convinced Geoffrey to go on the diet to change all that. Geoffrey "always comes up with these different things that I've never considered," Tarah explains and she wants to learn to initiate more. "I'm really working on it," she says.

One of the other challenges they faced going on the diet was trying to change Geoffrey's work habits so that he made their sex life more of a priority. "Geoffrey is a computer guy," Tarah explains. "He's on the computer 24/7, no kidding. We get home, he's on the computer. I make dinner, he's on the computer. I go to bed, he's on the computer. I go to bed at about ten, but he doesn't come to bed sometimes until four or even five." Tarah and Geoffrey certainly had their work cut out for them.

Unfortunately, after their second week things came to halt. Although Tarah "totally wanted to do the diet," she admitted that her husband "wasn't really into it." When I spoke to Geoffrey, he said that he had changed jobs that month and he was very stressed and preoccupied with his new position, which entailed more responsibility.

Yet despite their not being able to stick to the diet, they did benefit. "On the diet, I finally seduced Geoffrey," Tarah explains. "I put on music. I set the scene. I was so good. I was the best and he was totally excited—that was very positive." Tarah was also able to overcome her fear of giving Geoffrey oral sex and "was successful for the first time ever." They also said they didn't want to give up their menus—there were too many spices they still wanted to try!

I include Tarah and Geoffrey's story so you have a sense that the reality of your circumstances can conflict with being on the diet. But keep in mind that thirty-six of thirty-eight couples on the research team clearly succeeded. I believe that if you want all the many rewards that the diet has to offer, sticking to it and achieving that goal will not only be possible but invigorating, fun, and exciting!

"This one oral spice on the menu was amazing. I've tried to give Geoffrey oral sex before and I have not been successful. That was the first successful one, and he was totally excited."—TARAH

BEFORE THE DIET

"We're looking for connection through the chaos, but our focus is on the kids and it's a struggle. There's no time for us unless we fight for it. And most of the time we're too tired to fight for it."

—JULIA

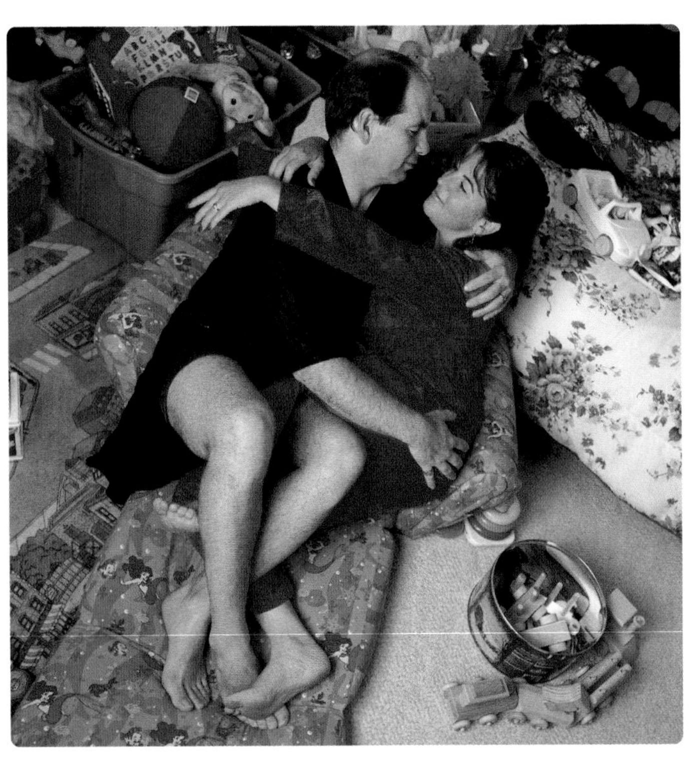

What Lola Wants, Lola Gets

JULIA & FRANK

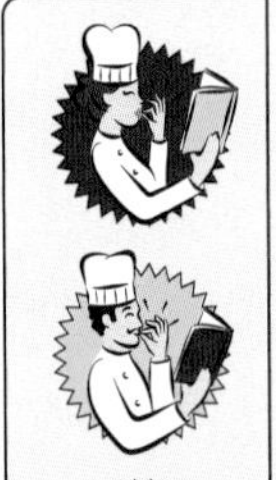

SHE: 30s, stay-at-home mother

HE: 30s, CEO of high-tech company

STATUS: together 9 years, married 8 years; 2 kids

Julia and Frank are one of those couples that moved from between a rock and a hard place to sheer nirvana—and one special catalyst was a saucy girl named Lola.

Just under a year before they started the Great American Sex Diet, they were questioning their marriage to such a degree that they were considering divorce. Frank, as CEO of

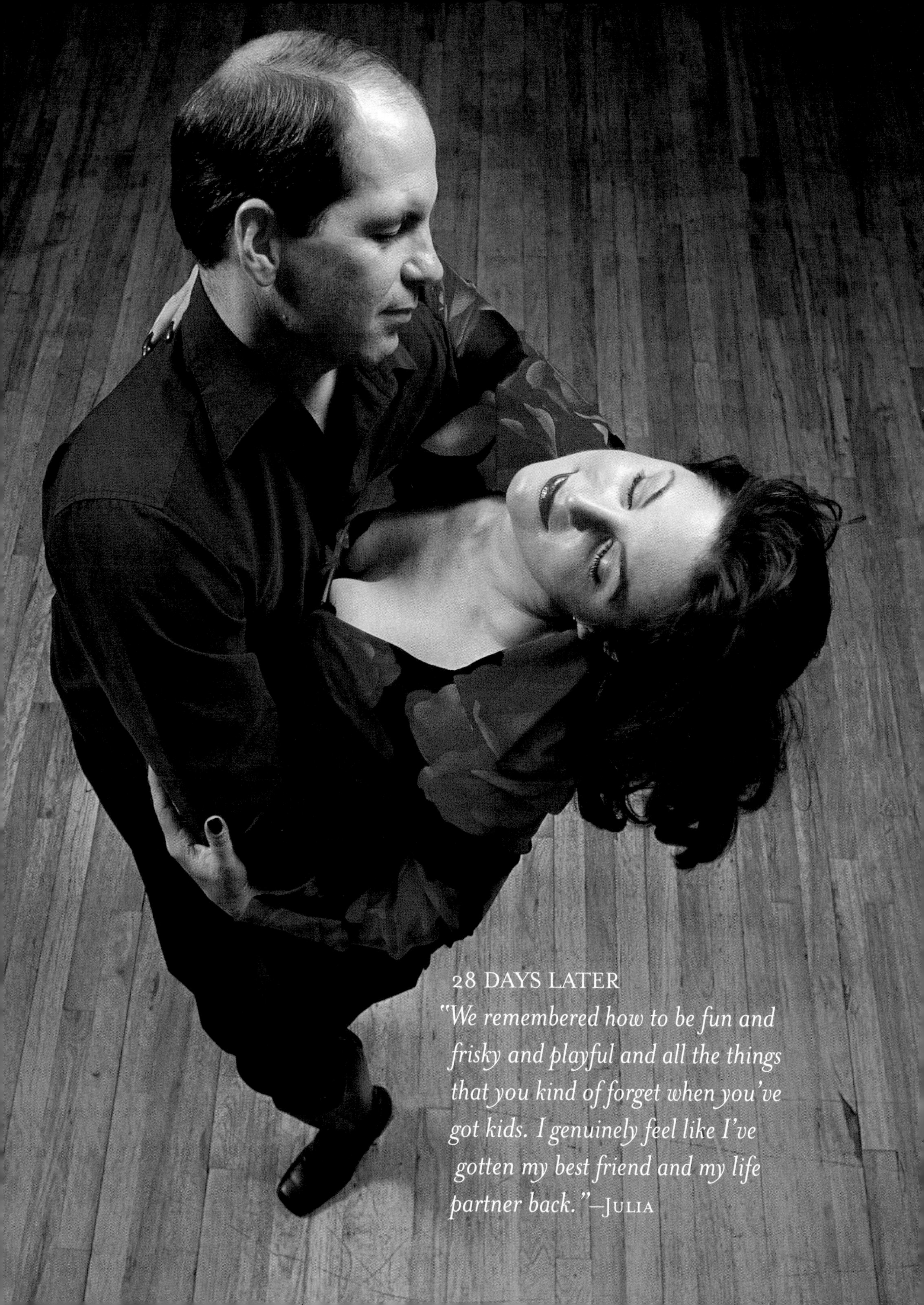

28 DAYS LATER

"We remembered how to be fun and frisky and playful and all the things that you kind of forget when you've got kids. I genuinely feel like I've gotten my best friend and my life partner back." —Julia

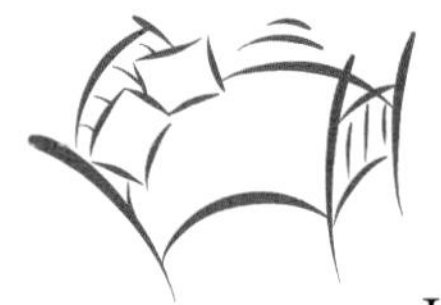

a demanding high-technology company, worked around the clock and had finally admitted to Julia that he dreaded coming home to the "chaos" of their family life. At the same time, Julia realized that the only times they were having sex was when she initiated. "We were like roommates," Julia recalls.

Their marriage and sex life weren't always this rocky. "It wasn't like this when we met," Julia explains. They were wild, daring, and adventurous, once getting caught making love high up in the mountains by a hovering plane! "It was a little Cessna," Julia says, "just catching the show! We loved the edge."

But this sense of wild abandon had dwindled in the past couple of years, and neither of them had seen neither hide nor hair of the infamous Lola, Julia's sexual alter ego that used to drive Frank wild. Julia explains how she internalized the stress of no longer connecting sexually: "I took it personally. I don't know if it's being a woman or what, but I began asking myself if there was something wrong with me." Julia, who used to be a dancer, also struggled with her body image. She'd gained weight and lost the "hard body" of her dancing years, and this contributed to her low self-esteem.

"I surprised Frank with the Lip Service spice. Oh my gosh, that was probably the best thing I ever did for him. He was in heaven."

—Julia

This strain went on a year and a half before Julia finally spoke up. After weeks had gone by without much sexual interest from Frank, Julia asked him, "Is there still anything between us?" And Frank said, "I haven't desired you for a long time." Hurt and confused, Julia left for the weekend. In the comfort of her friends' company, she began to reassess her marriage. What was her fault? What was Frank's? Could this marriage be saved?

She returned home and confronted Frank in her own way. "I came back and said, 'This is not my problem. I don't see any flaws in you, even though there are tons of them, because I love you. I don't see your receding hair. I don't see the scars. I don't see any of that. And if that's what you see in me, then it's your problem. I am not going to own it. I like the way I am.' And then I handed it all back to Frank, saying, 'It's on your shoulders. You have to get over it or you've got to get help, or you can leave.'"

A few days later Frank told Julia that he loved her. "That's what I desired in you . . . your spirit," he said. "And now the old Julia is back."

From that point on, they began to consciously work at their marriage, but as we all know, it's never easy. Frank still worked long, hard hours, and they were trying hard to find love among the chaos.

It was Julia's idea to try the diet and at first Frank was hesitant. Julia explains, "I was kind of hoping that he would stick with it as far as the scheduling goes and make it a priority. But I was a little leery." Frank remembers feeling like the diet would be "just one more thing I have to remember to do."

They started the diet and two weeks into it Frank was rushed to the emergency room. "We thought it was a heart attack," she says, "but thank God it wasn't." After that he had to go on a ten-day business trip. But when he returned, he saw how much the diet meant to Julia and they not only picked up where they left off, they zoomed ahead!

They loved the spices and the frequency. "I noticed that we were bummed out if we missed a night. We'd say, okay, we're going to have to catch up this weekend. Because we committed to it, we didn't want to blow it," says Julia. "There were weeks when we had sex more than four times, which was great. We had to get creative!"

Frank began initiating and surprising Julia, but one night in particular really topped the charts. As Frank described the evening, he gently tied Julia to the bed and then blindfolded her. Then he disappeared into the closet. "I walked into the closet and saw the Lola hairpiece hanging there and it just gave me the idea."

What happened next? Well, he slowly seduced her, all along letting her feel the hair from the wig brush against her. She was going crazy! Was she being seduced by her husband or by a woman?

As Frank says, "That evening went on for hours—just role playing and having fun!" Julia recalls, "He was even talking in a higher voice, pretending he was a woman. I was totally turned on! It was awesome, like the walls came down because that's something we would have never done before."

The sex diet not only returned Frank and Julia to the former passion of their wild, adventurous days, it also brought them closer together. "It changed the whole balance in the house," Julia explains. We now have that connection across a room. Now, even with the kids screaming I can look at him across the room and give him a smile and he smiles back."

BEFORE THE DIET

"After the kids and work and all this other stuff, we've lost that spark we once had. And we really want to get that back."

—CONRAD

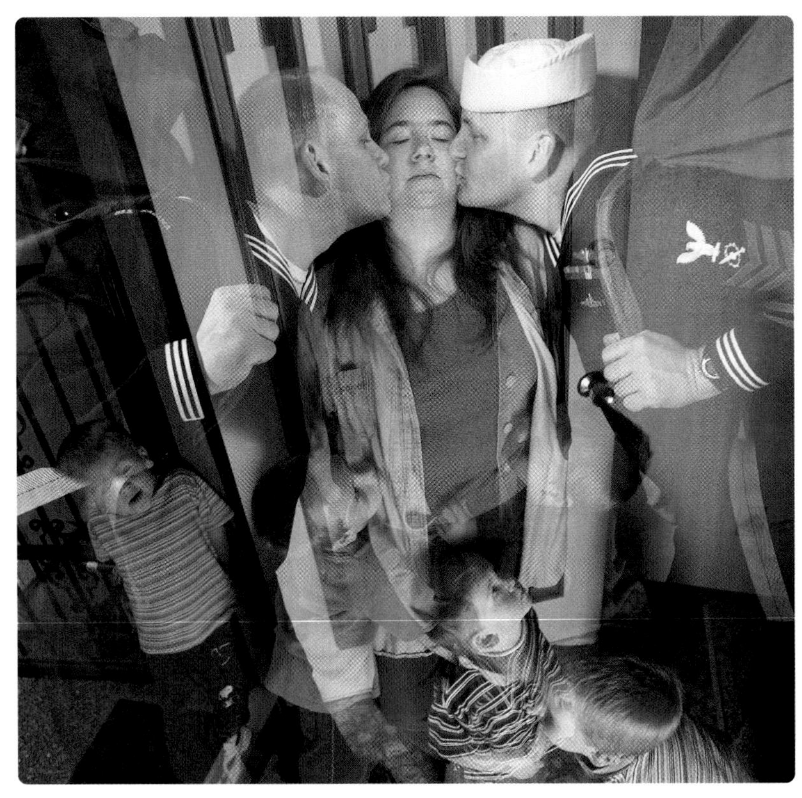

Batten Down the Hatches!

JULI & CONRAD

SHE: 30s, a homemaker and runs a cleaning service

HE: 30s, first class petty officer, U.S. Navy

STATUS: married 6 years, 3 kids

Conrad and Juli are one of those couples I could just hug all day. And to me, their voyage on the diet was nothing short of amazing. Just look at their after shot! They journeyed a tremendous emotional distance on the diet, arriving at a place of warmth, togetherness, and fabulous sex.

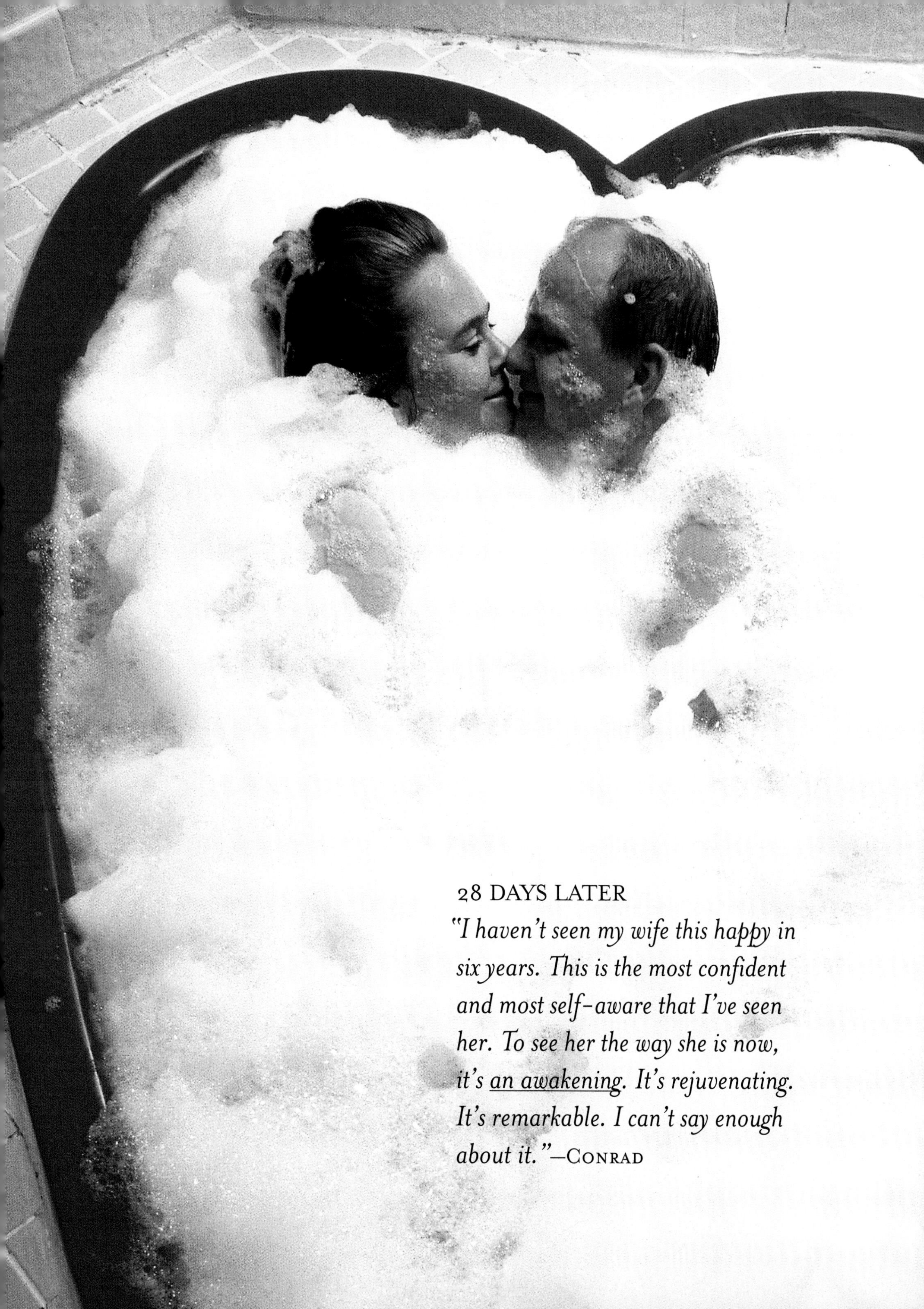

28 DAYS LATER

"I haven't seen my wife this happy in six years. This is the most confident and most self-aware that I've seen her. To see her the way she is now, it's <u>an awakening</u>. It's rejuvenating. It's remarkable. I can't say enough about it."—Conrad

As a first class petty officer in the U.S. Navy, Conrad is a true seaman—tough as nails on the outside with the heart of a lamb on the inside. He told me that when he and Juli first started dating, they had a certain magic—sometimes pulling off the highway to make love under an overpass! But when they got married, Juli got pregnant right away and they had three kids one after the other. After that, the magic seemed to dwindle and get lost in the shuffle. It sure sounded like a wild ride, but why did it have to end?

As they both explained, with the stress of very difficult pregnancies (Juli had morning sickness every day for the first three months), a harsh transition into motherhood, and Conrad's job, which requires him to spend up to three months at a time at sea, Juli grew depressed and totally lost her desire. They were having sex maybe once a month.

Then they decided to do the diet, excited that this might be a chance to resuscitate their intimate relationship. As Conrad says, "Juli knows that I have a pretty healthy sex drive and that she's also still in her prime." But they had a wall to climb. Before the diet, Juli had become totally shut down to sex. "I always want to try a different position, but she's not into that. She's really a control freak." He then told me that Juli can have sex only one way: on top, in a hunched-over position. He continues, "I'd like to try something different, but she talks about her weight. All I want is for her to trust me." She also shies away from either giving or receiving oral sex, which is also disappointing to Conrad.

> *"Oh, boy, I feel more in love. I feel more like we're one instead of two separate people. I'm more confident sexually. And when we didn't have sex, I missed it. The more I do it, the more I want it."*
>
> —Juli

It had also been three years since Juli had "made a move" on Conrad and it bothered him a lot that she rarely initiated. But Conrad believed in Juli. He knew that she used to love sex, and he wanted his "old Juli" to return. "I know she loves having orgasms," he says. "Sometimes she has more than one!"

But Juli felt overwhelmed by her depression. As she says, "I sit there all day long and tell myself negatives." I tried to reach out to

Juli by encouraging her to take baby steps. Then, once they were on the diet, the remarkable changes began. Conrad sums it up this way, "It's hard telling where we would be today without you and the influence of all the suggestions and creative ideas on the diet. The impact has just been huge. When I look back at how we were before, I don't understand how we were functionally compatible."

The diet simply changed their lives. Not only did they begin to have frequent sex, they had wild, uninhibited, sensual sex. Juli let go and became open to whole new dimensions of herself. "Now she can sit up on top of me, instead of scrunching over. She is not nervous about her body anymore. She's more confident. She really, truly enjoys her body now, versus thinking how much of a pain it is." This shift in Juli obviously made an enormous impact on Conrad. Juli agrees that she feels more confident sexually and that the diet really helped with her depression. The diet was "like the first step to opening my door."

This openness extended throughout all areas of her life. Whereas before she would often emotionally shut herself off from her family because of her depression, now she says she wants to "give more to my children and my husband."

Like so many couples, Conrad and Juli also began to really talk to each other, especially about sex. Conrad said, "I feel more comfortable talking about sex. I feel more intimate in that way." And naturally, being able to talk about sex, as well as have sex more often and more regularly, made them see how important it is in their lives. As Conrad said, "If you can find that one person and get that friction between the two of you, life is ecstatic. It's like wow. It's one of those things that you never want to lose."

They both appreciate and revel in all of these changes that came out of being on the diet. "There is no comparison to the Juli in the old body. I hadn't seen this Juli in six years," says Conrad. And Juli says adamantly, "I don't want to go back to my old ways. If I shut sex out of my life, then I'll go back to the way I was."

Juli and Conrad took their own special voyage on the diet, but it didn't take place at sea. It happened in their home, in between their own hot sheets!

BEFORE THE DIET

"There's a lot of stress that exists in our family. Cesar works really long hours, and I have to deal with the kids all day. I don't have much desire. We need to do something different and have a little fun."

—VALERIE

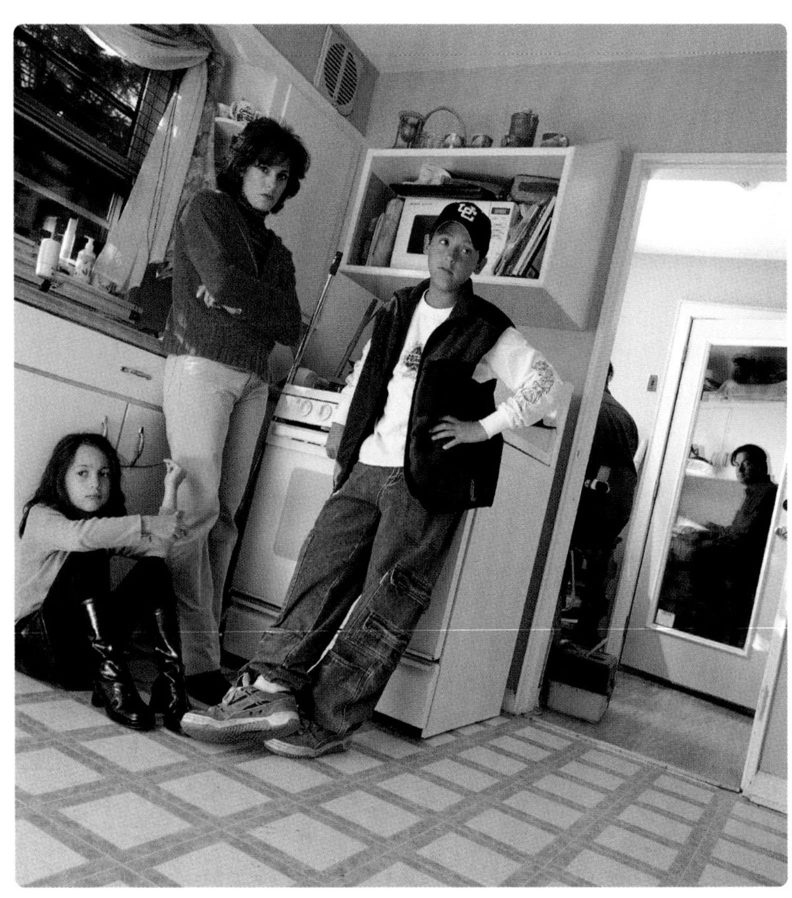

Letting Loose

VALERIE & CESAR

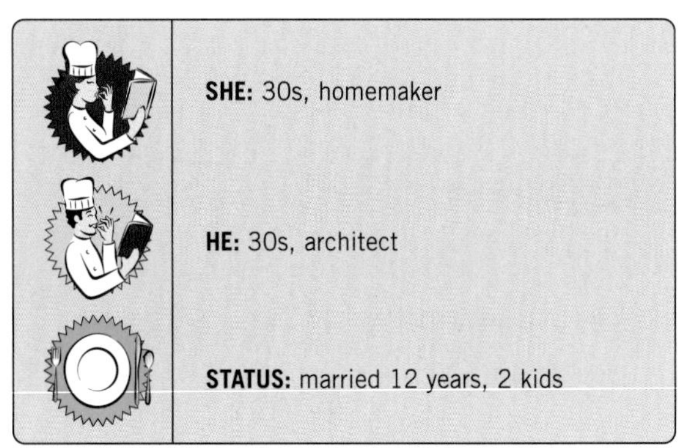

SHE: 30s, homemaker

HE: 30s, architect

STATUS: married 12 years, 2 kids

I was really moved by Valerie and Cesar's before photo. It's such a simple image, yet it says something powerful. As Valerie herself said, "It reflects the stress that existed in our family." So how do you cross the bridge from that kind of stress and distance to a place of togetherness, harmony, and marital happiness?

For Cesar and Valerie, that bridge was the

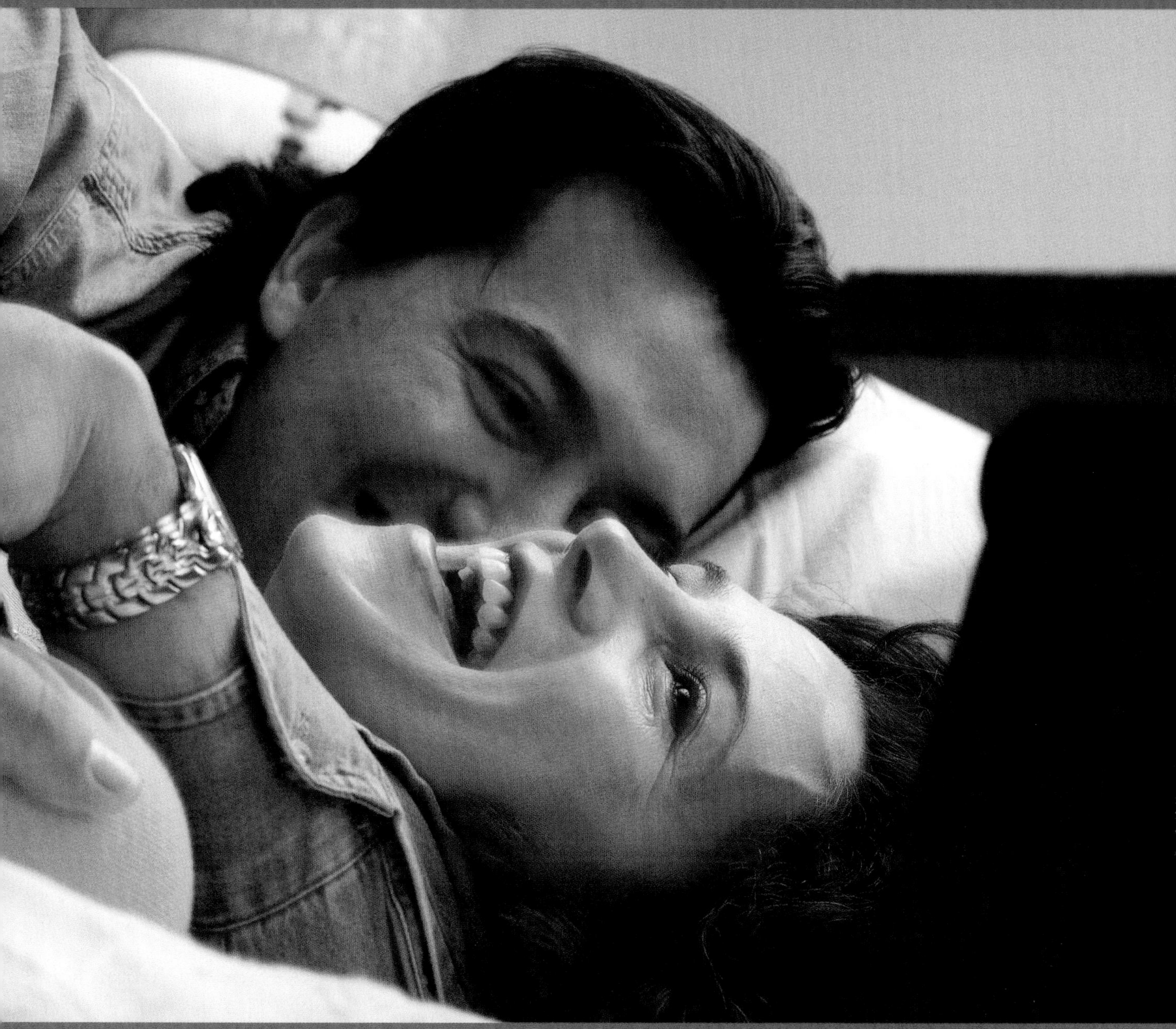

28 DAYS LATER

"Playfulness, communication, and affection emerged from being on the diet. A lot of the same stresses are there, but they're easier to make light of now. Intimacy definitely makes you feel closer and more relaxed. You just feel like the other person cares about you more."—Valerie

Great American Sex Diet. Married twelve years with two children, they have a long history together. Both of them wanted to jump-start their marriage—especially their sex life. They had been having sex only one or two times a month. Things had become so static that Cesar had become afraid to introduce anything new because he was so conditioned to being turned down by Valerie. He no longer even had the gumption to try.

When I spoke with Valerie, she was very forthright about being set in her ways. "I don't have any hang-ups, I just don't like to do a lot of things." She and Cesar had come to a standstill, unable to communicate and therefore unable to figure out a way to change. How was this otherwise loving couple going to move from this static place?

But once Valerie and Cesar actually began the diet, they found what they were looking for: a way to move Valerie out of her low desire. The commitment of the diet "made it easier to do this," she says. "That made me do it." And the results further convinced them. As Valerie said, "I see how positive the results are. Now when I have sex, I'm doing it for me and doing it for us, and doing it for the relationship."

The whole quality of their relationship changed. "We talk more to each other," Valerie explained. "Cesar is more helpful and he's doing things with a smile. A lot of the same stresses are there, but they're easier to make light of. So it's easier to cope with them." This kind of shift in a relationship happened with many couples. They begin to talk to each other, and presto, everything in their life becomes more manageable.

And though Valerie didn't become a sexual adventurer overnight, she did spread her wings. "I rented a movie which was steamy and sexy, and Cesar looks at me and says, 'Are you horny?' and I said, 'Yeah!' It

"What came out of the diet was that we were more affectionate with each other. The frequency really relieves a lot of stress and makes you more relaxed with each other."

—CESAR

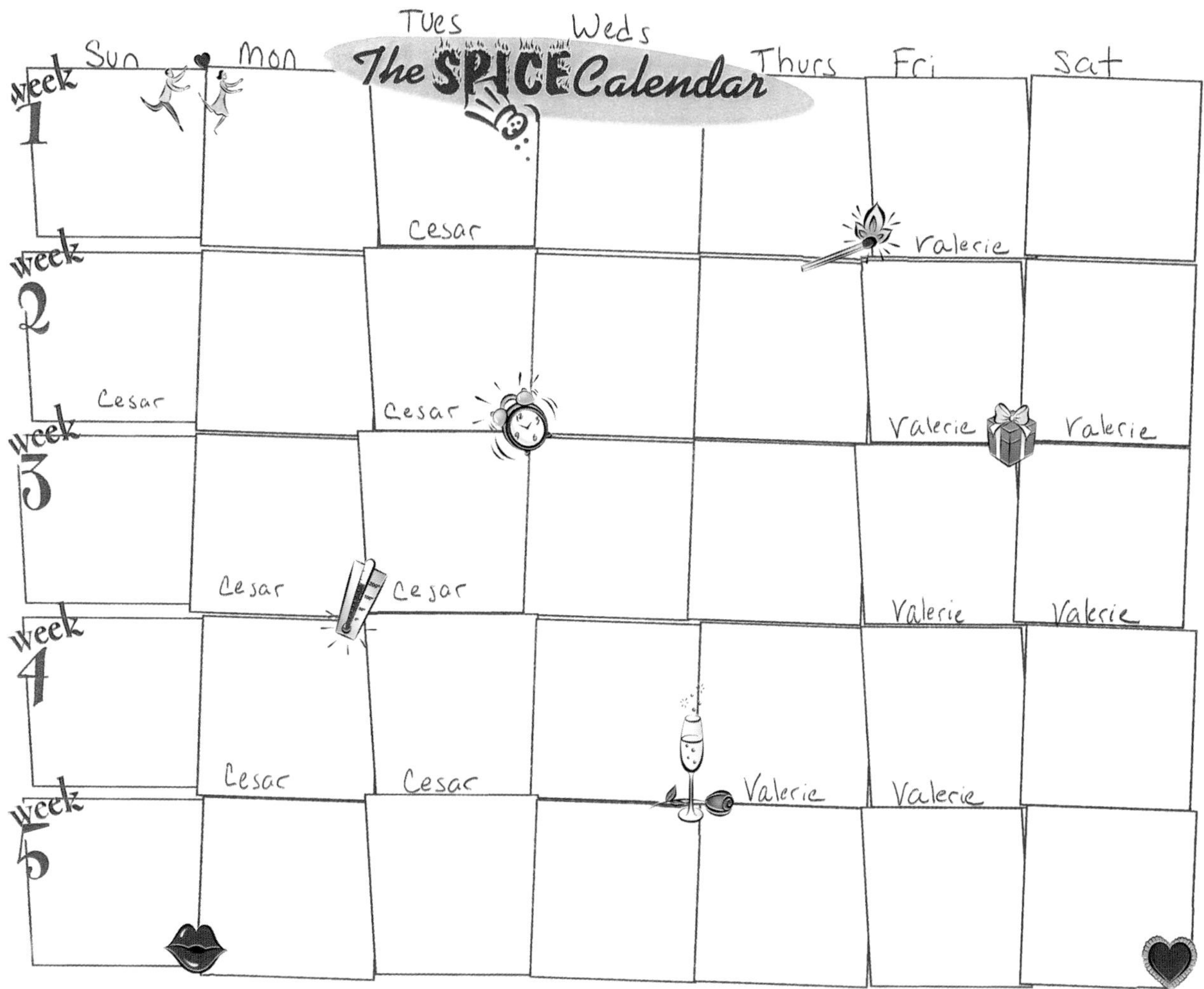

"The only thing that we did on our Spice Calendar was write down our names—your night, my night. We didn't write down any of the Anticipation Teasers but we verbalized them instead."—Valerie

was like foreplay!" Valerie also said she got off on "talking dirty." She told me, "I don't ordinarily talk dirty to him, but I did that, and I blindfolded him once."

Small steps, big changes. Sometimes that's all it takes to spice up a relationship.

"When you're having sex you feel better about the relationship and yourself."

—VALERIE

BEFORE THE DIET

"We have a very good relationship, and we have sex about three times a week. But I'd love to be more experimental in the bedroom and for Kara to initiate more."—Bob

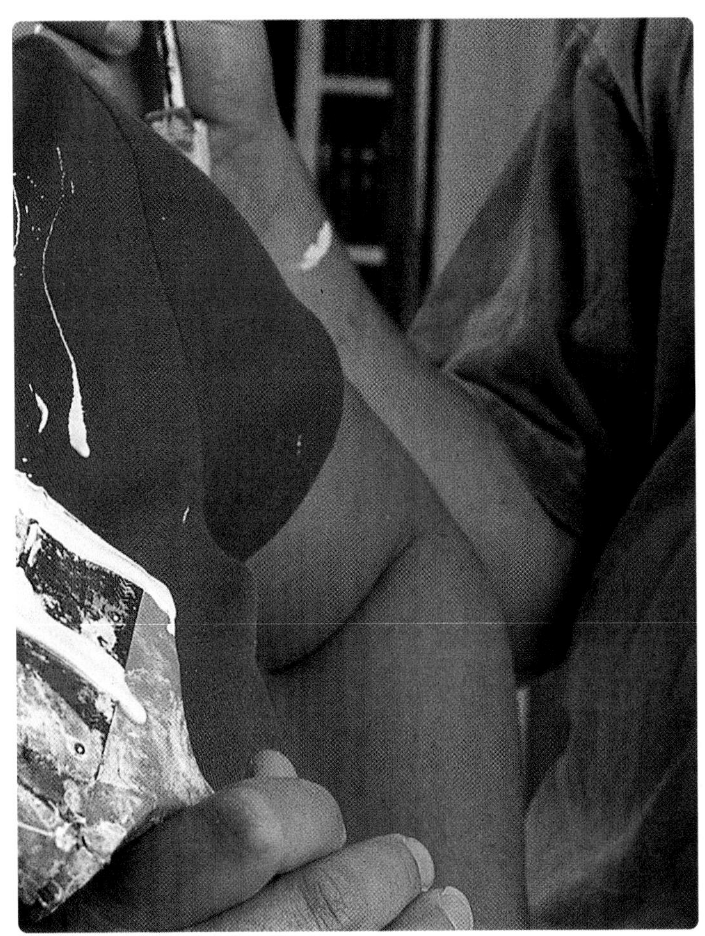

Guilty Pleasures

Kara & Bob

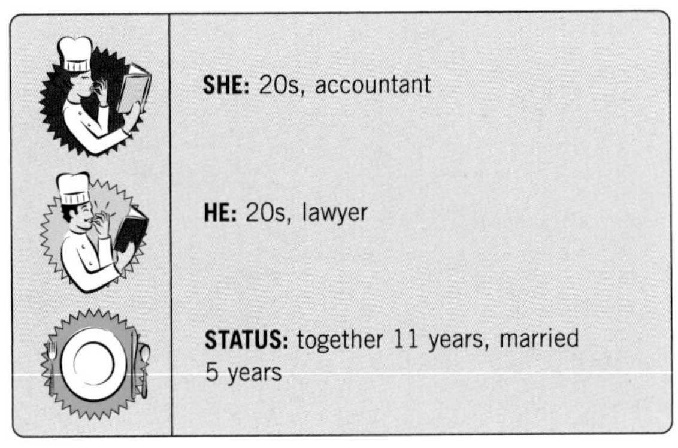

SHE: 20s, accountant

HE: 20s, lawyer

STATUS: together 11 years, married 5 years

You are probably wondering why you can't see the faces of this couple. Well, it's an interesting story.

Bob and Kara started dating when they were eighteen and describe their relationship as still very close and loving.

They've always had sex three or four times per week, but they had decided to try the diet

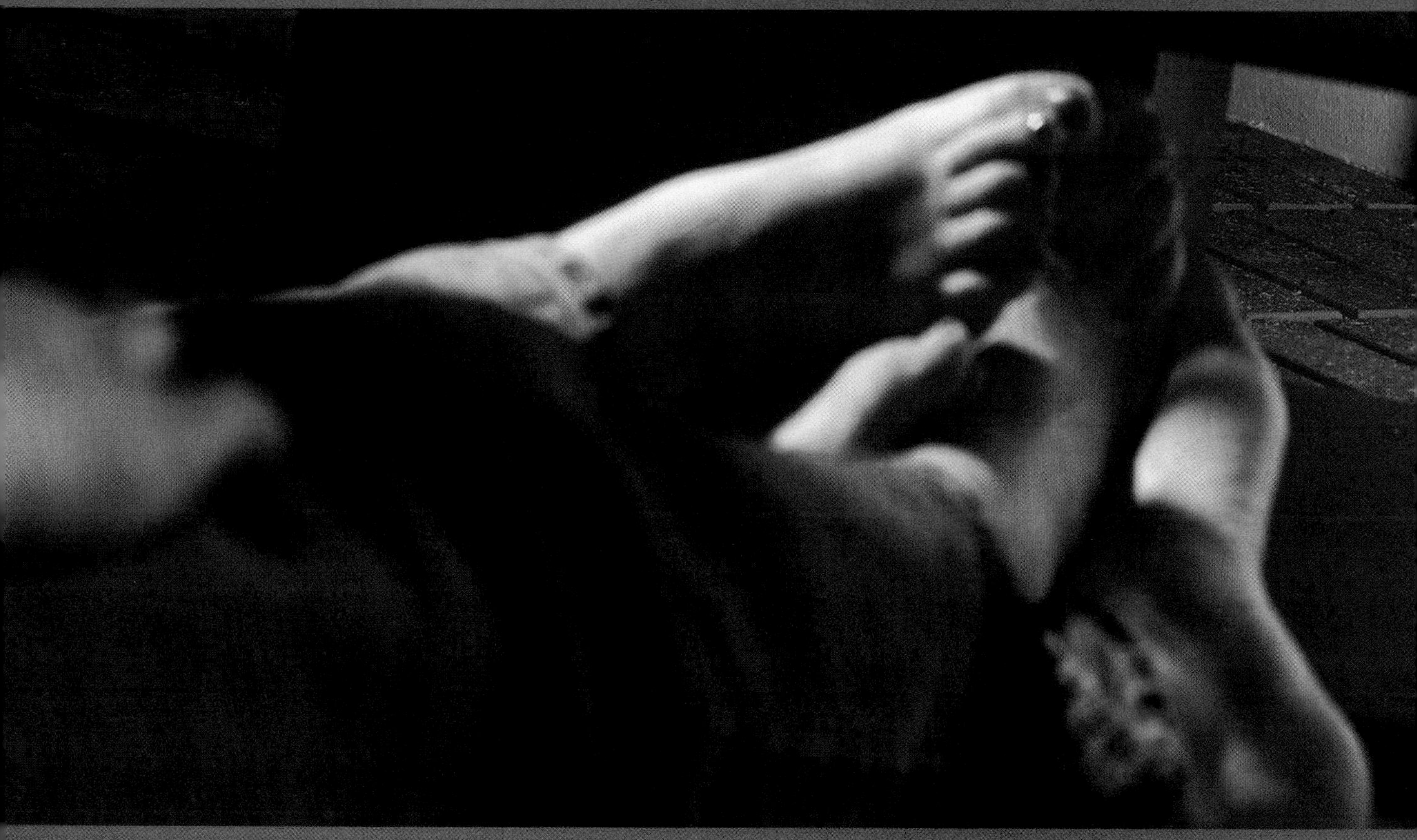

28 DAYS LATER

"The diet really opened up everything—good Lord! We got dirtier—and I thought we were dirty already! But we tried different positions, techniques, toys—everything was so new. The menu definitely opened Kara up a lot more."—Bob

as a way to break through other barriers. In particular, Kara, who had been a virgin when they married, felt very inhibited sexually.

For me, the degree of Kara's inhibitions is the most profound aspect of their story. Bob seemed especially concerned about wanting to encourage Kara to break down some of these boundaries. In fact, it was Bob who did most of the talking with me, and though I did speak with Kara, she always remained a bit reticent.

For Bob, the Great American Sex Diet "really opened up everything—good Lord—we even got dirty." One way in which Bob and Kara effected tremendous change was in Kara's willingness to touch herself. Bob recalls, "I had kept trying slowly, slowly to bring her hand down there and then she finally did it one time—whoa Nelly!" Bob says this was a big step for Kara. "She had tried doing it a few years ago and she had started gagging and almost threw up," he explains. "Because it was something her mom put in her mind."

Kara also experimented with toys. Bob remembers that Kara "used a vibrator on herself while I was in the shower—that drove me crazy."

One of the other big turning points was when Kara started to seduce Bob. He had always been the initiator . . . until one fateful day Bob returned from a ten-mile hike. After he had showered, Kara told him to lie down on the bed. She had oiled up her body and as she lay on top of him, she began rubbing up against him and then putting him inside her. "She was in total control," Bob says happily. "She didn't let me do anything . . . it was awesome."

Bob's deep satisfaction at seeing his wife open up was clear as he says reflectively, "She's done a lot of growing."

When I thanked Kara for sharing her story, she said shyly, "The diet really made me think. It's great to know there are different types of things to do sexually."

"When she did the Now This Is a Massage! spice on me, that was something totally different from what we've ever done before. She was in total control and didn't let me do anything. She was seducing me, and that was really cool. That was an awesome one!"

—Bob

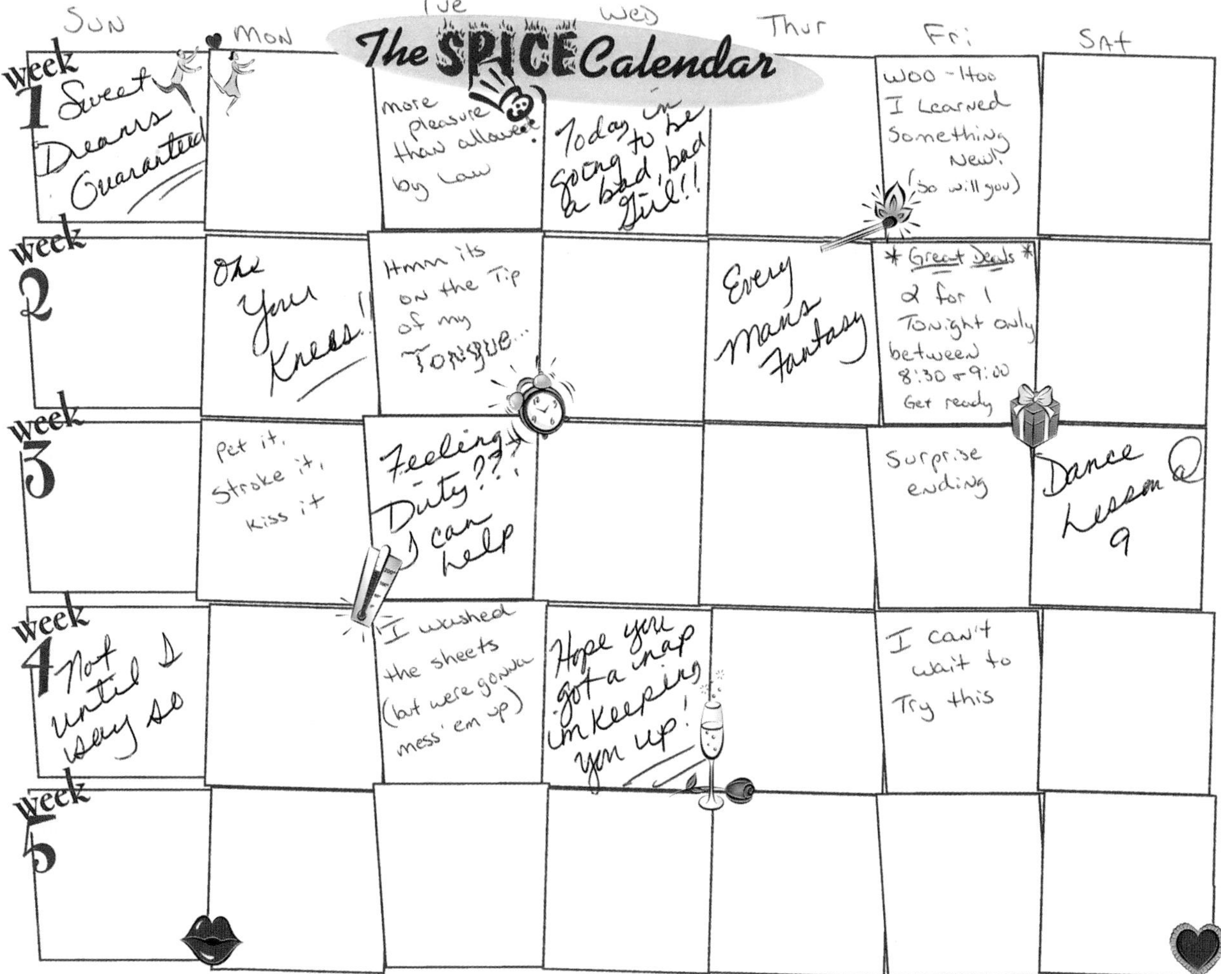

Kara was able to experiment because of her love and trust for her husband, but her deeper issues needed more time to heal and change. Twenty minutes after the final interview, Bob called to tell me that Kara was very upset. She didn't want her mother to know she had masturbated and she felt tremendous guilt and shame. The very next day Bob called to say they couldn't be in the book.

However, once they thought about it, they decided they would be comfortable with being in the book if they used pseudonyms and their faces were omitted from the before and after photos.

For me, including Kara and Bob became important because I have heard too many stories where negative beliefs about sex scar and limit someone's ability to feel the pleasure and joy of lovemaking. For this reason alone, I hope their story will show others that it is possible to move beyond fears and chart new horizons.

BEFORE THE DIET

"Every night, I come home, make dinner for the kids, help them with their homework, clean up, watch TV, and get the kids to bed. Then I try to go to sleep real quick to avoid sex. Night after night after night."

—JAYME

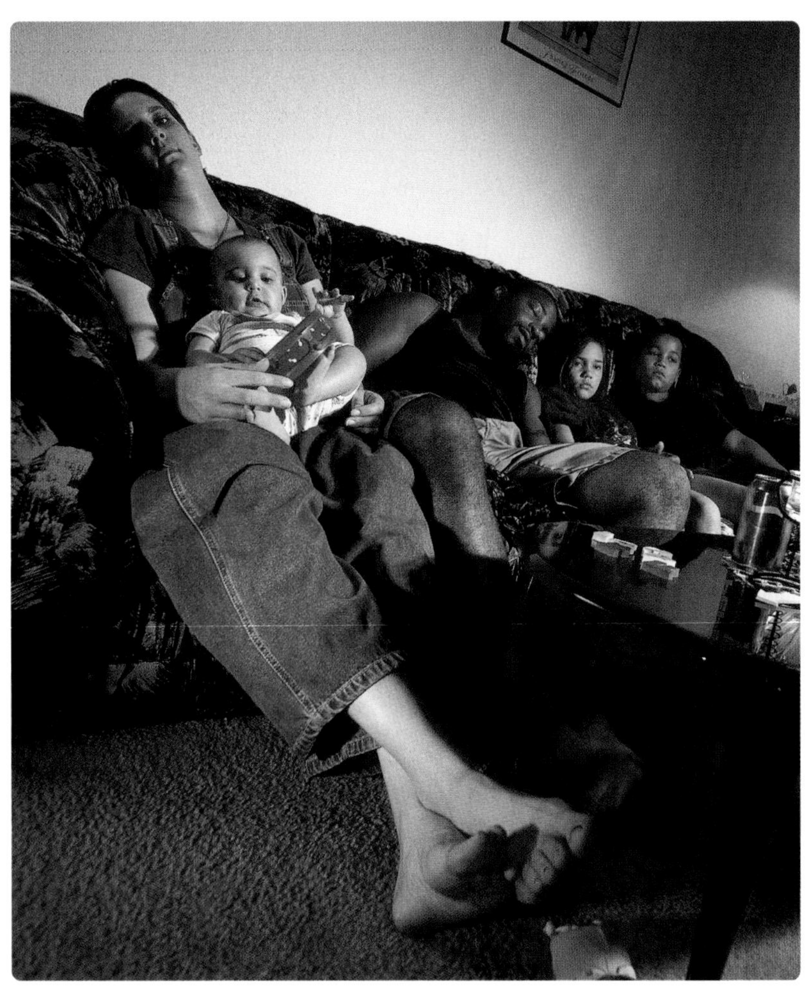

Changing Channels

JAYME & CHRISTOPHER

SHE: 20s, manager of adult boutique

HE: 20s, in construction

STATUS: together 4 years, married 3 years; 3 kids—1 together; 1 each from previous marriages

While on the diet, Jayme and Christopher discovered a new way to get in the mood for sex, and now they can't get enough of each other! This transformation is especially powerful given the fact that before they began the diet, Jayme had a distinct aversion to sex. Making matters even more significant is

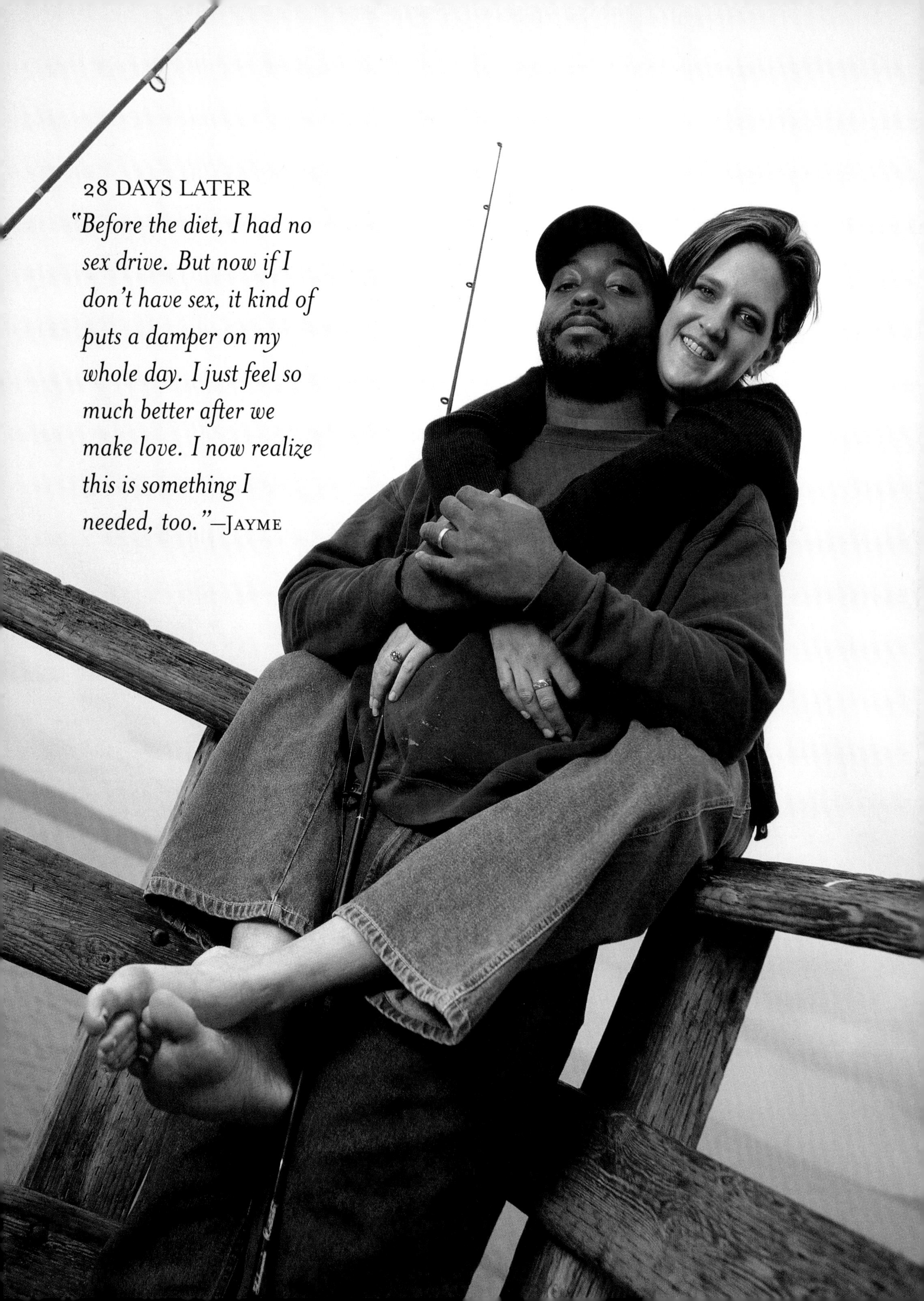

28 DAYS LATER

"Before the diet, I had no sex drive. But now if I don't have sex, it kind of puts a damper on my whole day. I just feel so much better after we make love. I now realize this is something I needed, too."—JAYME

Jayme's line of work: She's manager of an erotic boutique, specializing in toys, erotic videos, and other items to enhance people's sex lives. Before the diet, as she says, "I had no interest in sex. Nothing in the store is a turn-on for me, so I am hoping that the diet will bring more of a sexual desire out of me." But she really wanted to change her attitude. "I want to be able to be more sexually aware of myself."

Jayme and Christopher are a blended family. Together four years and married three, they each brought a child into the marriage and then they had another baby, who is now nine months old. Because they are an interracial couple, they are very aware of raising their children in a nonracist environment. She says, "I think it is very important to raise your kids in the type of environment where there is no prejudice and everybody loves each other as a whole. That is my goal for my kids."

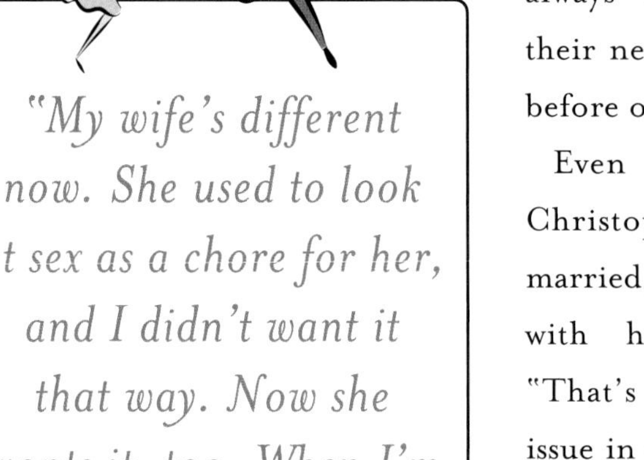

"My wife's different now. She used to look at sex as a chore for her, and I didn't want it that way. Now she wants it, too. When I'm falling asleep, she's like, 'Wake up! Wake up!' Before, I would've been the one saying that, but now she's the one. And it feels really good!"

—CHRISTOPHER

Like so many couples struggling to balance the demands of being parents and tending to their own relationship, Jayme and Christopher never have enough time to fit in their own needs. She continues, "Our kids are always around us and their needs tend to come before ours."

Even before she and Christopher met and married, Jayme struggled with her low desire. "That's always been an issue in our marriage and in our relationship. I try as best I can and he tries to be understanding. But it has been a strain. He always says, 'If you don't want to do it, I'm not going to make you, I'm not going to force you.'"

So they end up not having sex. Before the diet they were having sex maybe once or twice per month. Jayme says she doesn't want to be this way: "I think part of my problem is that by the end of the day, I'm so tired that it feels like an exercise to have sex with my husband. It takes a lot of energy. But I really don't want to feel like it's just part of our everyday routine." Another part of their everyday routine Jayme wanted to change was her habit of sitting in front of the TV: "Life is too short to be wasting time in front of the TV when you should be enjoying your other half and your children."

So how did they do on the diet? Great! One of the turning points actually occurred when Jayme was talking to me on the phone. She was explaining to me how one way she gets turned on is by watching erotic videos, but she had always felt too embarrassed and guilty to share this secret with her husband. Fortunately for her, Christopher happened to overhear our conversation and was blown away! After a long, open discussion, the two of them decided to try watching videos together—and, boy, did their sex life take off!

Jayme recalls, "I was embarrassed at first, but then I realized that they are something for a couple to enjoy together and there's nothing wrong with it. The erotic videos were just something for us to unwind with," Jayme explains. And how did Christopher respond to Jayme's movie requests? He went out and rented a slew of movies before she could say "two thumbs up!"

The frequency and the spices, combined with discovering the real joy of watching erotic videos together, really broke down barriers between Jayme and Christopher and especially enabled Jayme to reverse her low desire. For starters, she didn't feel the need to obsessively clean her house as a way to unwind from her day! And after several weeks on the diet, Jayme began to "crave" sex. As she says, "Before the diet, I had no sex drive. But now if I don't have sex, it kind of puts a damper on my whole day. I just feel so much better after we make love. I now realize this is something I needed, too."

And Christopher was thrilled with this change in his wife. As he says, "My wife's different now. She used to look at sex as a chore for her, and I didn't want it that way. Now she wants it, too. When I'm falling asleep, she's like, 'Wake up! Wake up!' Before, I would've been the one saying that, but now *she's* the one. And it feels really good!"

As Jayme and Christopher are the first to attest, sex is a powerful stimulant to change. And the diet was their instant catalyst. As Jayme says, "It brought us closer, and there's just more love."

"We'd always had our arguments, but now we hardly fight at all. He's more understanding about me and I'm more understanding about him. And now when we get together it's just more intimate."—Jayme

BEFORE THE DIET

"We have so many things that we do now—children, jobs, school, housework. At least for me, sex is one of the last things on my mind."

—AMOR

Total Surrender

AMOR & RAUL

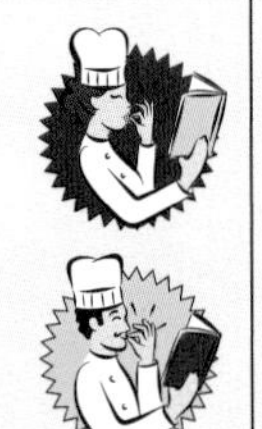

SHE: late 20s, hospital volunteer and student

HE: early 30s, government employee

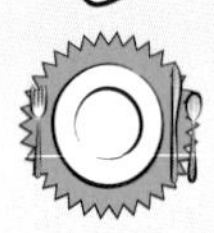

STATUS: married 10 years, 2 kids

Can you imagine having sex with your partner for years without ever experiencing the pleasure and release of an orgasm? Well, let me tell you the story of Amor and Raul, who achieved an enormous breakthrough on the Great American Sex Diet.

Very committed to each other and their two children, they have a full life and, as you can

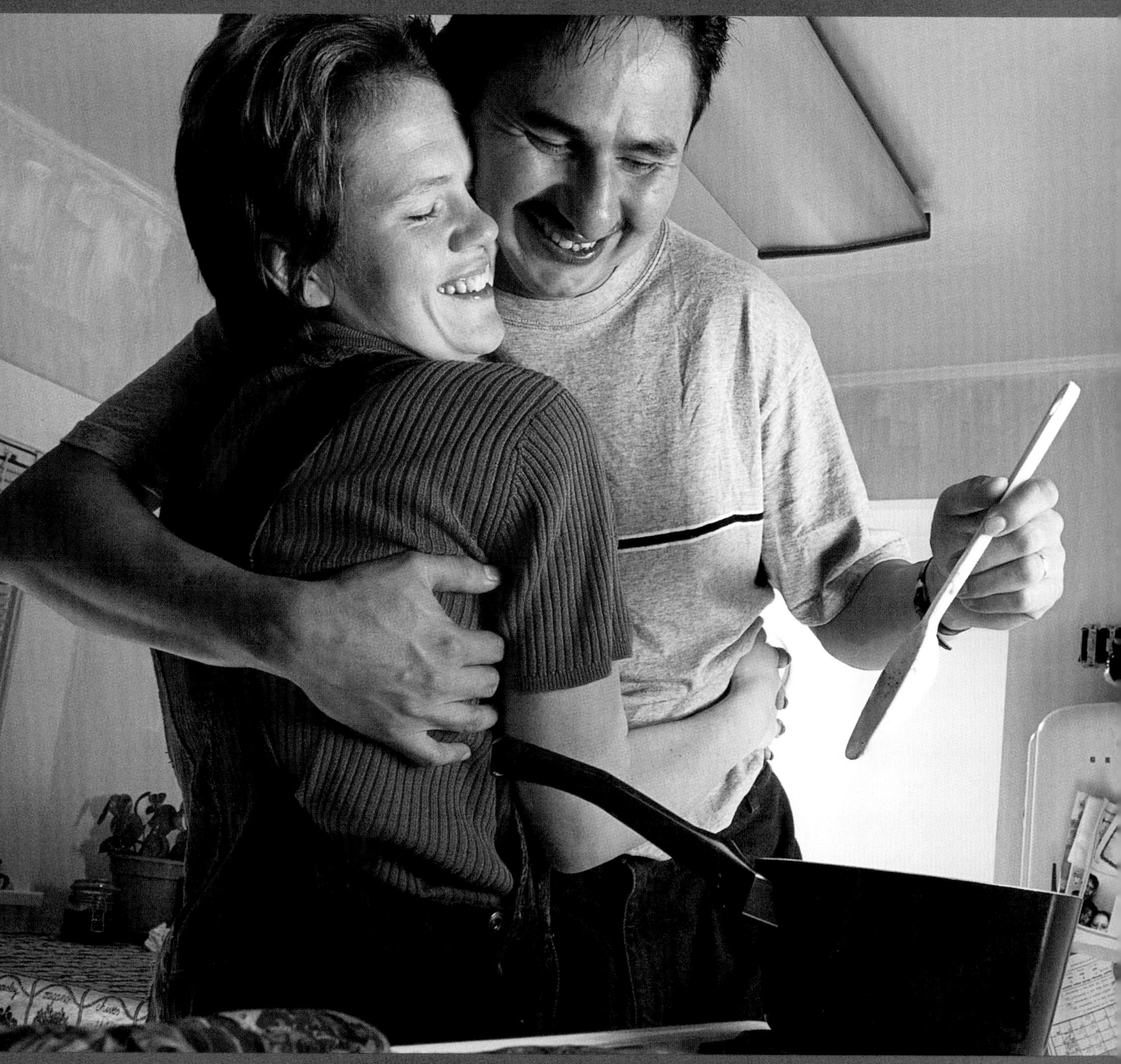

28 DAYS LATER

"We've learned that sex is important. You may not think so, but it is. It really does help a relationship. We're more talkative and more compassionate with each other. The diet brought us so much closer."—Amor & Raul

see from their before photo, their home is often the center of community for their many friends. But for all of their apparent love and conviction, I could tell that before the diet some important elements were missing. Some of what was missing was obvious to the naked eye: Raul was very affectionate and it was clear that he loves to touch and caress his wife. Yet she seemed to push him away—both physically and emotionally. When I asked Amor about it, she said, "I don't show him affection when it comes to hugging and kissing. And when it comes to sex, I just look at it as another task I have to do."

Yet despite this attitude, it was Amor's idea to do the diet. "I wanted to show Raul that I could do it," Amor explains. "And I wanted to be more willing to have sex and to understand why I only do it once a month." Up until last year Amor weighed 300 pounds. Raul loves Amor unconditionally no matter what the scale says, but the excess pounds bothered Amor tremendously. "The weight has a great deal to do with my low desire," she explains. "It's hard for somebody else to invade your body if you're not even happy with it."

"I had my very first orgasm on the diet and it was incredible! The frequency helped me just relax and get into it. Now I don't feel like I have a problem anymore. I stopped thinking, 'What's wrong with me?'"

—AMOR

Amor's discomfort with her weight seemed related to her awkwardness around her husband, but more than that, it spoke to her relationship with her own body. Before the diet she had never before experienced an orgasm in her life . . . not even through masturbation.

As they experimented with manual stimulation, toys, and different positions, Amor connected more and more to her body. And then—*bingo!*—she had her first orgasm. "The frequency helped me just relax and get into it and not see sex as something I had to do," Amor explains. "I normally think about all sorts of things when we make love, like how I need to study for a test or what I need to do the next day. But this time I just focused on the pleasure and tried not to think of other things. I had an orgasm for the first time in my life, and it was incredible!"

Amor's sweet release eased her mind as well as her body. "I don't feel like I have a problem

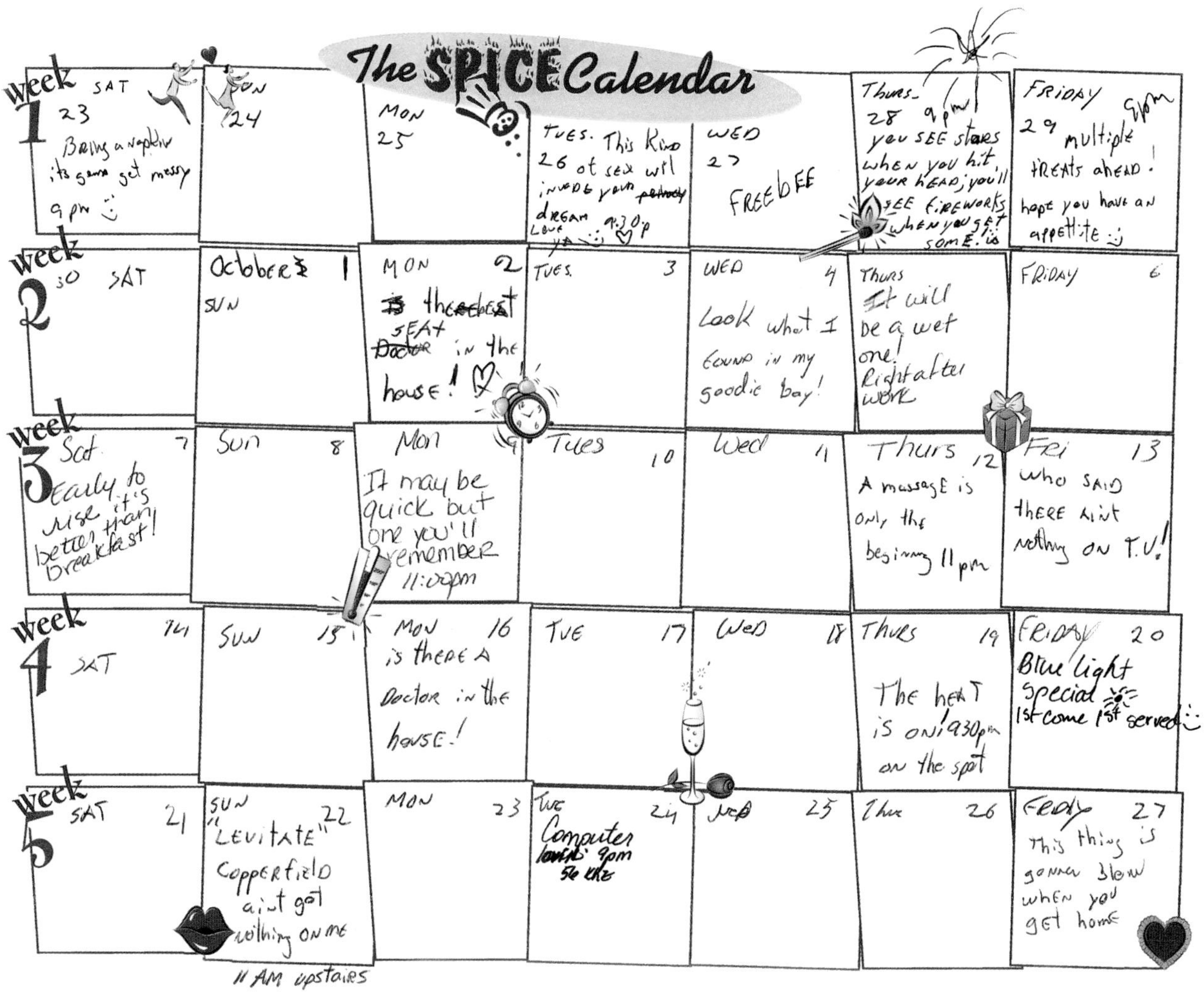

"The calendar was helpful to us, and it really did build anticipation. But we had trouble getting it filled out that first week. But after that it was great. It definitely worked!"—Raul

anymore," she says. "I stopped thinking, 'What's wrong with me?'"

Raul says that the diet "brought us closer together. We're more talkative and more compassionate with each other." He also remarks on the fact that Amor seduced him several times, which totally knocked his socks off: "I couldn't even tell you the last time she did that!"

Amor learned a valuable lesson on the diet. "When we're more intimate, our relationship's a lot easier," she says. "We have better communication and there's just not as much tension."

Except for *sexual* tension, that is! The frequency of their lovemaking and Amor's obvious desire for Raul impacted on him in a deeper way. As he says, "It made me feel like a man again."

BEFORE THE DIET

"Our love life has always been really fantastic, but we've hit a bump in the road and can't seem to get the juices flowing. We'd like to find the time to make love more often."

—ANNETTE

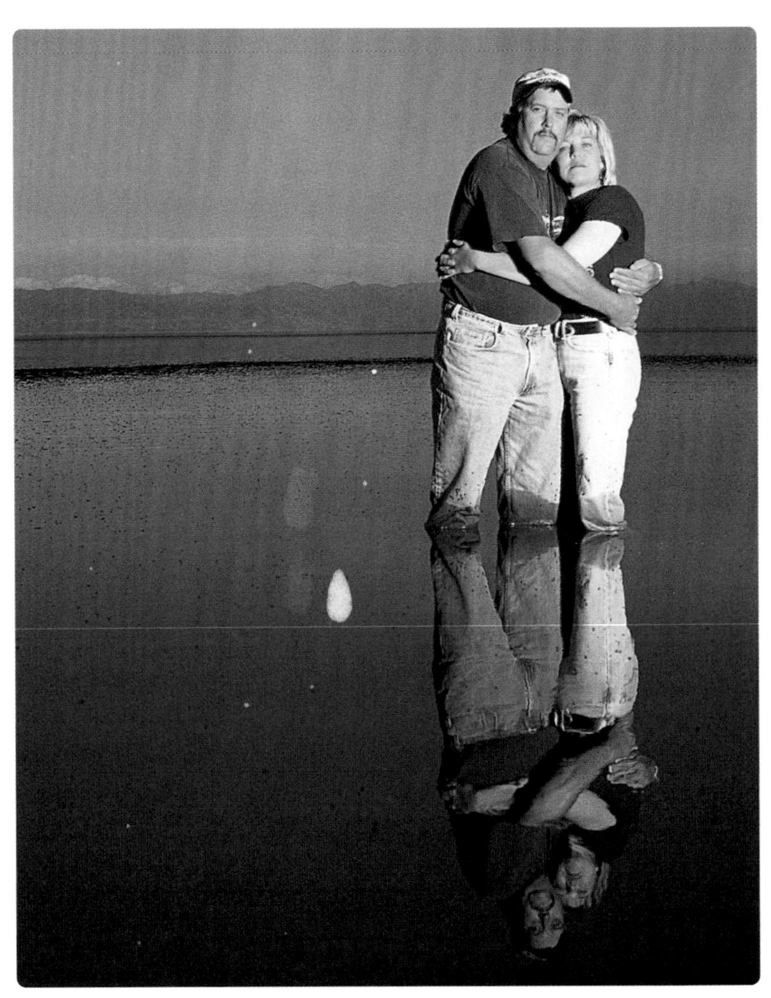

Wet & Wild

ANNETTE & SCOTT

SHE: 30s, works in the material control division at a power company

HE: 30s, works in the warehouse at a power company

STATUS: together 1½ years; she has 2 kids and he has 1

Most of us associate the Jacuzzi with sex, or at least with fooling around. Most of us, that is, except for Annette. Before going on the Great American Sex Diet, she had exclusively used her beautiful hot tub for relaxing. But as soon as she and her boyfriend Scott were unleashed on the diet, did they ever make a splash!

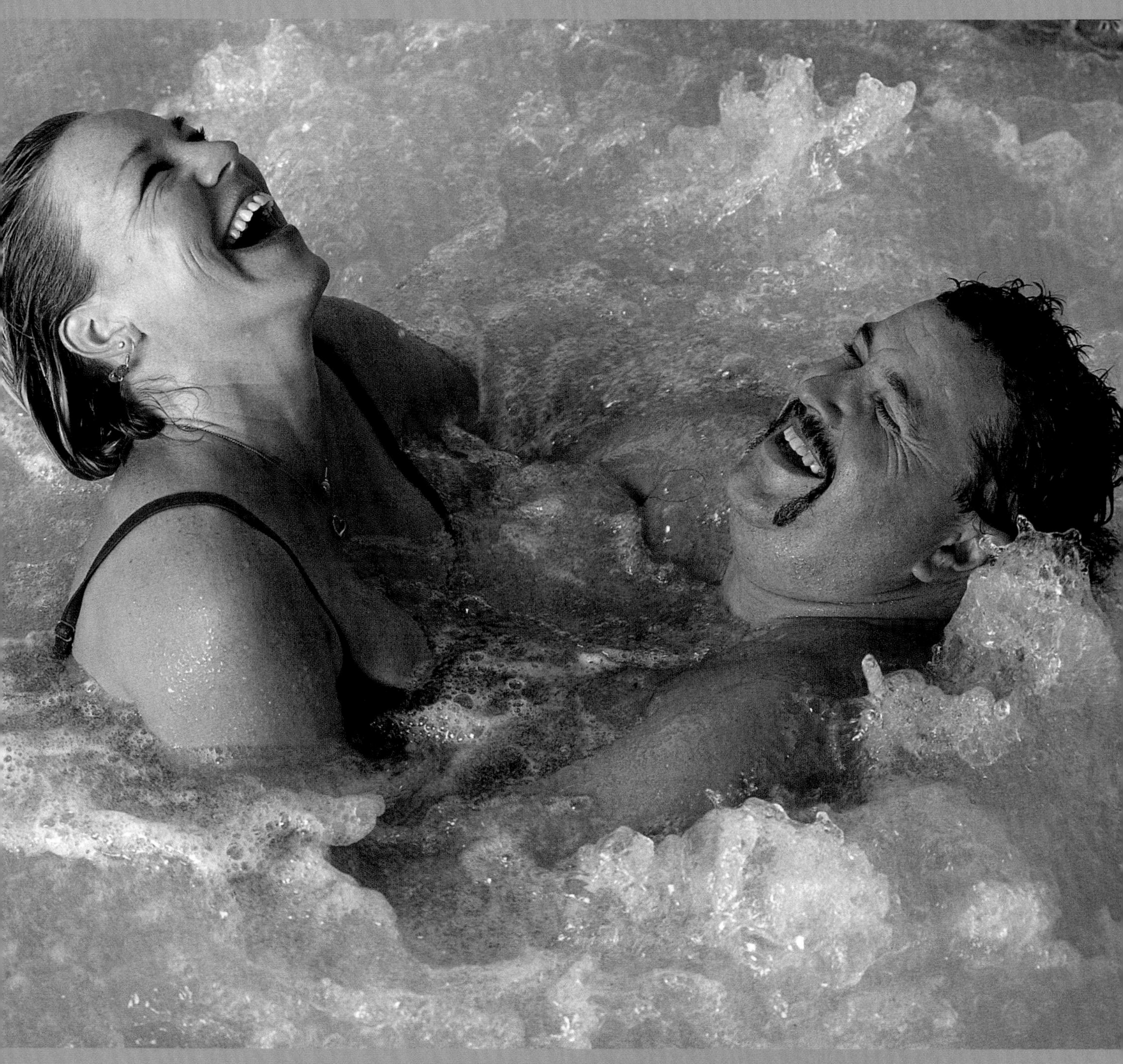

28 DAYS LATER

"The diet has really spiced things up for us. Not only did we make love more often, we got to try new things that were way out of the ordinary. We completely reinvented the hot tub!"—Annette

Though they've been together a relatively short time, they've known each other for years, having met at work. In fact, they considered each other best friends, confiding in each other at work every day. As Annette says of Scott, "I was going through a lot of trauma in my life and Scott taught me patience. He showed me how time heals everything." And though some of what Annette was confiding in Scott about was a dysfunctional relationship she was in at the time, Scott had no such distractions. As he admits, "When I met her I just looked at her and shook her hand and I felt our connection immediately." He knew he was in love. A true romantic, Scott kept his distance until Annette's other relationship had ended. But when Annette finally looked at Scott in a different light, boy, did that light turn on!

"I was like a sex maniac when we first got together," describes Annette. But within a year, "we were in a damn desert!" Both of them were alarmed and wanted to fix this problem. And so by the second weekend on the diet, they did just that! "All the kids were gone and we were going to take a trip," explains Annette, "but then we just decided to stay home and have sex." When I casually asked them how the weekend went, Scott said boldly, "It turned into a kind of marathon—we had sex four times in one day!"

I was even more amazed at their creativity. Not only did they constantly consult the menu for new ideas to surprise each other, they also filled in their calendar so completely they ran out of space and had to scribble their notes of passionate anticipation on a yellow legal pad and attach it to the back of the calendar! As Annette says, "It's so much fun to go back and read about what we did!" They even came up with their own spices to add to their menu: Creamy Breasts, Back-Up, and Sitting on the Ledge. Just take a look at Annette's notes!

One of their favorite spices was with water, and they did it—where else—in the Jacuzzi. As Annette says, "We completely reinvented the hot tub!" Scott adds, "Under the stars and everything! It was really nice for me to surprise her with something creative when we were splashing in the hot tub. I thought that was way cool."

Overall the diet made Annette feel "more aggressive and sexy. I liked being surprised, but I really liked surprising him, too." But Scott reminds me that the diet isn't over yet: "We're not done, not by a long shot. I still have a few more tricks up my sleeve."

My Spices
Annette
- The Heat is On
- The Velvet Stroke
- Actions speak louder than Words
- Finger Zinger
- Double your pleasure
- Blindfold w/Truffle (next couple of days)
- Lip Service
- Intensify his orgasm
- Make him tremble
- Seriously Sensitive
- Hidden Treasure

My own
- Stroking Wet
- Creamy Breasts
- Back-up
- sitting on the ledge

Scotts Spices
- 5 o'clock shadow
- Virtual reality
- Hoover has nothing on you
- Uncharted Territory
- The Swirl
- Ice Ice Baby
- Magic Fingers
- Panty Roulette
- Have you ever seen a nipple this hard
- Circuit training
- I'm famous for this
- The clock technique
- Thighs & Whispers
- Dangerous When wet

His Own
- on a ledge
- Snowy peaks

"Ohmigod, I read the menu a hundred times! I'd just keep going over it and over it. On my breaks at work, I'd take the Spice Menu out and decide which spices I wanted to surprise Scott with. Then I'd pick and choose and say, 'Okay, tonight I'm going to do this one!'"

—Annette

Fri 9/1

- woke up in morning Scott gave me up with one of those good deep G spot orgasms

- round 2 - I returned the favor in the hot tub - I don't know what to call this maybe "stroking wet"

- round 3 - Scott put me "on a ledge" I was about 3" above him, he was behind deep feeling!

- round 4 - This is one of my specialties well call this "you've heard of creamy thighs, now what about creamy breasts". sit him on the couch, kneel in front of him and rub lotion all over your body especially your chest. This will get him real hot, Then take him in your mouth tease him stroke him and get him real excited. then put him between your breasts, use your hands to make things tight. Stroke him with your breasts until he makes them creamy. He'll love it, and you'll love the visuals. What to add some spice wear nothing but high heels make the lotion show real good!

"We were supposed to go away for the weekend when we realized, 'Hey the kids are gone—we can have sex anywhere we want!' And so that's exactly what we did. We stayed home and had a sex marathon. We actually made love four times in twenty-four hours! I did so many spices, I couldn't even fit everything that we did on the calendar. I had to make notes on another sheet of paper to fit it all in. We had a great time!"—Annette

The SPICE Calendar

	SUN	MON	TUE	WED	THUR	FRI	SAT
week 1	Snowbird lots of fun	Photos (Brine Flyp)	Start the diet 8/22	My day date 9:30 "The Heat is on"!		This morning "actions speak louder than words"	My own Spice Back up against him in bed act like I'm tired. Start moving around see what comes up
week 2		I just got out of a hot bath I was hot, He suprises me with ice in his mouth all over my body	I "made him tremble"			See notes! Took the day off for love making	See notes Still at it
week 3	Very Very tired	Still tired (But can't wait for week 3)			Got naked in the Hot Tub. He bent me over, Then I made him sit on the edge		He did some trick with a hot drink Felt warm & Fuzzy!
week 4	I did the "finger zinger" to him	He used the finger zinger on me! Fun Joy!				The Velvet Stroke / Dangerous when wet	I was ready for this "G" Spot Orgasm
week 5	Got 2 goodies left "Blindfold" and double your pleasure combo	I don't think this diet will ever end!				My first Water Orgasm!	He was ready for this good old B.J.!

does it count if it was 7 times in 1 wk

Photos

"Planning the seductions on the Spice Calendar really built me up. You know how it is. You've got a hundred million things going on. But I could hardly wait until I could get in the hot tub and surprise her."—Scott

Sat 9/2
I started off with lip Service. It really does feel great!

This little trick Scott does is a real turn on he calls it Snowy Peaks. He slowly ~~as you~~ over you right below your Breasts Both of us put lotion on our hands he rubs my breasts while I stroke him. The visuals are fantastic. It gets more and more intense and erotic until ... all over the peaks. **CENSORED** ... about it it makes me hot. I have visuals of it all day!

BEFORE THE DIET

"The ring on the table has a lot of significance for me. It represents my hopes that we'll get engaged soon. I don't think he's ready for that yet, but we are still very much in love. We would like to try the diet to see if we can get back to the giddiness of the 'first kiss.'"

—Reneé

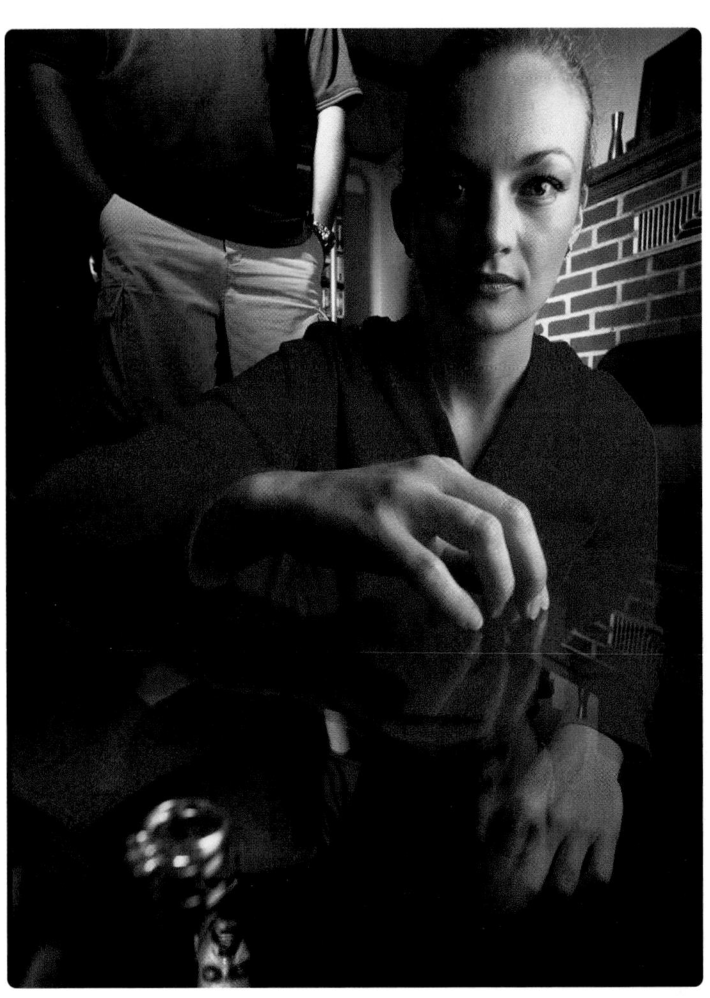

Swept Off Her Feet

Reneé & Jordan

SHE: 20s, controller for a furniture company

HE: 20s, works in telecommunications and is a musician

STATUS: together 3 years

Sometimes two people can seem outwardly perfect yet bubbling under the surface is a volcano ready to explode. This was the case with Reneé and Jordan. Upon first speaking with them, I was struck by their casual ease together. They seemed so happy and delighted with each other and immediately